The Heart of Africa

The Heart of Africa

Clinical Profile of an Evolving Burden of Heart Disease in Africa

EDITED BY

Simon Stewart PhD, NFESC, FAHA, FCSANZ

Mary MacKillop Institute for Health Research
Australian Catholic University
Melbourne, Victoria, Australia

Karen Sliwa MD, PhD, FESC, FACC

Hatter Institute for Cardiovascular Research in Africa
University of Cape Town
Cape Town, South Africa;
Soweto Cardiovascular Research Group
University of the Witwatersrand
Johannesburg, South Africa

Ana Mocumbi MD, PhD, FESC

Instituto Nacional de Saúde, Ministério da Saúde
Doenças Crónicas Não Transmissivéis Instituto
Maputo, Mozambique

Albertino Damasceno MD, PhD

Departamento de Medicina
Universidade Eduardo Mondlane
Maputo, Mozambique

Mpiko Ntsekhe MD, PhD, FACC

Division of Cardiology
University of Cape Town/Groote Schuur Hospital
Cape Town, South Africa

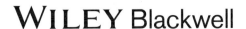

WILEY Blackwell

This edition first published 2016 © 2016 by John Wiley & Sons, Ltd

Registered Office

John Wiley & Sons, Ltd, The Atrium, Southern Gate, Chichester, West Sussex, PO19 8SQ, UK

Editorial Offices

9600 Garsington Road, Oxford, OX4 2DQ, UK

The Atrium, Southern Gate, Chichester, West Sussex, PO19 8SQ, UK

111 River Street, Hoboken, NJ 07030-5774, USA

For details of our global editorial offices, for customer services and for information about how to apply for permission to reuse the copyright material in this book please see our website at www.wiley.com/wiley-blackwell

The right of the author to be identified as the author of this work has been asserted in accordance with the UK Copyright, Designs and Patents Act 1988.

Library of Congress Cataloging-in-Publication Data

Names: Stewart, Simon, 1964–, editor. | Sliwa, Karen, editor. | Mocumbi, Ana, editor. | Damasceno, Albertino, editor. | Ntsekhe, Mpiko, editor.

Title: The heart of Africa : clinical profile of an evolving burden of heart disease in Africa / edited by Simon Stewart, Karen Sliwa, Ana Mocumbi, Albertino Damasceno, Mpiko Ntsekhe.

Description: Chichester, West Sussex ; Hoboken, NJ : John Wiley & Sons, Inc., 2017. | Includes bibliographical references and index.

Identifiers: LCCN 2016007512| ISBN 9781118336960 (pbk.) | ISBN 9781119097143 (Adobe PDF) | ISBN 9781119097006 (epub)

Subjects: | MESH: Heart Diseases–epidemiology | Epidemiologic Studies | Africa South of the Sahara–epidemiology

Classification: LCC RA645.H4 | NLM WG 210 | DDC 614.5/91096–dc23 LC record available at http://lccn.loc.gov/2016007512

A catalogue record for this book is available from the British Library.

Wiley also publishes its books in a variety of electronic formats. Some content that appears in print may not be available in electronic books.

Cover image: ©Simon Stewart

Set in 9/12pt Meridien by SPi Global, Pondicherry, India

Printed and bound in Malaysia by Vivar Printing Sdn Bhd

1   2016

Contents

Section 1: Maternal heart health
Karen Sliwa

Section 2: Infant and childhood heart disease
Ana Mocumbi

Section 3: Spectrum of cardiovascular risk and heart disease in sub-Saharan Africa
Simon Stewart

List of contributors

Editors

Simon Stewart PhD, NFESC, FAHA, FCSANZ
Mary MacKillop Institute for Health Research
Australian Catholic University
Melbourne, Victoria, Australia

Karen Sliwa MD, PhD, FESC, FACC
Hatter Institute for Cardiovascular Research in Africa
University of Cape Town
Cape Town, South Africa;
Soweto Cardiovascular Research Group
University of the Witwatersrand
Johannesburg, South Africa

Ana Mocumbi MD, PhD, FESC
Instituto Nacional de Saúde, Ministerio da Saude
Doencas Cronicas Nao Transmissiveis Instituto
Maputo, Mozambique

Albertino Damasceno MD, PhD
Departamento de Medicina
Universidade Eduardo Mondlane
Maputo, Mozambique

Mpiko Ntsekhe MD, PhD, FACC
Division of Cardiology
University of Cape Town/Groote Schuur Hospital
Cape Town, South Africa

Associate Editors

Ashley K. Keates BHSc (PH)
Mary MacKillop Institute for Health Research
Australian Catholic University
Melbourne, Victoria, Australia

Cressida J. McDermott BA (Hons)
Australian Catholic University
Melbourne, Victoria, Australia

Contributing Authors

John Anthony MBChB, FCOG, MPhil
Department of Obstetrics & Gynaecology
Groote Schuur Hospital
Cape Town, South Africa

Serigne A. Ba
Department of Cardiovacular Diseases
Cheikh Anta DIOP University
Hôpital A. le Dantec
Dakar, Senegal

Anthony Becker MBBCh, FCP(SA), PhD
Department of Medicine,
University of the Witwatersrand
Johannesburg, South Africa

Melinda Jane Carrington BA (Psych Hons), PhD
Mary MacKillop Institute for Health Research
Australian Catholic University
Melbourne, Victoria, Australia

Anastase Dzudie MD
Hospital General de Douala
Douala, Littoral, Cameroon

Denise Hilfiker-Kleiner PhD
Department of Cardiology and Angiology
Medical School Hannover
Germany

John Musuku BSc, MBcHb, MMed
Department of Paediatrics and Child Health
University Teaching Hospital
Lusaka, Zambia

Okechukwu Samuel Ogah MBBS, PhD, FESC, FACC
Division of Cardiology
University College Hospital
Ibadan, Oyo, Nigeria

Dike Bevis Ojji MBBS, PhD
Cardiology Unit
University of Abuja Teaching Hospital
Abuja, Nigeria

Mahmoud Sani MBBS, FWACP, FACP, FACC
Department of Medicine
Bayero University Kano/Aminu Kano Teaching Hospital
Kano, Nigeria

Krisela Steyn MD
Chronic Diseases of Lifestyle Unit
Medical Research Council
Tygerberg, South Africa

Tantchou Tchoumi Jacques Cabral MD, PhD
Cardiac Centre
St. Elizabeth Catholic General Hospital
Shisong, Cameroon

Friedrich Thienemann MD
Institute of Infectious Diseases and Molecular Medicine
University of Cape Town
Cape Town, South Africa

Kemi Tibazarwa MD, PhD
Department of Cardiovascular Medicine
Muhimbili National Hospital
Dar es Salaam, Tanzania

Peter Zilla MD, PhD, FCS(SA)
Christiaan Barnard Department of Cardiothoracic Surgery
University of Cape Town/Groote Schuur and Red Cross Children's Hospital
Cape Town, South Africa

Liesl Zühlke MD
Departments of Paediatric Cardiology and Medicine
University of Cape Town/Groote Schuur and Red Cross Children's Hospital
Cape Town, South Africa

Foreword

A PubMed search for articles on "heart disease in Africa" shows an exponential increase in the number of publications per year on this topic over the past 15 years (see figure). This rising production of new knowledge by African investigators together with external collaborators has been documented over the same period in the field of epidemiology and public health [1] and in other fields of health research in general [2]. The renaissance in health research that is underway in Africa has created the need for summaries of the new knowledge that are packaged for use by students, researchers, and policy makers in their day-to-day work.

Simon Stewart and his colleagues have compiled such a summary in this book on contemporary research in heart disease in Africa with the appropriate title "The Heart of Africa." The book is made up of summaries of original papers published by authors from Australia, Cameroon, Germany, Mozambique, Nigeria, Senegal, South Africa, Tanzania, and Zambia. Future editions of the book should benefit from a broader and more systematic selection of the emerging literature to include authors from a wider range of countries and languages of Africa.

This work is very well illustrated and referenced—with these occupying nearly half of the pages of the book, a feature that makes it valuable to researchers in this field. The Pan-African Society of Africa (PASCAR) endorses this laudable effort to compile recent publications on heart disease in Africa—with the ultimate aim of combating cardiovascular disease through the translation of the new knowledge into policy and practice.

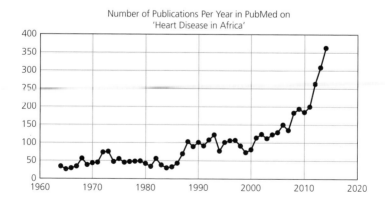

Number of Publications Per Year in PubMed on 'Heart Disease in Africa'

References

1 Nachega JB, Uthman OA, Ho Y-S, Lo M, Anude C, Kayembe P, Wabwire-Mangen F, Gomo E, Sow PS, Obike U, Kusiaku T, Mills EJ, Mayosi BM, IJsselmuiden C. Current status and future prospects of epidemiology and public health training and research in the WHO African region. *Int J Epidemiol* 2012;41:1829–1846.
2 Uthman OA, Wiysonge CS, Ota MO, Nicol M, Hussey GD, Ndumbe PM, Mayosi BM. Increasing the value of health research in the WHO African region beyond 2015: reflecting on the past, celebrating the present and building the future: a bibliometric analysis. *BMJ Open* 2015;5:e006340.

Bongani M. Mayosi MBChB DPhil
Department of Medicine
Faculty of Health Sciences
University of Cape Town
South Africa

Preface

When I first proposed the "heart of Africa" book more than 5 years ago, I had little idea of the enormous time and effort it would take to reach fruition. This is not a negative comment. It merely reflects the enormous efforts made by cardiology researchers and health care workers across the African continent to better understand and respond to an evolving epidemic of heart disease (and other forms of cardiovascular disease) in mostly vulnerable individuals and communities. While many high-income countries observe a relative decline in the population impact of heart disease and deal with the problem of an older patient population who readily survive earlier nonfatal encounters with the condition, Africa contends with a typically younger population with frequently advanced and readily fatal heart disease. Similarly, while high-income countries almost exclusively deal with noncommunicable forms of heart disease, Africa contends with both communicable and noncommunicable forms of heart disease. In clear contrast to regions such as Europe and North America, case complexity is often high, and available resources from the individual to societal perspective (particularly primary health care services) are often suboptimal.

Rather than provide a definitive guide to heart disease in Africa (an impossible task given the space required), this book presents the most salient research uncovering the evolving burden of communicable and noncommunicable forms of heart disease published within the past decade. The key features from each target manuscript were summarized and adapted for the book (i.e., they closely resemble what was originally published). Unless specific permission was sought and granted for reproduction, key tables and figures were redrawn and adapted from the originals by the editorial team. Addressing maternal and pediatric health to chronic forms of heart disease, a large portion of Africa's brightest and best cardiologic researchers present and review these key research papers (often their own), highlighting their most salient features. The book's content is designed to give anyone with an interest in heart disease in Africa an immediate sense of where we are tracking from a clinical to research perspective in responding to this evolving epidemic. In this respect, we expect the book to be of interest to health care workers, specialist clinicians, public health practitioners, and health policy makers alike. It will enable the reader to understand where Africa's relative strengths and weaknesses lie in dealing with a problem that will take decades to resolve, particularly given its close link to profound socioeconomic development and changes in cultural practices/norms over time.

With any luck, therefore, this will be the first of many books dedicated to understanding and responding to heart disease on the African continent. This will hopefully include a textbook describing the clinical management of the most common manifestations of heart disease from an African-specific perspective. Regardless of our sincere hopes and wishes, this will be a growth area for those dedicated to researching and treating heart disease and caring for the millions of Africans likely affected by its various forms in the decades to come. We hope you enjoy reading this book and are inspired to begin or continue your journey to improve multiple aspects of the heart health of Africa overall; the peoples and communities of Africa deserve nothing less.

Simon Stewart

Acknowledgments

The editors would like to thank all of the authors (and those who authored the highlighted research papers) for their contributions to this book. We have no doubt that many of these clinicians/researchers will be leading the fight against heart disease in Africa for many years to come. Their dedication and expertise as reflected by their contributions to this book are truly appreciated. We also wish to acknowledge the support of the Pan African Society of Cardiology (http://www. pascar.org/)—not only in terms of distributing copies of the book but in supporting its launch and other educational initiatives designed to improve standards of cardiovascular care and research in Africa. Finally, special mention must be made of our two associate editors (Ashley Keates and Cressida McDermott) who were instrumental in cowriting and editing the book. Without people like Kim and Cress, this book would simply not exist.

Sub-Saharan Africa and *The Heart of Africa*: A brief introduction

Africa is a large and diverse continent. For example, Sub-Saharan Africa (a major focus of this book) comprises 49 countries that are fully or partially located south of the Sahara Desert. Politically, it can be distinguished from North Africa, which is considered part of the Arab world [1]. Somalia, Djibouti, Comoros, and Mauritania belong geographically to Sub-Saharan Africa but are also part of the Arab world [2]. Africa's population currently sits at approximately 1.1 billion and this is expected to rise to 2.4 billion by 2050 [3]. More than 40% of the population comprises children and adolescents (<15 years of age) [4].

Reflective of its diversity, we the editors have done our very best to highlight research and receive contributions from as many countries as possible. Figure 1 shows how successful we were in this respect, while highlighting how and where we might improve in the future, both in terms of inviting contributions and supporting new clinical and research initiatives in cardiovascular health.

Despite estimates indicating a declining trend in poverty in Africa as a whole, Sub-Saharan Africa remains one of the most impoverished regions in the world, with approximately 47% of the population living on less than US$0.25 per day [5]. In addition, the region is adversely impacted by a significant burden of disease, owing largely to its lack of access to clean water and insufficient health care resources. Strikingly, while Sub-Saharan Africa bears 25% of the world's disease burden, it is home to only 3% of the global health workforce [6]. The two major infectious diseases plaguing Sub-Saharan Africa are malaria and HIV/AIDS. Malaria, an endemic illness in this region, accounts for the majority of cases worldwide [7]. Similarly, approximately 70% of all sufferers of HIV/AIDS worldwide are found in Sub-Saharan Africa [8]. However, recent advancements in education and prevention programs [9] as well as increases in the proportion of HIV-positive individuals receiving antiretroviral treatment [10] have led to 39% fewer AIDS-related deaths and a 33% reduction in HIV infections [8]. Although often associated with war, disease, famine, and poverty, Sub-Saharan Africa is one of the fastest developing regions in the world. It comprises six of the world's ten

The Heart of Africa: Clinical Profile of an Evolving Burden of Heart Disease in Africa, First Edition.
Edited by Simon Stewart, Karen Sliwa, Ana Mocumbi, Albertino Damasceno, and Mpiko Ntsekhe.
© 2016 John Wiley & Sons, Ltd. Published 2016 by John Wiley & Sons, Ltd.

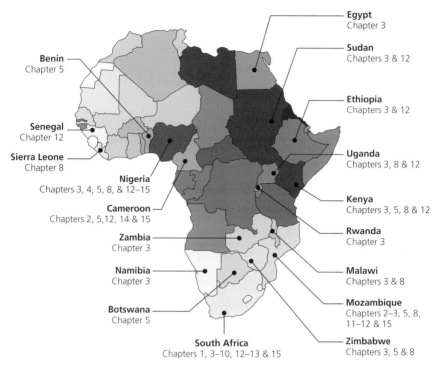

Figure 1 The different African countries highlighted in the research.

fastest growing economies [11]. This rise in economic growth is primarily attributed to increases in investments to infrastructure and resources, advancements in the telecommunication industry, and a steady expenditure per household [12].

References

1 Composition of macro geographical (continental) regions, geographical sub-regions, and selected economic and other groupings. 2013 [accessed June 2015]. Available from: http://unstats.un.org/unsd/methods/m49/m49regin.htm.

2 Barakat H. *The Arab World: Society, Culture, and State*. University of California Press, 1993.

3 United Nations Department of Economic and Social Affairs, Population Division. World Population Prospects: The 2006 Revision, Highlights, Working Paper No. ESA/P/WP.202. United Nations, 2007.

4 Central Intelligence Agency. *The World Factbook* 2008. Washington, DC: Central Intelligence Agency [accessed June 2015]. Available from: https://www.cia.gov/library/publications/download/download-2008/.

5 United Nations. *The Millennium Development Goals Report 2012*. New York: United Nations, 2012.

6 World Health Organization. *World Health Report 2006: Working Together for Health*. World Health Organization, 2006.

7 World Health Organization. *Malaria Fact Sheet no. 94* 2015 [accessed July 2015]. Available from: http://www.who.int/mediacentre/factsheets/fs094/en/.

8 United Nations. UN AIDS Fact Sheet 2014 [accessed July 2015]. Available from: http://www.unaids.org/en/resources/presscentre/factsheets/%23d.en.74010.

9 Desmond Tutu Foundation. *Desmond Tutu Foundation: What We Do* [accessed June 2015]. Available from: http://www.tutufoundationusa.org/what-we-do/.

10 The Joint United Nations Programme on HIV/AIDS (UN AIDS). Special Report: How Africa Turned AIDS Around. United Nations. 2013.

11 Africa's impressive growth. *The Economist*. 6 Jan 2011.

12 The World Bank. Africa's Growth Set to Reach 5.2 percent in 2014 with Strong Investment Growth and Household Spending [press release]. 7 April 2014.

SECTION 1
Maternal heart health

Karen Sliwa

University of Cape Town, South Africa; University of the Witwatersrand, Johannesburg, South Africa

S1.1 Maternal health: An African perspective

Globally, cardiac disease is emerging as an important indirect cause of maternal death. Cardiac conditions can be preexisting, such as rheumatic heart disease (RHD) or congenital heart disease (CHD), and can be unmasked by the increased hemodynamic load in pregnancy, or can be caused by pregnancy, for example, in the case of hypertensive disorders or peripartum cardiomyopathy (PPCMO). Maternal mortality has been difficult to track over time at the national level, particularly in low- and middle-income countries (LMIC) such as in Africa. Incomplete data sets, inexperience of physicians in applying the classifications, and misclassification of maternal deaths to other causes in countries with complete vital registration are common problems [1]. Nevertheless, Table S1.1 highlights the more than tenfold higher maternal mortality rates in South Africa relative to higher income countries [1]. However, many cases remain unreported due to lack of linkage to the causality of the pregnancy. Maternal death is rarely reported beyond 6 weeks postpartum, and the ICD-10 classification defining late maternal mortality (6 weeks to 1 year) is often not applied. Consequently, death due to PPCMO, which often presents only 3 to 5 months postpartum and is characterized by fatal left ventricular (LV) dysfunction and heart failure (HF), remains unreported. The same applies to a range of maternal conditions, including other common hypertensive disorders in pregnancy and right heart failure (RHF) in complex CHD. Unfortunately, therefore, in the African context, a number of important maternal conditions are not adequately recognized or addressed to improve maternal heart health outcomes. Appropriately, this first section and chapter of *The Heart of Africa* examines key components of the spectrum and nature of heart disease from a maternal and "start of life" perspective.

The Heart of Africa: Clinical Profile of an Evolving Burden of Heart Disease in Africa, First Edition.
Edited by Simon Stewart, Karen Sliwa, Ana Mocumbi, Albertino Damasceno, and Mpiko Ntsekhe.

Table S1.1 Comparison of maternal mortality per 100,000 live births worldwide. Source: Kassenbaum et al., 2014 [1]. Reproduced with permission of Elsevier.

	Maternal Mortality Ratio (per 100,000 live births)			Number of Maternal Deaths			Annualized Rate of Change in Maternal Mortality Ratio (%)		
	1990	2003	2013	1990	2003	2013	1990–2003	2003–2013	1990–2013
Worldwide	283.2 258.6, 306.9	273.4 251.1, 296.6	209.1 186.3, 233.9	376,034 343,483, 407,574	361,706 332,230, 392,393	292,982 261,017, 327,792	−0.3% −1.1, 0.6	−2.7% −3.9, −1.5	−1.3% −1.9, −0.8
Developed countries	24.5 23.0, 26.1	16.0 14.9, 17.0	12.1 10.4, 13.7	3827 3596, 4076	2341 2178, 2490	1811 1560, 2053	−3.3% −3.8, −2.8	−2.9% −4.2, −1.5	−3.1% −3.7, −2.5
Southern Africa	150.8 115.9, 182.6	490.4 367.8, 626.1	279.8 202.6, 381.5	2455 1886, 2973	8406 6305, 10733	4898 3547, 6679	9.1% 6.5, 11.8	−5.6% −8.1, −3.0	2.7% 1.2, 4.4
South Africa	134.0 93.3, 175.2	341.8 227.8, 431.0	174.1 96.3, 274.9	1403 977, 1835	3739 2492, 5262	1925 1065, 3041	7.2% 3.3, 11.1	−6.9% −11.1, −2.7	1.0% −1.6, 3.8

S1.1.1 Geographical context

Each of the studies surveyed in Section 1 were situated in South Africa; beginning in Cape Town, the section subsequently shifts to Soweto, which will become prominent as a primary landscape of this book. In order to set the studies in context, a brief overview of South Africa in general and Cape Town and Soweto in particular is now provided. South Africa, located at the southern tip of the African continent, has a population of 53,675,563, almost half of whom are aged below 25 [2]. Approximately 80% of the population is of African ancestry; the remainder are white (8.4%), of mixed ancestry (8.8%), or Indian/Asian (2.5%) [2]. Average life expectancy in South Africa is 60.8 years for men and 63.9 for women. In 2015 the infant mortality rate was reported as 33 deaths per 1,000 live births [2]. Around 64% of the population is urbanized [3], and this is growing at an annual rate of 1.59% [2]. Although the literacy rate is at 94% [4], 24.9% of the total population are unemployed [5]. HIV/AIDs is the leading cause of mortality in South Africa, followed by stroke, type 2 diabetes, and ischemic heart disease (IHD) [6].

Cape Town is the second most populous city in South Africa, with around 3.7 million inhabitants [7]. A combined 80% of the population describe themselves as of African or mixed ancestry, with 15.7% being white and 1.4% Indian/Asian [8]. The majority of the population (almost 70%) is aged between 15 and 64 years, with around a quarter below the age of 15. In 2015 nearly 36% of households were living below the poverty line, with an unemployment rate of 23.9% [9].

The South Western Townships, also known as Soweto, is an urban area that forms part of Johannesburg, Gauteng. With a population officially estimated to be around 1 million people (some unofficial estimates are double and even triple this amount), 99% of Soweto's inhabitants are of African ancestry [10]. All 11 of South Africa's official languages are spoken in Soweto, with isiZulu, Sesotho, and Setswana being the most prominent. With a historically high unemployment rate, Soweto has a mixed (but predominantly low) income profile and is known for its "matchbox" houses in some areas and its upmarket, expensive properties in others [11]. Soweto is serviced by the world-renowned Chris Hani Baragwanath Hospital. Unofficially labeled the largest hospital in the world (for beds) at one time, it remains the largest hospital in South Africa, with >3,000 beds and >6,500 staff members [12].

CHAPTER 1

Maternal heart health

Karen Sliwa[1], John Anthony[2], and Denise Hilfiker-Kleiner[3]

[1]University of Cape Town, South Africa; University of the Witwatersrand, Johannesburg, South Africa
[2]Department of Obstetrics & Gynaecology, Groote Schuur Hospital, Cape Town, South Africa
[3]Department of Cardiology and Angiology, Medical School Hannover, Germany

1.0 Introduction

In this chapter, we first report upon a recent single-center prospective cohort study from Groote Schuur Hospital [13] in which the majority of maternal deaths observed were attributable to various forms of cardiomyopathy (CMO), with only two being related to complications of sepsis and thrombosis affecting prosthetic heart valves. Significantly, 8 out of the 9 deaths reported in this patient cohort of 152 patients with 6-month follow-up would not have been reported if the definition of death within 42 days had been applied, thereby underestimating the number of cardiac deaths related to pregnancy as a result of late presentation and deaths occurring among women with familial CMO or PPCMO.

The last decade has seen a steady increase in the institutional maternal mortality rate for cardiac disease in South Africa [14]. While the maternal mortality rate was 3.73 % per 100,000 live births during the period 2005 to 2007, this rose to 5.64 in 2008 to 2010 and further still to 6 % during 2011 to 2013. After nonpregnancy-related infections, cardiac disease is the second most common cause of indirect maternal death, with complications of rheumatic heart disease (RHD) and CMO being the most significant contributors to cardiac deaths. The fact that more than half of those cases occurred postpartum is noteworthy; it implies that the maternal death rate in South Africa—already estimated to be 176/100,000 [1]—is probably grossly underestimated, as death could only be reported until 42 days postpartum.

Valvular heart disease (VHD) in pregnant women, whether due to congenital or acquired etiologies such as RHD, poses a particular challenge to clinicians and their patients. Significant valve disease increases the risks associated with pregnancy to both mother and fetus and requires a careful preconception risk assessment as well as specialised care during gestation to minimize maternal and fetal morbidity and mortality. Ideally, all women with VHD would undergo preconception evaluation, including advice on risk prediction and contraception, by a joint cardiac–obstetric team seeking advice from other specialties [15]. Of note, recent

The Heart of Africa: Clinical Profile of an Evolving Burden of Heart Disease in Africa, First Edition.
Edited by Simon Stewart, Karen Sliwa, Ana Mocumbi, Albertino Damasceno, and Mpiko Ntsekhe.

findings from the Global Rheumatic Heart Disease Registry (REMEDY) (see Section 2) indicated that of 1,825 women with RHD in child-bearing age, only 3.6% were using contraception [16].

PPCMO is a disease particularly common in African women. It develops in previously healthy women peripartum and carries a mortality rate of approximately 15%. In a recent publication we summarize the prevalence, clinical presentation, and natural history of PPCMO treated with standard HF medication [17]. Close collaboration with basic scientists from Hannover University, Germany, gave rise to unique translational research involving several animal models and human biological samples, providing breakthrough evidence [18] on the pathogenesis of human PPCMO. Treatment of mice (which serve as a model for human PPCMO) with bromocriptine, a dopamine antagonist inhibiting prolactin, prevented the development of the disease. Figure 1.1 summarizes the possible metabolic events leading to PPCMO.

Subsequent to this foundational research, a South African clinical trial in women with newly diagnosed PPCMO [19] was conducted. The trial showed significant clinical improvement in those treated with bromocriptine, compared to patients receiving only standard care. These initially positive results have since been confirmed via collaborative research in a German cohort [20], and this ongoing work was recently summarized in an invited review on this new treatment modality [21]. In conclusion, joint obstetric-medical-cardiac clinics will be the optimal approach for women presenting with cardiac disease in the peripartum period in sub-Saharan Africa. Appropriate guidance in referral to secondary and tertiary care hospitals with dedicated cardiac disease in maternity clinics should be implemented and is currently being explored in South Africa [13].

1.1 Spectrum of maternal cardiac disease in South Africa

Sliwa K, Libhaber E, Elliott C, Momberg Z, Osman A, Zühlke L, Lachmann T, Nicholson L, Thienemann F, Roos-Hesselink J, Anthony J. Spectrum of cardiac disease in maternity in a low resource cohort in South Africa. *Heart* 2014; 100(24):1967–74. [13]

1.1.1 Background
Data focusing on the spectrum and characteristics of cardiovascular disease (CVD) among women in LMIC are limited, especially among those who are pregnant [22,23]. In sub-Saharan Africa this significant clinical research gap is exacerbated by a shortage of physicians and health care resources.

1.1.2 Study aims
The aims of this study were to examine the spectrum and characteristics of CVD presenting in the prepartum and postpartum period, as well as describe maternal and fetal outcomes, in a representative cohort of African women in Cape Town, South Africa.

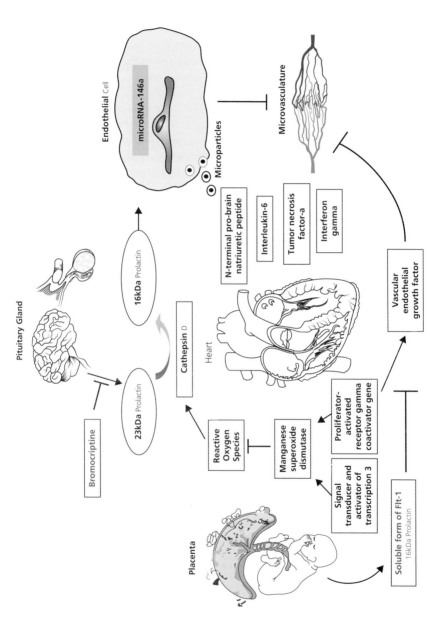

Figure 1.1 Basic mechanisms underlying peripartum cardiomyopathy.

1.1.3 Methods
1.1.3.1 Patient enrollment
During the period 1 July 2010 to 30 June 2012, 225 consecutive pregnant women with suspected or previously diagnosed CVD were assessed at their first visit to the joint cardiac–obstetric clinic, having been directed there via a referral algorithm from primary care and secondary care facilities in Cape Town and from within the tertiary hospital (see Figure 1.2). All referred patients were seen by a senior cardiology and obstetric consultant, and physicians from other disciplines (i.e., radiology, endocrinology, and anesthetics) were consulted. Patients were then assessed throughout their pregnancy, while those presenting postpartum were seen once at this clinic and subsequently managed at the general cardiac clinic or a dedicated CMO clinic, at Groote Schuur Hospital, Cape Town, South Africa. Patient appointments were scheduled according to standard management, which could entail a waiting period of up to 3 months. Patients with a history of CVD and a normal clinical inspection, along with minimal echocardiography changes, were seen only on one occasion early and subsequently referred to second-level obstetric care. Most patients were referred from peripheral hospitals; therefore, records were not available to document maternal and fetal outcomes. Those patients who presented with signs, symptoms, or a World Health Organization (WHO)

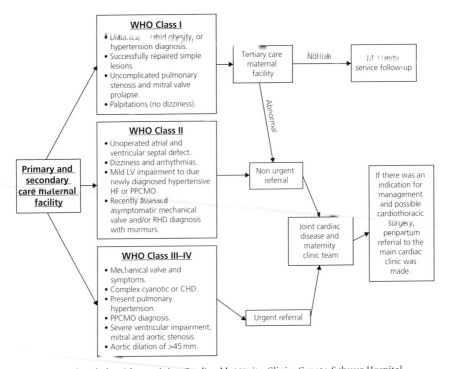

Figure 1.2 Referral algorithm to joint Cardiac Maternity Clinic, Groote Schuur Hospital.

classification stage of II–IV underwent clinical visits at <28 weeks (second trimester), 28 to 37 weeks (third trimester), onset of labor until hospital discharge (peripartum period), and at 6 weeks and 6 months postpartum.

1.1.4 Results

As detailed in Table 1.1, patients of African ancestry were significantly more likely to present with advanced disease (WHO II–IV) than those of other ethnic groups (p<0.0001). Patients in the modified WHO class II–IV exhibited significantly higher heart rate (p<0.0001) and gravidity (p=0.0002) than those in WHO class I. Comorbidity, including HIV infection, was associated with more severe cardiac disease (p<0.0001). Overall, 73 (32.4%) patients were classified as

Table 1.1 Patients' demographic and clinical characteristics according WHO functional class.

	WHO I (n = 73)	WHO II–IV (n = 152)	All (n = 225)
Age (years)	28.8±7.0	28.5±6.1	28.6±6.4
Ethnicity			
African ancestry	23 (31.5%)	79 (52.0%)	101 (44.9%)
Mixed	15 (20.6%)	56 (36.8%)	72 (32.0%)
Caucasian	19 (26.0%)	15 (9.9%)	34 (15.1%)
Other	16 (21.9%)	2 (1.3%)	18 (8.0%)
Medical history			
Hypertension	2 (2.7%)	10 (6.6%)	12 (5.3%)
Hypercholesterolemia	0 (0%)	3 (2.0%)	3 (1.3%)
HIV infection	2 (2.7%)	36 (23.7%)	38 (16.9%)
Syphilis	0 (0%)	1 (0.7%)	1 (0.4%)
TB	0 (0%)	4 (2.6%)	4 (1.8%)
Clinical history			
Previously known CVD	40 (54.8%)	53 (34.9%)	93 (41.3%)
Previous CVD operation	27 (37.0%)	30 (19.7%)	57 (25.3%)
NYHA Class I–II	73 (100%)	120 (78.9%)	193 (85.8%)
NYHA Class III–IV	0 (0%)	32 (21.1%)	32 (14.2%)
Systolic BP (mm Hg)	118±13	119±16	119±15
Diastolic BP (mm Hg)	75±10	74±11	74±11
Heart rate (beats/min)	78±12	90±19	86±18
Weight (kg)	72.5±12.5	72.1±18.6	72.1±16.8
Obstetric history			
<12 weeks	3 (4.1%)	4 (2.6%)	7 (3.1%)
12 to 24 weeks	32 (43.8%)	52 (34.2%)	84 (37.3%)
>24 weeks	31 (42.5%)	66 (43.4%)	97 (43.1%)
Median gravida (range)	2 (1–6)	2 (1–7)	2 (1–7)
Median para (range)	1 (0–4)	1 (0–5)	1 (0–5)
Nulliparous	29 (39.7%)	36 (23.6%)	65 (28.9)
Twin pregnancies	0 (0%)	3 (2.0%)	3 (1.3%)

WHO class I; of these, 27 (37.0%) had been referred for other reasons such as history of palpitations or the need for pre-conception counseling, 26 (35.6%) presented with minor or operated CHD and no significant residual structural abnormality, 16 (21.9%) had RHD, and 4 (5.5%) had chronic hypertension with no end-organ damage. The remaining 152 (67.6) patients were placed in WHO class II–IV and required close follow-up; of these, 21 (13.8%) presented with PPCMO, 15 (9.9%) with prior CHD surgical correction, 15 (9.9%) with prior surgery for RHD, 11 (7.2%) with idiopathic dilated CMO, 9 (5.9%) with hypertension-related CMO, 8 (5.3%) with atrial septal defect, 6 (4.0%) with ventricular septal defect, 5 (3.3%) with ventricular arrhythmias, 4 (2.6%) with Takayasu's disease, 4 (2.6%) with Marfan's disease, 3 (2.0%) with coarctation, and 3 (2.0%) with constrictive pericarditis. Notably, IHD was absent in this cohort. Figure 1.3 displays the distribution of patients per disease group.

As shown in Table 1.2, 122 (80.3%) patients presented prepartum, including 66 (54.1%) presenting for the first time with a gestational age entry at >24 weeks. Patients of African ancestry were more likely to present postpartum (p=0.009). Overall, 30 (19.7%) patients presented in the postpartum period with severe functional impairment as measured by NYHA class (p<0.001) and displayed significantly higher NTproBNP levels (p<0.0001) and heart rate (p<0.001). Patients presenting with developing symptoms of PPCMO had significantly larger LV dimensions and with a markedly lower left ventricular ejection fraction (LVEF) (44.7±11.8% versus 54.5±12.4%; p<0.003). Of the women diagnosed with CVD prepartum, 27% received diuretics, 7.5% beta blockers, and 7.3% warfarin while pregnant.

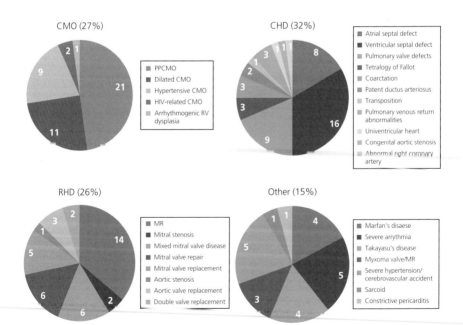

Figure 1.3 Case distributions according to disease categories.

Table 1.2 Patients' demographic and clinical characteristics.

	Presenting Prepartum (n = 122)	Presenting Postpartum (n = 30)	All (n = 152)
Age (years)	28.2 ± 6.2	29.6 ± 5.8	28.5 ± 6.1
Ethnicity			
African ancestry	55 (45.1%)	24 (80.0%)	79 (51.9%)
Mixed	50 (41.0%)	6 (20.0%)	56 (36.8%)
White	15 (12.3%)	0 (0%)	15 (9.9%)
Other	2 (1.6%)	0 (0%)	2 (1.3%)
Language			
Afrikaans	40 (32.8%)	3 (10.0%)	43 (28.3%)
English	29 (23.8%)	4 (13.3%)	33 (21.7%)
isiXhosa	41 (33.6%)	17 (56.6%)	58 (38.2%)
isiZulu	9 (7.4%)	3 (10.0%)	12 (7.9%)
Education level			
Year 1–7	36 (29.5%)	10 (33.3%)	46 (30.3%)
Year 8–11	73 (59.8%)	19 (63.3%)	92 (60.5%)
Income per month (ZAR)			
<300	39 (32.0%)	17 (56.7%)	56 (36.8%)
300–999	31 (25.4%)	7 (23.3%)	38 (25.0%)
1,000–9,999	48 (39.3%)	6 (20.0%)	54 (35.5%)
General medical history (%)			
Hypertension	10 (8.2%)	0 (0%)	10 (6.6%)
HIV infection	26 (21.3%)	10 (33.3%)	36 (23.6%)
TB	3 (2.5%)	1 (3.3%)	4 (2.6%)
CVD family history	21 (17.2%)	2 (6.7%)	23 (15.1%)
PPCMO/CMO family history	10 (8.2%)	1 (3.3%)	11 (7.2%)
Heart valve replacement	16 (13.1%)	0 (0%)	16 (10.5%)
Obstetric history			
Presenting with prepartum			
12 to 24 weeks	52 (42.6%)	0 (0%)	52 (34.2%)
>24 weeks	66 (54.1%)	0 (0%)	66 (43.4%)
Nulliparous	32 (26.2%)	4 (13.3%)	36 (23.7%)
Parous	90 (73.8%)	26 (86.7%)	116 (76.3%)

1.1.4.1 Cardiac outcomes

Only one patient who was diagnosed with CVD prepartum had no postpartum visit. Therefore, follow-up data were available for 142 (93.4%) patients. Maternal mortality rate was 9 of 152 (OR 5.92%, 95% CI 2.15, 9.65%) within the 6-month postpartum follow-up period. Of these, 7 (77.8%) patients died due to familial CMO or PPCMO, with 2 cases of prosthetic valve complications. All patients who died had been assessed as WHO class III or IV. Significantly, 8 (88.9%) of 9 patients died 42 days postpartum. Overall, 30 patients had a poor outcome as predefined using a combined endpoint of death, low LVEF, or remaining in New York Heart Association (NYHA) Class III or IV. Of the women diagnosed with CVD prepartum, 41 (33.6%) developed signs and symptoms of heart disease while pregnant, leading to admission in 20% of cases. At the final follow-up, 13 (10.7%) of the patients were found to be in NYHA Class III or IV. Of the 30 patients diagnosed with CVD postpartum, 3 (10.0%) died before their 6-month visit. Of the remaining patients, 12 (44.4%) felt minimally to moderately better compared to their first presentation, 3 (11.1%) were unchanged, and 12 (44.4%) felt minimally or moderately worse.

1.1.4.2 Fetal and obstetric outcome

Mean gestational stage was 36.7 ± 4.2 years with a significantly longer gestational period in patients presenting with antenatal cardiac disease versus those presenting postpartum (p=0.04). Eleven patients developed gestational hypertension during pregnancy. Overall, there was a high operative delivery rate, with 46 (30.3%) of 152 patients having received a cesarean section. No significant differences in obstetric outcome were revealed between the modified WHO Class II, III, and IV disease categories. Perinatal death occurred in 1 (0.7%) out of 152 patients (0.66; 95% CI 0.00, 1.94) due to one fetal death, translating to a perinatal mortality of 7/1,000 live births. In addition, there were two miscarriages and two medically indicated terminations. Mean birth weight for the entire cohort was 2850.8 ± 552.7 g, with 33/148 born weighing <2500 g and 46/148 born preterm (<37 weeks' duration).

1.1.5 Study interpretation

Overall, this study revealed a pattern of disease that was markedly different from that of developed countries in terms of RHD, the CMOs, and CHD. Maternal mortality occurred in 9 of 152 (5.9%) patients. This was significantly higher than that reported in a recent study undertaken by the European Society of Cardiology [24]. Most deaths were due to forms of CMO, with only two deaths being related to complications attributable to sepsis and thrombosis affecting prosthetic heart valves. These data point to the need for care to be intensified covering the postpartum period, including earlier referral to the general cardiac or CMO clinic and adequate counseling about the risks of future pregnancy and contraceptive services. A recent systematic review of the burden of antenatal heart disease in South Africa reported a prevalence of heart disease ranging from 123 to 943 per 100,000 deliveries, with RHD being the most common abnormality, followed by CMO [25]. These data also revealed that 18% of women who survived and attended follow-up clinics experienced symptoms that were worse after the pregnancy, with 44% displaying moderate-to-severe disability. There were no stillbirths and only one neonatal death. Although 30% of the patients delivered before 37 weeks, the mean gestational age at delivery fell just short of 37 weeks and the mean birth weight was 2.85 kg. In the future, echocardiography-based screening of patients may further improve identification and referral of high-risk cases, although the cost-effectiveness of this intervention has yet to be established [26,27]

1.1.6 Study limitations

As with all observational studies of this kind, particularly when focused on a single center and community, the wider generalizability of observed associations (with the inherent caveat around inferring causality) and outcomes needs to be considered. Despite the study's relatively large size and detailed clinical phenotyping, its data should still be interpreted with some caution.

1.1.7 Study conclusion

In conclusion, these data derived from a South African maternal cohort revealed a disease pattern markedly different from that seen in developed countries. Joint obstetric–cardiac care is related to the survival rates of pregnant mothers, even those with complex diseases, and their offspring. The greatest risk of adverse outcomes is attributable to late presentation and advanced cardiac failure, with death commonly occurring outside the 42-day maternal mortality reporting period. The perinatal outcome in an environment of intensive surveillance and management was found to be generally good.

1.2 Initial evaluation of bromocriptine treatment for PPCMO in South Africa

Sliwa K, Blauwet L, Tibazarwa K, Libhaber E, Smedema JP, Becker A, McMurray J, Yamac H, Labidi S, Struhman I, Hilfiker-Kleiner D. **Evaluation of bromocriptine in the treatment of acute severe peripartum cardiomyopathy: a proof-of-concept pilot study.** *Circulation* 2010; 121:1465–73. [28]

1.2.1 Background

As shown in recent studies focusing on PPCMO, only 23 to 54% of patients show recovery of cardiac function within 6 months [29–32]. Previous reports suggest that enhanced oxidative stress in a mouse model for PPCMO (mice with a cardiac-specific deletion for signal transducer and activator of transcription-3) triggers the activation of cathepsin D, a ubiquitous lysosomal enzyme that subsequently cleaves serum prolactin into its antiangiogenic and proapoptotic 16-kDa form [18]. This is associated with endothelial inflammation, impaired cardiomyocyte metabolism, and reduced myocardial contraction, suggesting that oxidative stress, inflammation, and prolactin may be interconnected and responsible for initiating PPCMO. Although these preliminary results suggesting beneficial effects of bromocriptine treatment in patients with acute PPCMO appear promising, concerns have been raised about the risk of thrombotic complications, including cerebral vascular incident and acute myocardial infarction (AMI) [33–36] and potential negative consequences for the children of these mothers, who are unable to breast-feed [37].

1.2.2 Study aims

The aim of this study was to initially assess the efficacy of bromocriptine on recovery of LV function, symptom status, and other clinical measures in patients presenting within the first month postpartum with new-onset symptomatic PPCMO and a LVEF <35%. A further aim was to identify prolactin, mainly its 16-kDa angiostatic and proapoptotic form, as a key factor in the pathophysiological development of PPCMO.

1.2.3 Methods

1.2.3.1 Patient enrollment

The study was conducted at the Chris Hani Baragwanath Hospital in Soweto, South Africa, where 93 pregnant patients suspected of having PPCMO were screened for confirmation. Patients were included in the study if they presented with a negative HIV status and CHF that developed during the final month of pregnancy or the first month postpartum. They were excluded if they presented with clinical conditions other than CMO that could increase plasma levels of inflammatory markers; a systolic blood pressure (BP) of <160 or <95 mm Hg or a diastolic BP of >105 mm Hg; significant liver disease; impaired renal dysfunction; a history of psychiatric disorder or peptic ulcer disease; or any other clinical conditions that in the opinion of the investigators precluded inclusion (e.g., IHD or malignancy). Clinical assessment, signs and symptoms, blood analysis, and echocardiography were recorded at baseline and at 6-month follow-up.

1.2.3.2 Pharmacotherapy

All patients received treatment with the loop-diuretic furosemide and the angiotensin-converting enzyme (ACE) inhibitor enalapril. Enalapril and carvedilol doses were titrated upward as tolerated during the first 4 weeks after diagnosis and then remained unchanged throughout the remainder of the study period. Carvedilol was added after resolution of overt HF. Patients who presented with LV thrombus or a LVEF of <25% received anticoagulation therapy with warfarin for 6 months. Furosemide dose was decreased as indicated according to clinical assessment during the 6-month study period. Ten patients were randomized to standard therapy (PPCMO-Standard) as described above, and the other 10 were randomized to standard therapy and received bromocriptine (PPCMO-Bromocriptine) 2.5 twice daily for 2 weeks followed by 2.5 mg daily for 6 weeks thereafter. After baseline visits, monthly outpatient visits were organized for medication response assessment and evaluation. Patients who were receiving bromocriptine underwent cardiac MRIs at 4 to 6 weeks after diagnosis to detect mural thrombi. All newborns of the study patients were assessed every 6 months with standard growth-monitoring charts issued by the South African Department of Health and maintained by primary physicians.

1.2.4 Results

Overall, 20 (21.5%) consecutive patients out of the 93 patients screened were enrolled in the study. As shown in Table 1.3, both the PPCMO-Standard and the PPCMO-Bromocriptine groups were found to have a similar age, parity, systolic

Table 1.3 Patients' demographic and clinical characteristics.

	PPCMO-Standard n = 10	PPCMO-Bromocriptine n = 10
Demographic characteristics		
Age (years)	28 ± 10	24 ± 6
Parity	2 (IQR 1–6)	1.5 (IQR 1–3)
Clinical characteristics		
Systolic BP (mm Hg)	110 ± 19	116 ± 23
Diastolic BP (mm Hg)	76 ± 18	70 ± 16
Heart rate (beats/min)	108 ± 15	102 ± 13
NYHA class		
II/III	5 (50.0%)	5 (50.0%)
IV	5 (50.0%)	5 (50.0%)
Echocardiographic presentations		
LV end-diastolic diameter (mm)	59 ± 5	55 ± 10
LV end-systolic diameter (mm)	52 ± 6	46 ± 9
LVEF (%)	26.9 ± 7.6	27.2 ± 8.1
Mitral regurgitation (grade)	1.9 ± 0.6	2.1 ± 0.6
Mitral effective regurgitant orifice (cm^2)	0.44 ± 0.18	0.45 ± 0.13
Laboratory presentations		
Hemoglobin (g/dL)	11.8 ± 1.9	13.0 ± 2.2
Creatinine (μmol/L)	66 (IQR 5, 96)	71 (IQR 6-109)
High-sensitivity C-reactive protein (mg/L)	6.0 (IQR 4.0, 115)	7.8 (IQR 1.1, 58)
Prolactin (μg/L)	30.0 (IQR 5.1, 233)	49.9 (IQR 3.8, 135)
Log N-terminal pro b-type natriuretic peptide	8.54 ± 1.24	8.54 ± 1.24

and diastolic BP, heart rate, NYHA Class, LV end-diastolic diameter, and LV end-systolic diameter.

1.2.4.1 Pharmacotherapy

At 6 months, the median daily enalapril dosage for the PPCMO-Standard group was 10 mg/day compared to 5 mg/day for the PPCMO-Bromocriptine group. Similarly, the median carvedilol dosage among the PPCMO-Standard group was 12.5 mg twice daily compared to 6.25 mg twice daily for the PPCMO-Bromocriptine group. For both groups, the median furosemide dosage was 80 mg/day (IQR 80, 120 mg).

1.2.4.2 Baseline and 6-month echocardiographic parameters

The study groups did not significantly differ in systolic and diastolic BP, heart rate, or LV end-diastolic and end-systolic dimension changes from baseline to 6 months. However, LVEF recovery was greater in the PPCMO-Bromocriptine group compared with the PPCMO-Standard group (31% versus 9%; p = 0.012), as was improvement of mitral regurgitation (MR) (p = 0.013), along with several other parameters shown in Table 1.4.

Table 1.4 Patients' baseline and 6-month echocardiographic changes according to group.

	Baseline		6 Months	
	PPCMO-Standard	PPCMO-Bromocriptine	PPCMO-Standard	PPCMO-Bromocriptine
Clinical parameters				
Systolic BP (mm Hg)	110±19	116±23	115±9	118±13
Diastolic BP (mm Hg)	76±18	70±16	73±6	74±9
Heart rate (beats/min)	108±15	102±13	79±15	64±7
Echocardiographic parameters				
LV end-diastolic diameter (mm)	59±5	55±10	56±12	51±9
LV end-systolic diameter (mm)	52±6	46±9	45±11	34±10
LVEF (%)	27±8	27±8	36±11	58±11
MR (grade)	1.9±0.6	2.1±0.6	1.5±1.0	0.22±0.44
Mitral effective regurgitant orifice (cm²)	0.44±0.18	0.45±0.13	0.34±0.18	0.11±0.03
Left atrial diameter (cm)	3.83±0.62	3.54±0.25	3.93±0.83	3.36±0.53
Mitral E velocity (cm/s)	89±23	86±19	85±24	66±24
Mitral A velocity (cm/s)	33±6	32±7	45±12	48±19
Mitral E velocity/A velocity ratio	2.73±0.68	2.82±0.76	1.94±0.67	1.63±1.13
Deceleration time (ms)	136±30	118±26	168±36	197±59
Mitral medial annular (E') tissue Doppler imaging. velocity (cm/s)	6.5±1.1	7.0±1.3	7.3±2.5	12.4±2.4
E/E' (medial annular velocity)	14.0±4.0	12.5±3.0	12.4±6.4	5.4±2.5
Mitral lateral annular (E') tissue Doppler imaging. velocity (cm/s)	6.6±0.97	7.2±1.1	7.3±2.5	12.4±2.5
E/E' (lateral annular velocity)	13.8±4.2	12.0±2.0	12.1±3.9	5.4±2.5

1.2.4.3 Natriuretic peptide levels

Log N-terminal pro b-type natriuretic peptide change was found to differ between the groups, with a borderline statistically significant (positive) difference present in the PPCMO-Bromocriptine group as compared with the PPCMO-Standard group (p=0.05).

1.2.4.4 Outcomes and infant findings

In the PPCMO-Standard group, 4 patients died prior to the 6-month follow-up, due to HF (n=3) and sudden cardiac death (n=1). Alternatively, only 1 patient died in the PPCMO-Bromocriptine group at 7 days due to severe HF; all remaining patients survived to 6 months. Furthermore, all 9 surviving PPCMO-Bromocriptine patients were found to have recovered to NYHA Class I at the 6-month follow-up. In contrast, 3 PPCMO-Standard patients were assessed as NYHA Class II and 3 as NYHA Class III at 6 months. With respect to the infant outcomes, a total of 21 children were assessed throughout the study, all displaying normal growth curves when recorded on the WHO standard weight-for-age growth charts. Although all

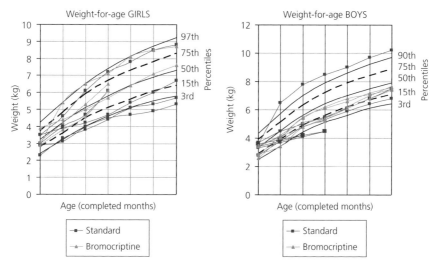

Figure 1.4 Comparison of infant growth curves according to maternal treatment group.

children were alive at the 6-month follow-up, weight-for-age data at 6 months were available for 13 children. However, there was no significant difference in the children's growth curves at 3 months according to study group (see Figure 1.4).

1.2.5 Study interpretation

This key study showed that the addition of bromocriptine to standard HF therapy in women with PPCMO was associated with significantly greater improvements in NYHA functional class, LV systolic and diastolic function, and degree of functional MR than was observed with standard therapy alone. Moreover, bromocriptine appeared to be well tolerated with no thrombotic complications observed, and although its use prevented lactation and breast-feeding in the PPCMO patients, the growth and survival of their infants were normal. In addition, both forms of prolactin promote inflammation [38], a reaction that seems to be associated with PPCMO in this African cohort, given that most patients displayed increased serum levels of the inflammatory marker high-sensitivity C-reactive protein [30]. Positive effects of bromocriptine on BP, vascular resistance, and plasma norepinephrine levels have been described [39]. However, it has been shown to increase stroke volume index and to decrease LV filling pressure [39,40]. The mortality rate in the PPCMO-Standard group was higher than in the group receiving bromocriptine, a finding that diverges from data previously reported [29,30,41,42]. This difference may be due to variations in inclusion criteria, as patients in this study were enrolled within 24 hours after diagnosis.

1.2.6 Study limitations

This trial involved a number of limitations that require comment. First, as a pilot study, the cohort was small, albeit with sufficiently encouraging results to prompt larger and more definitive studies in the future. Second, blinding of the study was not possible as the PPCMO-Standard group continued to nurse their infants while the PPCMO-Bromocriptine group could not breast-feed due to bromocriptine-induced cessation of lactation. Although this was a small study with only short-term follow-up, these results suggest no disadvantage to the infant of a PPCMO patient who could not breast-feed for this reason. However, at the time of this report a larger study was currently underway in Germany testing this concept. The European Cardiac Society via the EURObservational Research Programme is currently collecting information on 1,000 patients with PPCM from >40 countries, which will also include a large number of women who have received bromocriptine.

1.2.7 Study conclusion

In conclusion, the addition of bromocriptine to standard HF therapy appeared to improve cardiac function in women presenting with PPCMO, with no ill effects evident in their infants. Despite the small sample size, which consequently cannot be taken as representative of the population at large, these results are very encouraging.

1.3 Health outcomes associated with PPCMO in South Africa

Blauwet LA, Libhaber E, Forster O, Tibazarwa K, Mebazaa A, Hilfiker-Kleiner D, Sliwa H. **Predictors of outcome in 176 South African patients with peripartum cardiomyopathy.** *Heart* 2013; 99(5):308–13. [17]

1.3.1 Background

As described above, PPCMO is known to cause HF among pregnant women several months before and 6 months after delivery. Even though most PPCMO patients experience a higher rate of recovery of LV function than observed in those with other forms of nonischemic CMO [43], only 23 to 54% patients are reported to recover at 6 months [29–31,43,44]. Case series have demonstrated that poor outcomes are predicted by LV dilation, LV thrombus, LV systolic dysfunction, and body mass index (BMI), as well as renal and liver dysfunction [31,44–48]. However, the association between HF and BMI, renal function, and liver dysfunction has not been previously assessed in patients with PPCMO.

1.3.2 Study aims

The aim of this study was to determine whether those variables previously linked to poor outcomes in PPCMO (outlined above) are indeed predictors of outcome in a large cohort of PPCMO patients in Soweto, South Africa.

1.3.3 Methods
1.3.3.1 Patient enrollment

Patients being referred to the Chris Hani Baragwanath Hospital in Soweto, South Africa, from local clinics, secondary hospitals, and the Department of Obstetrics at the same hospital were studied. Each patient underwent assessment for preexisting cardiac signs and symptoms during first presentation at the cardiac unit and at the 6-month follow-up; this was confirmed by examining the obstetric card carried by each patient. Blood analysis, echocardiography, and clinical assessment were also performed at baseline and at follow-up. Inclusion criteria comprised age between ≥16 and ≤40 years old, symptoms of CHF that developed during the last month of pregnancy or the first 5 months postpartum and no other identifiable cause of HF, LVEF ≤45% by transthoracic echocardiography, and sinus rhythm. Patients were excluded if they presented with significant organic VHD, a systolic BP >160 mm Hg or diastolic BP >100 mm Hg, clinical conditions other than CMO that could increase plasma levels of inflammatory markers, severe anemia (hemoglobin <9 g/dL), and/or IHD or malignancy. Of the 176 patients who were included in the study, 164 (93.2%) received treatment with furosemide, 141 (80.1%) were treated with ACE inhibitor, 113 (64.2%) were prescribed digoxin, and 100 (56.8%) were prescribed carvedilol after resolution of overt HF. ACE inhibitors and carvedilol doses were titrated upward as tolerated throughout the 6-month study period.

1.3.4 Results

1.3.4.1 Cohort profile

In total, 176 consecutive patients diagnosed with PPCMO and fulfilling the inclusion criteria were enrolled in the study. All patients were of African ancestry. The mean age was 30.7 ± 6.9 years, mean parity was 2 (range 1–7); mean BMI was 25.6 ± 5.2 kg/m², and most of the women (82%) presented as NYHA Class III or IV. Table 1.5 compares the patients' characteristics from baseline to 6-month follow-up, demonstrating that while the mean LV end systolic dimension decreased significantly from 51.3 ± 7.6 mm to 42.3 ± 9.5 mm (p < 0.0001), mean LVEF increased significantly from 27.3 ± 8.1 mm to 43.3 ± 12.5 mm (p < 0.0001). Over the same period, mitral inflow E/A decreased significantly from 2.01 ± 0.86 ms to 1.51 ± 0.65 ms, and mitral inflow deceleration time increased significantly from 140.0 ± 66.1 ms to 185 ± 67.9 ms (p < 0.0001 for both). Hemoglobin, renal function, and liver function test results had also improved at 6 months.

1.3.4.2 Health outcomes

During 6-month follow-up, 9 (5.1%) patients were lost to follow-up, 3 (1.7%) moved to remote areas where follow-up could not occur, and 2 (1.1%) did not undergo echocardiographic assessment at 6 months. Of the remaining 162 (80.1%) patients, 45 (27.8%) met the prespecified combined endpoint of death, or (if still alive) remained in NYHA Class III/IV and/or had a residual LVEF <35% at 6 months. Univariate analysis of baseline profiling revealed that this prespecified composite endpoint was predicted by increased LV end systolic diameter, mitral inflow E/A, aspartate transaminase, and alanine transaminase; and decreased systolic BP, LVEF, mitral inflow deceleration time, and total cholesterol. Of the 141 patients who survived, 30 (21.3%) had fully recovered LV function (LVEF ≥55%) at 6 months. When comparing the baseline characteristics of the patients

Table 1.5 Patients' baseline and 6-month follow-up characteristics.

	Baseline (n = 176)	6-Month Follow-up (n = 141)
Age (years)	30.7 ± 6.9	—
Median parity (range)	2 (1–7)	—
BMI (kg/m²)	25.6 ± 5.2	—
Systolic BP (mm Hg)	111 ± 17	113 ± 17
Diastolic BP (mm Hg)	72 ± 13	72 ± 12
Heart rate (beats/min)	97.3 ± 19.1	—
NYHA functional class		
I/II	33 (18.8%)	128 (90.8%)
III/IV	143 (82.3%)	13 (9.2%)
Echocardiography		
LV end-diastolic diameter (mm)	59.5 ± 7.3	54.0 ± 8.6
LV end-systolic diameter (mm)	51.8 ± 7.6	42.3 ± 9.5
LVEF (%)	27.1 ± 8.1	43.3 ± 12.5
E-velocity (ms)	0.89 ± 0.25	0.80 ± 0.22
A-velocity (ms)	0.49 ± 0.20	0.57 ± 0.18
E/A	2.02 ± 0.89	1.51 ± 0.65
Deceleration time (ms)	134.5 ± 63.2	185.1 ± 67.9
LV thrombus	19 (10.8%)	0 (0%)
Laboratory		
Hemoglobin (g/dL)	11.1 ± 1.9	12.8 ± 1.52
Creatinine (mmol/L)	84.1 ± 20.5	76.4 ± 23.5
Urea (mmol/L)	5.4 ± 2.9	4.4 ± 1.6
Total protein (g/L)	77.9 ± 11.4	82.2 ± 8.9
Albumin (g/L)	40.1 ± 18.5	43.7 ± 13.5
Total bilirubin (μmol/L)	17.3 ± 26.8	11.0 ± 8.6
Direct bilirubin (μmol/L)	9.2 ± 23.2	4.5 ± 4.9
Indirect bilirubin (μmol/L)	8.2 ± 7.3	6.1 ± 4.4
Alkaline phosphatase (U/l)	117.9 ± 51.0	97.4 ± 36.4
Aspartate transaminase (U/l)	45.0 ± 46.8	26.4 ± 12.9
Alanine transaminase (U/l)	54.7 ± 67.1	24.5 ± 14.0
γ-glutamyl transpeptidase (U/l)	72.4 ± 49.4	52.8 ± 40.8

who fully recovered to those of the patients who did not, it was found that predictors of LV recovery included older age, increased hemoglobin levels, and decreased LV end systolic diameter, LV end diastolic dimension, and creatinine levels.

1.3.5 Study interpretation

These data confirm previous reports that a relatively high proportion of surviving patients with PPCMO (around 4 in 5 cases) have residually poor LV function (i.e., minimum cardiac recovery) at 6 months [31,47]. Baseline predictors of poor outcome in this series of patients included increased LV end systolic diameter, lower BMI, and lower total cholesterol levels. Older age appears to be a novel predictor of LV recovery, while younger age, lower BMI, increased LV end systolic diameter and LV end diastolic diameter, and higher NYHA class all seem to be predictors of mortality. As previously reported, increased LV end systolic diameter at diagnosis was a significant predictor of outcome, even when adjusted for other variables in multivariate analysis [44]. However, in contrast with previous reports, LVEF and LV end diastolic diameter at diagnosis, NYHA class, and presence of LV thrombus were not predictors of poor outcome [30,31,44,45,47,48]. Numerous studies have shown an association between cholesterol and mortality in patients with chronic HF [49–51]. As the cohort experienced a relatively low number of deaths, multiple logistic regression analysis of mortality was not performed. Future studies are therefore necessary to further clarify and validate predictors of mortality among this patient population. More awareness of CVD in pregnant women is urgently required. The team has developed a web-based data entry platform that contains a number of videos for women from low socioeconomic backgrounds providing information on common cardiac conditions in pregnancy. This data entry platform can be accessed under www. hedu-africa.org (Figure 1.5).

1.3.6 Study limitations

As noted earlier, as in all observational studies of this kind, particularly when focused on a single center and community, the wider generalizability of observed associations (with the inherent caveat around inferring causality) and outcomes needs to be considered. In particular, this was a selected population attending a specialist program focusing on PPCMO, and there is a need to confirm observations in other parts of Africa—noting the creation of a prospective registry for this very purpose.

1.3.7 Study conclusion

In conclusion, high LV end systolic diameter and low total cholesterol were found to be associated with poor outcomes in a large cohort of African women with PPCMO. Conversely, lower LV end systolic diameter and older age were related to high levels LV function recovery.

S1.2 Maternal health in Africa: The way forward

Given residually high levels of maternal ill health and mortality, there is urgent need to refocus on this major health issue throughout the African continent; particularly given high mortality rates in the content of the relatively (to other African countries) well-developed maternal health care system in South Africa. Much of the death and disability at this stage of life is cardiac related and highly preventable with more structured surveillance and proactive management of underlying cardiovascular issues (particularly hypertension). In response to these

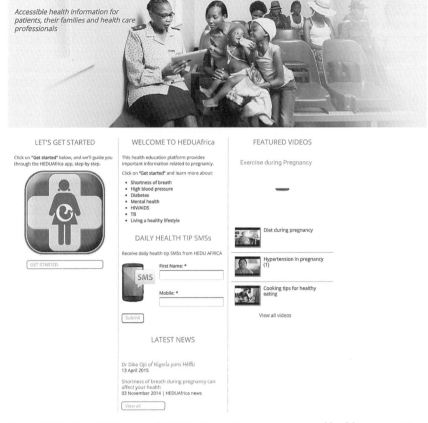

Figure 1.5 The Health Education (HEDU) Initiative to improve maternal health outcomes in South Africa.

data, ongoing research is focusing on harnessing information technology to provide important health messages to African women to improve their overall and maternal heart health. If successful, these will have a profound impact on maternal outcomes and, of course, on the short- and longer-term health prospects of the next generation of African children (see Section 2 below). More specific efforts are also underway to more actively quantify the distribution and number of cases of PPCMO via an Africa registry, along with ongoing efforts to better understand and treat this potentially devastating condition.

References

1 Kassebaum NJ, Bertozzi-Villa A, Coggeshall MS, Shackelford KA, Steiner C, Heuton KR, et al. Global, regional, and national levels and causes of maternal mortality during 1990–2013: a systematic analysis for the Global Burden of Disease Study 2013. *Lancet.* 2014;384(9947):980–1004.

2 Central Intelligence Agency. *The World Factbook: South Africa.* Washington, DC: Central Intelligence Agency; 2015 [updated September 4, 2015; accessed September 2015].

3 The World Bank. World Development Indicators: Urban Population [dataset] 2013. Available from: http://data.worldbank.org/indicator/SP.URB.TOTL.IN.ZS/countries.

4 The World Bank. World Development Indicators: Literacy Rate [dataset] 2013. Available from: http://data.worldbank.org/indicator/SE.ADT.LITR.ZS/countries.

5 The World Bank. World Development Indicators: Unemployment [dataset] 2015 [September 2015]. Available from: http://data.worldbank.org/indicator/SL.UEM.TOTL.ZS/countries.

6 World Health Organization. South Africa: WHO Statistical Profile. 2015. Available from: http://www.who.int/gho/countries/zaf.pdf?ua=1.

7 City of Cape Town. City of Cape Town: Facts and Figures. 2015 [updated September 2015; accessed September 2015]. Available from: https://www.capetown.gov.za/en/visitcapetown/Pages/Factsandfigures.aspx.

8 Statistics South Africa. Census 2011 Municipal Report: Western Cape. Statistics South Africa, 2012. Available from: http://www.statssa.gov.za/census/census_2011/census_products/WC_Municipal_Report.pdf.

9 Statistics South Africa. City of Cape Town 2015 [accessed September 2015]. Available from: http://www.statssa.gov.za/?page_id=1021&id=city-of-cape-town-municipality.

10 Statistics South Africa. South African National Census of 2011. South Africa, 2012.

11 City of Johannesburg. Johannesburg Growth and Development Strategy: Region D. South Africa, 2015 [accessed June 2015]. Available from: http://joburg.org.za/index.php?option=com_content&task=view&id=174&Itemid=168&limitstart=1.

12 Chris Hani Baragwanath Hospital. *Chris Hani Baragwanath Hospital: General Information Soweto,* South Africa [accessed July 2015]. Available from: https://www.chrishanibaragwanathhospital.co.za/.

13 Sliwa K, Libhaber E, Elliott C, Momberg Z, Osman A, Zuhlke L, et al. Spectrum of cardiac disease in maternity in a low-resource cohort in South Africa. *Heart.* 2014;100(24):1967–74.

14 Soma-Pillay K, Sebe, Sliwa K. The importance of cardiovascular pathology contributing to maternal death in South Africa: Confidential Enquiry into Maternal Deaths in South Africa, 2011–2013. *Cardiovasc J Afr.* 2016 (available online, February 2016).

15 Sliwa K, Johnson MR, Zilla P, Roos-Hesselink JW. Management of valvular disease in pregnancy: a global perspective. *Eur Heart J.* 2015;36(18):1078–89.

16 Zuhlke L, Engel ME, Karthikeyan G, Rangarajan S, Mackie P, Cupido B, et al. Characteristics, complications, and gaps in evidence-based interventions in rheumatic heart

The Heart of Africa: Clinical Profile of an Evolving Burden of Heart Disease in Africa, First Edition.
Edited by Simon Stewart, Karen Sliwa, Ana Mocumbi, Albertino Damasceno, and Mpiko Ntsekhe.
© 2016 John Wiley & Sons, Ltd. Published 2016 by John Wiley & Sons, Ltd.

disease: the Global Rheumatic Heart Disease Registry (the REMEDY study). *Eur Heart J.* 2015;36(18):1115–22a.

17 Blauwet LA, Libhaber E, Forster O, Tibazarwa K, Mebazaa A, Hilfiker-Kleiner D, et al. Predictors of outcome in 176 South African patients with peripartum cardiomyopathy. *Heart.* 2013;99(5):308–13.

18 Hilfiker-Kleiner D, Kaminski K, Podewski E, Bonda T, Schaefer A, Sliwa K, et al. A cathepsin D-cleaved 16 kDa form of prolactin mediates postpartum cardiomyopathy. *Cell.* 2007; 128(3):589–600.

19 Sliwa K, Blauwet L, Tibazarwa K, Libhaber E, Smedema JP, Becker A, et al. Evaluation of bromocriptine in the treatment of acute severe peripartum cardiomyopathy: a proof-of-concept pilot study. *Circulation.* 2010;121(13):1465–73.

20 Haghikia A, Podewski E, Libhaber E, Labidi S, Fischer D, Roentgen P, et al. Phenotyping and outcome on contemporary management in a German cohort of patients with peripartum cardiomyopathy. *Basic Res Cardiol.* 2013;108(4):366.

21 Hilfiker-Kleiner D, Sliwa K. Pathophysiology and epidemiology of peripartum cardiomyopathy. *Nat Rev Cardiol.* 2014;11(6):364–70.

22 Mocumbi AO, Sliwa K. Women's cardiovascular health in Africa. *Heart.* 2012;98(6):450–5.

23 Sliwa K, Mayosi BM. Recent advances in the epidemiology, pathogenesis and prognosis of acute heart failure and cardiomyopathy in Africa. *Heart.* 2013;99(18):1317–22.

24 Roos-Hesselink JW, Ruys TP, Stein JI, Thilen U, Webb GD, Niwa K, et al. Outcome of pregnancy in patients with structural or ischaemic heart disease: results of a registry of the European Society of Cardiology. *Eur Heart J.* 2013;34(9):657–65.

25 Watkins DA, Sebitloane M, Engel ME, Mayosi BM. The burden of antenatal heart disease in South Africa: a systematic review. *BMC Cardiovasc Disord.* 2012;12:23.

26 Mayosi BM, Flisher AJ, Lalloo UG, Sitas F, Tollman SM, Bradshaw D. The burden of non-communicable diseases in South Africa. *Lancet.* 2009;374(9693):934–47.

27 Sliwa K, Zilla P. Rheumatic heart disease: the tip of the iceberg. *Circulation.* 2012;125(25):3060–2.

28 Sliwa K, Blauwet L, Tibazarwa K, Libhaber E, Smedema JP, Becker A, et al. Evaluation of bromocriptine in the treatment of acute severe peripartum cardiomyopathy a proof-of-concept pilot study. *Circulation.* 2010;121:1465–73.

29 Fett JD, Christie LG, Carraway RD, Murphy JG. Five-year prospective study of the incidence and prognosis of peripartum cardiomyopathy. *Mayo Clin Proc.* 2005;80:1602–6.

30 Sliwa K, Forster O, Libhaber E, D. FJ, Sundstrom JB, Hilfiker-Kleiner D, et al. Peripartum cardiomyopathy: inflammatory markers as predictors of outcome in 100 prospectively studied patients. *Eur Heart J.* 2006;27:441–6.

31 Elkayam U, Akhter MW, Singh H, Khan S, Bitar F, Hameed A, et al. Pregnancy-associated cardiomyopathy. clinical characteristics and a comparison between early and late presentation. *Circulation.* 2005;111:2050–5.

32 Brar SS, Khan SS, Sandhu GK, Jorgensen MB, Parikh N, Hsu JW, et al. Incidence, mortality, and racial differences in peripartum cardiomyopathy. *Am J Cardiol.* 2007;100:302–4.

33 Iffy L, Lindenthal J, McArdle JJ, Ganesh V. Severe cerebral accidents postpartum in patients taking bromocriptine for milk suppression. *Isr J Med Sci.* 1996;32:309–12.

34 Hopp L, Weisse AB, Iffy L. Acute myocardial infarction in a healthy mother using bromocriptine for milk suppression. *Can J Cardiol.* 1996;12:415–8.

35 Loewe C, Dragovic LJ. Acute coronary artery thrombosis in a postpartum woman receiving bromocriptine. *Am J Forensic Med Pathol.* 1998;19:258–60.

36 Dutt S, Wong F, Spurway JH. Fatal myocardial infarction associated with bromocriptine for postpartum lactation suppression. *Aust N Z J Obstet Gynaecol.* 1998;38:116–7.

37 Fett JD. Caution in the use of bromocriptine in peripartum cardiomyopathy. *J Am Coll Cardiol.* 2008;51.

38 Hilfiker-Kleiner D, Sliwa K, Drexler H. Peripartum cardiomyopathy: recent insights in its pathophysiology. *Trends Cardiovasc Med.* 2008;18(5):173–9.

39 Francis GS, Parks R, Cohn JN. The effects of bromocriptine in patients with congestive heart failure. *Am Heart J.* 1983;106(1):100–6.

40 Goldberg LI. The role of dopamine receptors in the treatment of congestive heart failure. *J Cardiovasc Pharmacol.* 1989;14(suppl 5):S19–S27.

41 Sliwa K, Skudicky D, Candy G, Bergemann A, Hopley M, Sareli P. The addition of pentoxifylline to conventional therapy improves outcome in patients with peripartum cardiomyopathy. *Eur J Heart Fail.* 2002;4:305–9.

42 Sliwa K, Fett J, Elkayam U. Peripartum cardiomyopathy. *Lancet.* 2006;368:687–93.

43 Cooper LT, Mather PJ, Alexis JD, Pauly DF, Torre-Amione G, Wittstein IS, et al. Myocardial recovery in peripartum cardiomyopathy: prospective comparison with recent onset cardiomyopathy in men and nonperipartum women. *J Card Fail.* 2012;18:28–33.

44 Duran N, Gunes H, Duran I, Biteker M, Ozkan M. Predictors of prognosis in patients with peripartum cardiomyopathy. *Int J Gynaecol Obstet.* 2008;101:137–40.

45 Goland S, Bitar F, Modi K, Safirstein J, Ro A, Mirocha J, et al. Evaluation of the clinical relevance of baseline left ventricular ejection fraction as a predictor of recovery or persistence of severe dysfunction in women in the United States with peripartum cardiomyopathy. *J Card Fail.* 2011;17:426–30.

46 Habli M, O'Brien T, Nowack E, Khoury S, Barton JR, Sibai B. Peripartum cardiomyopathy: prognostic factors for long-term maternal outcome. *Am J Obstet Gynecol.* 2008;199:415e1–5.

47 Amos AM, Jaber WA, Russell SD. Improved outcomes in peripartum cardiomyopathy with contemporary. *Am Heart J.* 2006;152:509–13.

48 Witlin AG, Mabie WC, Sibai BM. Peripartum cardiomyopathy: a longitudinal echocardiographic study. *Am J Obstet Gynecol.* 1997;177:1129–32.

49 Afsarmanesh N, Horwich TB, Fonarow GC. Total cholesterol levels and mortality risk in nonischemic systolic heart failure. *Am Heart J* 2006;152:1077–83.

50 Horwich TB, Hamilton MA, Maclellan WR, Fonarow GC. Low serum total cholesterol is associated with marked increase in mortality in advanced heart failure. *J Card Fail.* 2002;8:216–24.

51 May HT, Muhlestein JB, Carlquist JF, Horne BD, Bair TL, Campbell BA, et al. Relation of serum total cholesterol, C-reactive protein levels, and statin therapy to survival in heart failure. *Am J Cardiol.* 2006;98:653–8.

SECTION 2

Infant and childhood heart disease

Ana Mocumbi

Instituto Nacional de Saúde, Maputo, Mozambique

S2.1 Infant and childhood heart disease in Africa

Heart disease in the young imposes a substantial burden on the families, health systems, and societies of Africa. The number of children affected is high, considering the occurrence of CHD, which is at least the same as that found in developed countries, and the occurrence of a variety of acquired diseases that are preventable but neglected. Few children receive a timely diagnosis in Africa. Moreover, only a small number of those benefit from treatment, leading to early deaths and chronic incapacity [1,2]. Pediatric cardiovascular care is a major area of need in Africa, given the high fertility rates and the fact that half the population is under the age of 15 years. The provision of pediatric cardiac services is too expensive for most developing countries, where problems other than cardiac diseases take priority in budget allocation [3]. Consequently, access to pediatric cardiovascular care in Africa is limited, as reflected in the scarcity of trained pediatric cardiologists and specialized services available in some countries in the continent (see Table S2.1). The numerous difficulties in applying and performing surgery in Africa include a lack of human resources, poor financing, low levels of patient education, and a dearth of sustainability strategies. Although most CHD can be treated through a single procedure, significantly improving life expectancy and quality of life, surgery for the type of acquired diseases particularly prevalent in Africa can be highly demanding in terms of technical expertise and medical follow-up. This includes interventional cardiology, multiple drugs, and surgery. It is on this basis, and in consideration of all the inherent challenges that must be overcome to improve the heart health of children in Africa, that this section of the book describes recent studies on the epidemiology, characterization, and management of heart disease in the African setting, focusing on specific aspects of pediatric cardiology care in the continent.

The Heart of Africa: Clinical Profile of an Evolving Burden of Heart Disease in Africa, First Edition.
Edited by Simon Stewart, Karen Sliwa, Ana Mocumbi, Albertino Damasceno, and Mpiko Ntsekhe.
© 2016 John Wiley & Sons, Ltd. Published 2016 by John Wiley & Sons, Ltd.

Table S2.1 Demographics and availability of pediatric cardiovascular care services according to three African countries [4–6].

Country	Cameroon	Mozambique	Zambia
Demographics			
Population	19,599,000	23,391,000	13,089,000
Population <15 years	41%	4%	46%
Life expectancy (years)	51	49	48
Availability of pediatric cardiovascular care			
Pediatric cardiologists	4	3	2
Hospitals with pediatric cardiologist	3	3	1
Catheterization labs	1	2	1
Catheterization labs performing pediatric interventions	1	1	0
Pediatric cardiac surgeons	0	2	1
Centers with pediatric cardiac surgery	0	2	1

S2.1.1 Geographical context

After the South Africa–centric Section 1, the second section of this book spreads out across the African continent, particularly the southern, southeastern, and central regions. Chapter 2 introduces us to Mozambique, which will also appear in several subsequent sections, and to Cameroon, which becomes a focus once more in Section 6. In Chapter 3, the neighboring Malawi and Zimbabwe are featured, with a brief return to urban South Africa and finally to Mozambique. This chapter also highlights the multicenter REMEDY study, which included patients from an impressive array of 12 African countries.

Mozambique is a large and culturally diverse country located on the southeast coast of Africa, bordered by the Indian Ocean. Currently home to approximately 25 million people, Mozambique has an estimated population growth rate of 2.45% per annum [4]. Indigenous tribal groups such as the Makhuwa, Tsonga, Lomwe, and Sena compose 99.96% of the population, with the remainder identifying as European, Euro-African, or Indian [4]. Although the official language of Mozambique remains Portuguese, several indigenous languages are also in use. A striking 45% of Mozambicans are below the age of 15, with an additional 21% aged between 15 and 24 years and a population median age of 16.9 years [4]. Just over half of the population is estimated to live below the poverty line, with a literacy rate of 59%, and 32% described as urbanized [5]. Mozambique has a high underlying infant mortality rate (approximately 70 deaths per 1,000 live births), while average life expectancy sits at 53 years [5]. Access to health care in Mozambique is scarce, with a rate of 0.04 physicians and 0.07 hospital beds per 1,000 persons [4].

The Republic of Cameroon is situated in Central Africa, with an estimated 23,739,218 inhabitants [6]. Often referred to as 'Africa in miniature' for its cultural and geological diversity, Cameroon is home to multiple different ethnic groups, including Cameroon highlanders, Equatorial Bantu, Kirdi, Fulani, Northwestern Bantu, Eastern Nigritic, and other Africans, while non-Africans form less than 1% of the population [6]. With English and French as its official languages, Cameroon is also host to 24 major African language groups [6]. Children aged below 15 years compose over 40% of the population, with an infant mortality rate of approximately 54 deaths per 1,000 live births and an average life expectancy of 58 years. Although unemployment in Cameroon is relatively low at 4%, underemployment affects approximately 70% of working residents [7], and close to 40% of the total population are estimated to live below the poverty line [8]. Further, despite spending more on health than any other sub-Saharan African country with the exception of South Africa, the Cameroonian health system is rife with inequality, and its health outcomes are paradoxically lagging behind its neighbors [9].

Located in Southern Africa, the Republic of Malawi is one of the continent's smallest countries. With a current population of just under 18 million (rising by 3.32% per annum) [10], Malawi has the eighth-highest fertility rate worldwide, at 5.6 children per woman [11]. Native ethnic groups, predominantly the Chewa (32.6%), Lomwe (17.6%), and Yao (13.5%), make up the majority of the populace and several languages are in use, the most common being Chichewa, while English remains the official language [10]. Only 16% of Malawi's residents are regarded as urbanized, while the most recent available estimates report over half of the population to live below the poverty line [12]. Malawi faces a critical shortage of health personnel and resources, with a rate of 0.02 physicians per 1,000 persons and only a third of the WHO's recommended nursing ratio [13].

Also situated in Southern Africa, Zimbabwe is three times larger than Malawi, although its population is smaller, at just over 14 million people [14]. Nearly all (99.4%) of Zimbabwe's inhabitants are of African ancestry; the majority ethnic group is the Shona, with a significant minority consisting of Ndebele people [14]. Zimbabwe is home to 16 official languages, the most widely spoken being Shona [14]. A striking three-quarters of the population lives below the poverty line [12], and this figure rises in rural residents, who represent two-thirds of the population [12,15]. Due largely to the critical economic situation, Zimbabwe is grappling with a severe shortage of health care resources and personnel, particularly affecting specialty areas and midwifery [16]. In recent years the infant mortality rate in Zimbabwe has improved to approximately 26 deaths per 1,000 live births in 2015 [17], while total life expectancy at birth has increased by 13 years since 2000 [18]. However, 2012 estimates reveal that healthy life expectancy in both sexes is 9 years below overall life expectancy at birth, representing 9 years of full health lost through morbidity and disability [18].

CHAPTER 2

Congenital heart disease

Ana Mocumbi[1], Tantchou Tchoumi Jacques Cabral[2], John Musuku[3], and Serigne A. Ba[4]

[1] Instituto Nacional de Saúde, Maputo, Mozambique
[2] St. Elizabeth Catholic General Hospital, Shisong, Cameroon
[3] University Teaching Hospital, Lusaka, Zambia
[4] Cheikh Anta DIOP University, Dakar, Senegal

2.0 Introduction

In the African context, CHD is a significant cause of mortality among infants and young children, despite most affected children presenting with simple defects with left-to-right shunt physiology [2,19–21]. Moreover, the few studies that have explored the epidemiology of CHD in Africa report its high association to HF [22,23]—see Section 6 on HF in the adult population. Unsurprisingly perhaps, the incidence of CHD in Africa appears comparable to that found in Western nations [24], although the profile of diagnosed defects may differ. For example, left obstructive lesions are rarely diagnosed in African settings [25], which could indicate a genuine difference in the occurrence of these conditions or may merely reflect the lack of awareness of health professionals during the neonatal period. Hypocalcemia, resulting from vitamin D deficiency, has been suggested as a cause of the observed low prevalence of obstructive aortic lesions [26]. In some African countries, cases of CHD outnumber acquired cardiac disease in children below the age of 15 years [21]. This is undoubtedly due to late diagnosis and referral to specialist care, which commonly occurs after the first year of life in Kenya [19] and Mozambique [2]. The tragic consequence is that a significant number of patients miss the crucial window for optimal surgical interventions. Moreover, in many settings, affected children do not reach a referral center with capacity for catheterization or surgery until they are already affected by irreversible complications such as fixed pulmonary hypertension (PH), arrhythmia, or sequelae of thromboembolism [1,2,27]. Cardiac evaluation at birth, in postnatal clinics, and in immunization centers would be necessary to allow for early detection and possible prevention of these deaths. This chapter focuses on the diagnosis, management, and follow-up of structural heart disease in children. It particularly focuses on data describing the epidemiology of CHD, the challenges of diagnosis in the context of limited resources in the setting of

The Heart of Africa: Clinical Profile of an Evolving Burden of Heart Disease in Africa, First Edition.
Edited by Simon Stewart, Karen Sliwa, Ana Mocumbi, Albertino Damasceno, and Mpiko Ntsekhe.
© 2016 John Wiley & Sons, Ltd. Published 2016 by John Wiley & Sons, Ltd.

high demand, and current strategies to enhance access to management of these conditions. The latter includes humanitarian initiatives, north-south collaboration projects, and improvement of health systems in selected countries. Specific aspects of the management of CHD in the context of resource-poor settings are also discussed.

2.1 CHD management and its challenges in Mozambique

Mocumbi AO, Lameira E, Yaksh A, Paul L, Ferreira MB, Sidi D. Challenges on the management of congenital heart disease in developing countries. *International Journal of Cardiology* 2011; 148(3):285–8. [2]

2.1.1 Study background

CHD is defined as the abnormality of cardiovascular function or structure that is present at birth, with approximately 8 per 1,000 babies diagnosed in developed countries. In these countries, CHD is detected prenatally and a diagnosis is established in 40%–50% of patients within 1 week and in 60% within 1 month after birth [28], conferring all the advantages of proactive management and counseling. These data contrast sharply with the health care reality in sub-Saharan Africa, where only a minority of children benefit from available treatments, with late diagnoses, unskilled personnel, and/or lack of surgical facilities negatively influencing their health outcomes.

2.1.2 Study aims

The aim of this study was to describe the characteristics and spectrum of CHD diagnosed at a newly created referral unit for CVD in Maputo, Mozambique (the Instituto do Coração), as a reflection of the typical challenges of its management in LMIC. This unit provided specialist treatment to the entire Mozambique population, as it was the only institution performing cardiac surgery and cardiac catheterization procedures during the study period of April 2001 to December 2007.

2.1.3 Study methods
2.1.3.1 Patient enrollment

All echocardiographically confirmed cases of patients with CHD who approached the Instituto do Coração were included in the study. Affected patients were diagnosed by the local team and operated on 3 to 6 months after diagnosis. Age at diagnosis, age at surgery, surgery type, early complications, follow-up, and mortality were recorded for all patients. Surgeries were performed by expatriate surgeons who visited the institution periodically as part of humanitarian missions while local personnel were being trained for these roles.

2.1.3.2 CHD classification according to complexity

As a considerable number of patients included in this study had more than one heart defect, a hierarchical system of classification was created to accommodate each patient into one diagnostic category. Simple defects included atrial septal defects, persistence of ductus arteriosus, and ventricular septal defects; moderate defects included aortic stenosis, ostium primum atrial septal defect, pulmonary stenosis, and Tetralogy of Fallot. Complex defects included complete atrioventricular septal defect, congenitally corrected transposition of great arteries, double outlet right ventricle, pulmonary atresia, tricuspid atresia, other cyanotic CHD, and other single ventricle physiology.

2.1.4 Study findings

Overall, a total of 534 patients with a cardiac malformation were studied. Of these, 282 (52.8%) patients were diagnosed under the age of 2 years and 179 (33.5%) were diagnosed between the ages of 2 and 17 years. Complications at diagnosis occurred in 155 (29%) patients with the most common complication being severe polycythemia (9.2%), followed by HF (8.8%), fixed PH (8.4%), infective endocarditis (1.7%), and stroke (0.8%) (see Table 2.1). The most frequently presented physiologic defect was left-to-right shunts in 354 (66.3%) patients, primarily caused by large ventricular septal defect (26.6%), atrial septal defect type ostium secundum (14.2%), and restrictive ventricular septal defect (10.5%). More than half (56.9%) of congenital defects were categorized as simple, with the remainder comprising moderate (22.3%) and complex defects (20.8%). The five most common defects were (a) ventricular septal defects found in 201 (37.6%) patients, (b) Tetralogy of Fallot in 85 (15.9%), (c) atrial septal defect in 77 (14.4%), (d) complete atrioventricular septal defect in 32 (6%), and (e) double outlet right ventricular (RV) found in 29 (5.4%) patients.

2.1.4.1 Surgical procedures

Overall, 481 (90.1%) patients presented with cardiac abnormalities that required surgical correction. However, contraindication to surgery was also determined to be present in 96 (20%) patients. Specifically, 45 (46.9%) patients presented with fixed PH, 24 (25%) with associated malformations, 9 (9.4%) with severe malnutrition, 9 (9.4%) with CMO, 5 (5.2%) with severe neurological impairment and/ or neurological deficit, and 4 (4.2%) with HIV infection. Of note, 13 (2.7%) patients refused surgery, 27 (5.6%) died during the surgical preparation phase, and 40 (8.3%) were lost to follow-up. In total, therefore, 196 (40.8%) patients underwent surgery. Mean age at surgery was 8±10 years. The complexity of cardiac malformations subject to surgical correction in these patients was as follows: 101 (51.5%) simple defects, 66 (33.7%) moderate defects, and 29 (14.8%) complex defects. Overall, 8 (4.1%) patients required early reoperation due to bleeding and 8 (4.1%) died within 30 days after the surgical procedure. The most common postsurgical complications were postpericardectomy syndrome

Table 2.1 Patients' demographic and clinical characteristics, defects, and classification of CHD.

Characteristic	Patients (n = 534)
Median age at diagnosis (years)	4
Women	296 (55.4%)
Dysgenetic syndrome	54 (10.1%)
Major noncardiac abnormality	8 (1.5%)
Complications at diagnosis	
Fixed PH	45 (8.4%)
HF	47 (8.8%)
Infective endocarditis	9 (1.7%)
Severe polycythemia	49 (9.2%)
Stroke	4 (0.8%)
Left-to-right shunts	354 (66.6%)
Aortopulmonary window	1 (0.2%)
Atrial septal defect type ostium primum	2 (0.4%)
Atrial septal defect type ostium secundum	76 (14.2%)
Atrial septal defect type sinus venosus	1 (0.2%)
Complete atrioventricular septal defect	47 (8.8%)
Large persistent ductus arteriosus	26 (4.9%)
Large ventricular septal defect	142 (26.6%)
Restrictive ventricular septal defect	56 (10.5%)
Ventricular septal defect with RV obstruction	3 (0.6%)
Right-to-left shunts	103 (19.3%)
Pulmonary atresia with ventricular septal defect	7 (1.3%)
Pulmonary atresia without ventricular septal defect	3 (0.6%)
Tetralogy of Fallot	85 (15.9%)
Ventricular septal defect with Eisenmenger	8 (1.5%)
Other defects	
Aortic aneurisms in Marfan syndrome	5 (0.9%)
Congenital MR	2 (0.4%)
Heterotaxy/isomerism	5 (0.9%)
Pulmonary stenosis	8 (1.5%)
Single ventricle	9 (1.7%)
Situs inversus with double discordance	3 (0.6%)
Transposition of the great arteries	21 (3.9%)
Tricuspid atresia	9 (1.7%)
Truncus arteriosus	2 (0.4%)
Other	13 (2.4%)
Simple defects	304 (56.9%)
Atrial septal defect	77 (14.4%)
Persistent ductus arteriosus	26 (4.9%)
Ventricular septal defect	201 (37.6%)

Table 2.1 (continued)

Characteristic	Patients (n = 534)
Moderate defects	119 (22.3%)
Aortic valve abnormality	1 (0.2%)
Ostium primum atrial septal defect	2 (0.4%)
Pulmonary stenosis	8 (1.5%)
Tetralogy of Fallot	85 (15.9%)
Other	23 (4.3%)
Complex defects	111 (20.8%)
Complete atrioventricular septal defect	32 (6%)
Congenitally corrected transposition of the great arteries	1 (0.2%)
Double outlet right ventricle	29 (5.4%)
Pulmonary atresia	1 (0.2%)
Tricuspid atresia	9 (1.7%)
Truncus arteriosus	2 (0.4%)
Other cyanotic CHD	25 (4.7%)
Other single ventricle physiology	12 (2.2%)

(n = 22, 11.2%), residual ventricular septal defect (n = 4, 2%), severe pulmonary insufficiency (n = 4, 2%), neurological defects (n = 2, 1%), paroxysmal cardiac arrhythmias (n = 2, 1%), and renal failure (n = 2, 1%).

2.1.5 Study interpretation

Specialist care is required for the diagnosis of CHD regardless of the location. This poses a particular challenge to resource-poor African countries. Individuals diagnosed with CHD and fortunate enough to access specialist centers typically face large amounts of travel, as well as an added complication for those with limited personal resources. This commonly leads to a delayed diagnosis, often occurring only when affected individuals present with other complications such as HF, infective endocarditis, pulmonary vascular obstructive disease, and/or severe cyanosis. As in previous studies in similar populations [29,30], this was certainly the case in Mozambique; providing the correct management and care for affected patients residing in the diverse regions of sub-Saharan Africa was a challenge. The concerning number of patients presenting with late and/or irreversible complications of CHD highlights the scarcity of surgical facilities and pediatric cardiologists in the region relative to the urgent clinical need for them, particularly before the Instituto do Coração in Maputo was established. The fact that a majority of patients presented with late complications related to simple cardiac defects not only reflects the fact that minor defects may be asymptomatic and undetected without screening, it also confirms the lack of awareness of untrained health professionals upon presentation of affected children.

Overall, this study found a predominance of simple acyanotic defects such as ventricular septal defect, atrial septal defect, and patent ductus arteriosus; and that Tetralogy of Fallot was the most significant cyanotic malformation [21,25]. The low frequency of aortic stenosis and coarctation of the aorta evident in the current cohort may be due to missed diagnosis, given the often inadequate human and technical resources for diagnosis during the neonatal period. Significantly, not all affected individuals could be operated on due to lack of available surgical teams and the state of presentation at the time of diagnosis. Four percent of case fatalities were reported prior to surgery, which is unfortunately attributable to the long waiting period from diagnosis to surgery; the majority of the patients did not receive operations until 3 to 6 months following diagnosis. Almost 10% of the study cohort was lost to follow-up prior to surgery, undoubtedly due to a lack of understanding of the risks involved. Moreover, some parents refused surgery for their children after a clinical improvement was noted following the application of medical therapy. These concerning figures underline the urgent need for education strategies for the parents of children diagnosed with CHD to ensure optimal health outcomes. Instituto do Coração was the first institution to perform open-heart surgery and interventional cardiac catheterization in Mozambique; the large volume of successfully treated patients highlights the historical and contemporary opportunities to extend the reach of cardiac surgery for a broad range of CHD cases in a large and vulnerable population.

2.1.6 Study limitations

As in all observational studies of this kind, particularly when focused on a single center and region, the wider generalizability (in this case wider Africa) of observed cases and outcomes needs to be considered. However, this study is notable for focusing on a national center for treating CHD. Notably, it is likely that undetected cases of CHD and fatalities occurring in outlying regions of the country (particularly given the geographic profile of Mozambique) would not have reached the Instituto do Coração and been subsequently documented.

2.1.7 Study conclusions

In conclusion, the management of CHD in LMIC, such as Mozambique, are vastly different from that applied in high-income countries. Treating cardiologists operating in scarce specialist centers are often confronted with patients who are in no state for a successful operation due to delayed diagnosis and development of associated complications. At the same time, a lack of education means that many individuals who would benefit from surgery refuse it. Given the paucity of surgical options for CHD in Mozambique and other parts of sub-Saharan Africa, there is an urgent need to increase the scope and reach of early detection strategies to apply more proactive management. As always, this includes investment in primary health care units to increase the number of timely referrals from those communities remote to specialist services.

2.2 CHD management and its challenges in Cameroon

Tchoumi JCT, Ambassa JC, Chelo D, Djimegne FK, Giaberti A, Cirri S, Kingue S, Butera G. **Pattern and clinical aspects of congenital heart diseases and their management in Cameroon.** *Bulletin de la Societe de Pathologie Exotique* 2011; 104(1):25–28. [31]

2.2.1 Study background

As discussed above, CHD poses a particular problem to resource-poor countries in sub-Saharan Africa, associated with typically late presentations of HF, which reflect low detection and treatment rates in childhood. Unfortunately, Cameroon is no exception [32]. Consequently, a similar strategy to that used in Mozambique was adopted to increase access to surgery for CHD. Specifically, the clinical research paper highlighted in this chapter describes the experiences of the Cardiac Centre in Shisong, in the northern part of Cameroon, in dealing with CHD presentations.

2.2.2 Study aims

The aim of the study was to examine the incidence, clinical characteristics, and management of CHD in Cameroon.

2.2.3 Study methods

Prior to the implementation of this study, partnerships were formed between Associazione Bambini Cardiopatici Nel Mondo, La Chaîne de l'Espoir, Cuore Fratello, Mécénat Français, Policlinico San Donato in Milan, Saint Elizabeth Catholic General Hospital, and Tertiary Sisters of Saint Francis, to improve health outcomes relating to CHD in the region. Specifically, these partnerships facilitated the application of surgical procedures and training of specialist physicians to improve the management of patients with CHD in Cameroon.

2.2.3.1 Patient enrollment

During the period January 2006 to November 2009, patients who were referred to the Cardiac Centre of Saint Elizabeth Catholic General Hospital in Shisong, the Mother and Child Centre of Chantal Biya's Foundation at Yaoundé, and the pediatric, neonatology, and cardiac departments of the *Douala General Hospital* were enrolled in the study. Patients who presented with cyanosis, failure to thrive, clubbing, growth retardation, frequent respiratory tract infections, and/or cardiac murmur (to detect trivial CHD) were excluded from the study. Each patient's clinical characteristics were recorded and a transthoracic Doppler echocardiogram was performed.

2.2.4 Study findings

In total, 505 patients were enrolled in the study, with 140 (27.7%) patients derived from the Cardiac Centre in Shisong, 266 (52.7%) from the Mother and Child Foundation in Yaoundé, and 99 (19.6%) from the General Hospital in Douala (see Figure 2.1). Overall, there were more women (55%) than men and the mean age was 10.0 ± 9.7 years.

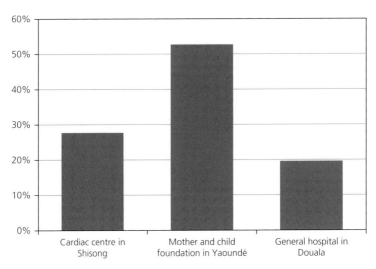

Figure 2.1 Distribution of study patients from the three participating referral centers.

Table 2.2 CHD patients' transthoracic Doppler-echocardiography presentations according to the three referral centers.

Pathology	Douala (n = 99)	Shisong (n = 140)	Yaoundé (n = 266)
Anomalous venous pulmonary return	—	2 (1.4%)	▬
Arterial duct	—	17 (12.1%)	32 (12.0%)
Atrioventricular cushion defect	12 (12.1%)	10 (7.1%)	—
Coarctation of the aorta	—	2 (1.4%)	—
Common arterial trunk	—	2 (1.4%)	11 (4.1%)
Congenital mitral valve regurgitation	—	2 (1.4%)	—
Double outlet right ventricle	—	3 (2.1%)	—
Ebstein disease	—	—	5 (1.9%)
Isolated interatrial communication	22 (22.2%)	4 (2.9%)	12 (4.5%)
Isolated pulmonary artery stenosis	22 (22.2%)	4 (2.9%)	24 (9.0%)
Isolated ventricular septal defect	34 (34.3%)	54 (38.6%)	112 (42.1%)
Left isomerism	—	2 (1.4%)	—
Tetralogy of Fallot	17 (17.2%)	37 (26.4%)	24 (9.0%)
Transportation of great arteries with ventricular septal defect	—	—	11 (4.1%)
Tricuspid atresia	—	2 (1.4%)	—

2.2.4.1 Transthoracic Doppler-echocardiography presentations

As shown in Table 2.2, the distribution of cases differed across the three participating centers ($p < 0.05$ for all comparisons). For example, in the Cardiac Center in Shisong, there were significantly more cases of Tetralogy of Fallot (26.1%), arterial duct (12.4%), double outlet RV (2.1%), tricuspid atresia (1.6%), anomalous venous pulmonary return (1.5%), congenital mitral valve regurgitation (1.2%), left isomerism (1.2%), and coarctation of the aorta (1.1%) when compared with the other two centers. At the Mother and Child Foundation in Yaoundé, there were more cases of isolated ventricular septal defect (42%), common arterial trunk (4%), transportation of great arteries with ventricular septal defect (4%), and Ebstein disease (2%). Finally, in the General Hospital in Douala, more patients presented with atrioventricular cushion defect (12%), isolated interatrial communication (22%), and isolated pulmonary artery stenosis (22%).

2.2.4.2 Surgical and postsurgical management
Once diagnosed with CHD, presenting patients were recorded on a waiting list for surgery in order of disease severity and type. Those requiring surgery were on the waiting list for more than 3 months before operation, and around 10% of patients died before their scheduled surgery. Surgical procedures were completed and paid for by not-for-profit organizations. In total, 56 open-heart procedures were completed in the Cardiac Center in Shisong with a success rate of 100%.

2.2.5 Study interpretation
The majority of the current findings were consistent with previous studies conducted throughout Africa. Ventricular septal defect was revealed as the most common CHD diagnosis in Cameroon, while Tetralogy of Fallot and ventricular septal defects were often associated with severe growth retardation, cyanosis, and clubbing, echoing previous studies conducted in Zimbabwe [33] and Nigeria [34]. The incidence and prevalence of CHD found in Cameroon were comparable with the rates revealed in Nigeria [25], even though a previous study based in Egypt reported a relatively low prevalence of CHD [35]. Notably, the high number of partnerships formed to complete this study allowed all open-heart surgeries to be successfully completed. Yet despite this encouragingly high success rate, there remains an urgent need for future studies to explore the impact of education and prevention strategies in order to decrease late detection of CHD and subsequently high mortality prior to the opportunity for surgery, as well as the high number of patients for whom surgery is no longer viable.

2.2.6 Study limitations
The same caveats that apply to the study from Mozambique described in Section 2.1.6 also apply to this study, with the difference that the focus is on multiple institutions rather than a single center.

2.2.7 Study conclusions
In conclusion, these data revealed a high prevalence of ventricular septal defects and other forms of CHD in Cameroon. Without the large number of partnerships forged for the implementation of specialist surgical services, mortality rates would have undoubtedly been higher. As in other sub-Saharan African countries, the support of surgical management of CHD applied as a national program of intervention is urgently required to decrease mortality rates among Cameroonian children. Importantly, such programs must be supported by cost-effective detection and education strategies to optimize health outcomes.

CHAPTER 3

Acquired heart disease

Ana Mocumbi[1], Liesl Zühlke[2], and Peter Zilla[2]

[1] Instituto Nacional de Saúde, Maputo, Mozambique
[2] University of Cape Town/Groote Schuur and Red Cross Children's Hospital, Cape Town, South Africa

3.0 Introduction

Progress in the practice and science of cardiology has produced a considerable reduction in the incidence, morbidity, and mortality associated with acquired CVD in developed countries, but these benefits have not reached the majority of individuals living in developing countries. This relates partly to the lack of preventive and therapeutic measures for common "neglected" conditions, which almost exclusively affects the poorest individuals of developing countries. Indeed, several cardiovascular conditions are restricted to or predominantly affect African children. These conditions result from uncontrolled infections, are linked to poverty, and/or occur in areas without established research facilities and surveillance systems. Their epidemiology and significance is thus often unappreciated or dwarfed by the statistics on acute infectious diseases. Among acquired diseases, acute rheumatic fever, RHD, tuberculous pericarditis, CMO, HIV-related complications, and parasitic diseases must be mentioned. Acute rheumatic fever with pancarditis is often fatal and chronic RHD is the chief cause of valvular disease in the continent. Moreover, due to inadequate primary and secondary prophylaxis, Africa is home to the highest prevalence and most malignant forms of chronic RHD in the world. As the vertical transmission of HIV infection still occurs in many parts of the continent, cardiac complications are often found in young people, particularly tuberculous pericarditis and myocarditis. Notably, depending on the geographic location and economic characteristics of the regions, diseases such as endomyocardial fibrosis (EMF), Takayasu's Disease, and nutritional CMO's may affect children and adolescents in variable proportions. In this chapter we discuss four studies describing the spectrum and particularities of diagnosis and management of these conditions in Africa.

The Heart of Africa: Clinical Profile of an Evolving Burden of Heart Disease in Africa, First Edition.
Edited by Simon Stewart, Karen Sliwa, Ana Mocumbi, Albertino Damasceno, and Mpiko Ntsekhe.
© 2016 John Wiley & Sons, Ltd. Published 2016 by John Wiley & Sons, Ltd.

3.1 The spectrum of pediatric cardiac disease in Malawi

Kennedy N, Miller P. **The spectrum of pediatric cardiac disease presenting to an outpatient clinic in Malawi.** *BMC Research Notes* 2013; 6(53):1–4. [36]

3.1.1 Study background

Specialized services focused on children with underlying heart disease are scarce in Malawi due to the increasing burden of infectious diseases. Health services are poorly distributed with inadequate resources to treat children diagnosed with diarrhea, HIV/AIDS, malaria, malnutrition, pneumonia, or heart disease [37]. Despite the decline in the proportion of Malawian children dying before their fifth birthday (Millennium Goal 4 [38]), there is still a need for programs to concentrate on the burden of noncommunicable diseases. Although a number of African studies have illustrated the spectrum of pediatric cases of cardiac disease, prior to this report there were no published data from Malawi [21,33,39–41].

3.1.2 Study aims

The aim of this study was to describe the spectrum of pediatric cardiac disease in the Queen Elizabeth Central Hospital in Blantyre, Malawi, established in 2008.

3.1.3 Study methods

3.1.3.1 Patient enrollment

During the period January 2009 to February 2011, all children referred to the pediatric cardiac clinic of the Queen Elizabeth Central Hospital with an abnormal echocardiogram were included in the study and recorded in a database. All inpatients referred from other hospitals were excluded. Diagnosis was confirmed by echocardiograms performed by specialists, with ethical approval obtained prior to commencement of the study.

3.1.4 Study findings

A total of 250 children were included in the study. The majority of the patients were boys (n = 152, 60.8%). As shown in Table 3.1, slightly more patients presented with CHD (55.6%) than with acquired forms of heart disease. The most commonly presenting forms of CHD were ventricular septal defect (24%), Tetralogy of Fallot (10%), patent ductus arteriosus (7.2%), atrioventricular septal defect (5.2%), and other cyanotic conditions (4.4%). Other cyanotic CHD included double outlet RV in 5 patients and transposition with ventricular septal defect in 3 patients. The most commonly presenting forms of acquired heart disease were RHD (22.4%), dilated CMO (13.6%), other CMO (3.2%), EMF (2%), pericarditis (2%), and secondary PH (1.2%). Other CMOs included noncompacted LV (n = 3), Hurler syndrome (n = 2), and single cases of Duchenne and hypertrophic CMO. Attributable causes of pericarditis included pneumococcal

Table 3.1 Patients' spectrum of diagnosis.

Diagnosis	Patients (n = 250)
CHD	
Aortic stenosis	2 (0.8%)
Atrial septal defect	5 (2%)
Atrioventricular septal defect	13 (5.2%)
Coarctation of the aorta	1 (0.4%)
Marfan syndrome with aortic regurgitation	1 (0.4%)
Patent ductus arteriosus	18 (7.2%)
Pulmonary stenosis	3 (1.2%)
Tetralogy of Fallot	25 (10%)
Ventricular septal defect	60 (24%)
Other cyanotic CHD	11 (4.4%)
Acquired heart disease	
Dilated CMO	34 (13.6%)
EMF	5 (2%)
Pericarditis	5 (2%)
RHD	56 (22.4%)
Secondary PH	3 (1.2%)
Other CMO	8 (3.2%)

pericarditis (n = 1), acute tuberculosis (TB) (n = 2), and constrictive pericarditis (n = 2). Secondary PH included single cases of upper airway obstruction, HIV infection, and schistosomiasis. Of those with dilated CMO (n = 34), 22 (64.7%) patients had a known HIV status, with 3 (13.6%) children presenting as HIV positive. During the study period, 40 patients were referred for cardiac surgery in South Africa. However, of these, only 24 (60%) underwent the recommended operation.

3.1.5 Study interpretation

The spectrum of pediatric cases of cardiac disease in Malawi was consistent with that described in previous studies [21,33,39–41]; however, the age at presentation was extremely late. Almost half of study patients presented with an acquired form of heart disease and just over half presented with RHD. As up to 70% of children presenting with RHD in regions of the world without access to surgery will die by the age of 25 years [42], this result sheds some light on the high infant mortality rates and the early adult morbidity and mortality rates observed in the region. The other most commonly presenting form of acquired heart disease in the current study was dilated CMO. Out of the 22 patients with a known HIV status, only 3 were HIV-positive. Heart disease is known to be associated with HIV infection [43] (see Chapter 9), and there is a deficiency in detecting potential heart disease in HIV-positive children in Malawi. With regard to the patients presenting with CHD (see Chapter 2), consistent with previous studies from around Africa [21,33,39,40] the conditions documented in the current cohort were predominantly less complex (i.e., those associated with more favourable 1-year survival rates) than fatal cases.

3.1.6 Study limitations

Various limitations in this study should be noted. In particular, the study cohort was subject to certain biases and thus is unlikely to be representative of the broader population. First, the extremely poor state of transport in Malawi prevents many sufferers of heart conditions from seeking adequate health care. Second, inpatients referred from other hospitals were excluded from the study. Consequently, the included sample was restricted to residents of the immediate surroundings, and the current results are thus likely to underestimate the true spectrum of pediatric heart disease in the broader region. On the other hand, because the majority of patients resided within 10 km of the Queen Elizabeth Central Hospital, the findings do provide valuable data on heart disease in that particular area.

3.1.7 Study conclusions

In conclusion, the most common presentation of acquired heart disease in this cohort was RHD, while the most frequently observed type of CHD was ventricular septal defect. A wider population-based prevalence study is urgently required to obtain more accurate data in Malawi and to determine the full degree of pediatric heart disease. Unfortunately, the current results support the notion that untreated heart disease contributes to markedly high infant mortality and premature adult morbidity rates.

3.2 Adolescent heart disease and vertically acquired HIV infection in Zimbabwe

Miller RF, Kaski JP, Hakim J, Matenga J, Nathoo K, Munyati S, Desai SR, Corbett EL, Ferrand RA. **Cardiac disease in adolescents with delayed diagnosis of vertically acquired HIV infection.** *Clinical Infectious Diseases* 2013; 56(4):576–82. [44]

3.2.1 Study background

There are an estimated 2.5 million HIV-infected children aged less than 14 years worldwide, with approximately 90% presenting in sub-Saharan Africa. The majority of these cases arise from mother-to-child transmission [45]. When HIV-positive children seek medical care in older childhood and early adolescence, they often present with an association between HIV infection and lung disease and/or heart disease [46,47]. Previous studies suggest that heart disease and HIV infection are well described in high- and low-resource populations, and that the most common cardiac abnormalities are decreased LV fractional shortening, dilated CMO, increased LV wall thickness/mass, LV diastolic dysfunction, and pericardial effusion [43,48–55]. However, data on HIV-infected children and cardiac abnormalities in this setting are limited. For details on the interaction between HIV infection and heart disease in adulthood, see Chapter 9.

3.2.2 Study aims
The aim of this study was to determine the clinical and echocardiographic characteristics and features of heart disease among previously studied HIV-infected adolescents receiving treatment in Harare, Zimbabwe [47].

3.2.3 Study methods
3.2.3.1 Patient enrollment and data collection
Patients aged 10 to 19 years attending the HIV outpatient clinics at Parirenyatwa Hospital and Harare Central Hospital were included in the study [47]. Individuals were excluded from the study if they resided outside Harare, had HIV infection that was horizontally acquired (transmitted sexually or through blood transfusion), were pregnant or too ill to participate, or had recently diagnosed TB, pulmonary Kaposi sarcoma, or an intercurrent acute lower respiratory tract infection. HIV was considered vertically acquired when there was a known maternal HIV infection, maternal or sibling death, and when there was no history of frequent early childhood infections, pubertal delay, or stunting [47,56]. Ethics approval was obtained as well as informed consent from the guardians of all eligible patients prior to study enrollment. Profiling included demographic characteristics in addition to symptoms and stage of HIV infection, and receipt of Highly active antiretroviral therapy (HAART). Clinical examination (to obtain weight and height), echocardiographic readings, and measurements of CD4 counts were performed as well as the recording of pulse oximetry, heart rate, and presence or absence of ankle edema.

3.2.4 Study findings
3.2.4.1 Demographic and clinical characteristics
As shown in Table 3.2, nearly half of the cohort were aged 16 to 19 years (47.3%), followed by 27.3% aged 13 to 15 years, and 25.5% aged <13 years. Overall, 70.9% were receiving ART for a mean duration of 20 months (IQR 5 to 40 months). The median CD4 count was 402 cells/µL (IQR 196–590) for those taking ART and 351 cells/µL (IQR 77–535) for those not taking such therapy (p=0.16). The most common signs and symptoms among patients were shortness of breath on exertion (42.7%) and chest pain on exertion (39.1%). There was no cigarette smoking in the study cohort and no patients were receiving digoxin, β-blockers, vasodilators, diuretics, calcium channel blockers, or ACE inhibitors. RHD, sickle cell disease, and CHD were also not present, although patients had a previous dilated CMO diagnosis.

Table 3.2 Patients' demographic and clinical characteristics.

Characteristic	Patients (n = 110)
Age (years)	
<13	28 (25.5%)
13–15	30 (27.3%)
16–19	52 (47.3%)
Profile	
Men	52 (47.3%)
Height for age (*z* score)	−2.22 (IQR −3.05 to −1.3)
Weight for age (*z* score)	−1.84 (IQR −3 to −0.94)
BMI (kg/m²)	−0.69 (IQR −1.81 to 0.11)
Taking ART	78 (70.9%)
Regimen	
2 nonnucleoside reverse-transcriptase inhibitors + 1 nonnucleoside reverse-transcriptase inhibitor	70 (63.6%)
2 nonnucleoside reverse-transcriptase inhibitor S + protease inhibitor	6 (5.5%)
Unknown	2 (1.8%)
Signs and symptoms	
Shortness of breath on exertion	47 (42.7%)
Chest pain on exertion	43 (39.1%)
Palpitations	10 (9.1%)
Ankle edema	7 (6.4%)
NYHA class	
I	69 (62.7%)
II	18 (16.4%)
III	21 (19.1%)
IV	2 (1.8%)
Tachycardia at rest (heart rate >100 beats/min)	31 (28.2%)
Arterial oxygen saturation at rest <92%	16 (14.6%)
CD4 count (cells/µL)	384 (IQR 171–578)

3.2.4.2 LV systolic impairment and dilatation

Of patients presenting with LV systolic impairment and dilatation (n = 12, 10.9%), 3 (2.7%) exhibited concurrent mild mitral valve regurgitation while 3 (2.7%) displayed LV end-diastolic dysfunction.

3.2.4.3 LV diastolic dysfunction and hypertrophy

In total, 4 (3.6%) patients presented with a ratio of <1 between early- and late-diastolic trans-mitral ventricular filling velocities, while 23 (20.9%) had a ratio of >2. More than half of the cohort (67.3%) presented with left ventricular hypertrophy (LVH), with 7 patients (6.4%) presenting with concentric hypertrophy.

3.2.4.4 PH and RV dilatation

Overall, 8 (7.3%) patients presented with an estimated pulmonary artery systolic pressure of >25 mm Hg. Of these, 4 (5%) patients exhibited an estimated pulmonary artery systolic pressure of >30 mm Hg, and an additional 32 (29%) patients without elevated estimated pulmonary artery systolic pressures presented with isolated RV dilatation.

3.2.5 Study interpretation

The principal finding of this study was the significant burden of heart disease among HIV-positive adolescents with vertically acquired HIV infection receiving health care. Echocardiogram measurements showed that more than half the study cohort presented with LVH. A nonpredicted result was that almost 30% of the patients had RV dilatation without an elevated estimated pulmonary artery systolic pressure; this condition is often associated with chronic lung disease [47] and as reported in Zimbabwe and the United States, is typically ascribed to cor pulmonale [57–59]. However, this study found no association between echocardiogram evidence of LV diastolic dysfunction, RV dilatation, and LVH and various clinical variables, although it did reveal relationships between LV diastolic dysfunction and women, the presence of stunting, and RV dilatation. These findings are supported by a previous study conducted in Thailand [53]. Early diagnosis of HIV infection is crucial to the subsequent development of heart disease (see Chapter 9), and international recommendations clearly suggest that affected patients (and/or their guardians) and treating physicians need to consider the risk of developing heart disease and the possibility of slowing its progression by applying HAART [60].

3.2.6 Study limitations

As with the other observational studies described above, the same caveats around the generalizability and accuracy of observed case presentations (particularly noting issues relating to ready access to specialist care in LMIC) apply.

3.2.7 Study conclusions

In conclusion, there is an association between vertically acquired HIV infection and heart disease among adolescents that requires further investigation. A majority of the patients in Harare, Zimbabwe, demonstrated evidence of LVH; however, only a minority presented evidence of impaired LV diastolic dysfunction. There is an urgent need for future studies to focus on the availability of health care resources and to implement appropriate prevention and treatment strategies.

3.3 Primary prevention of acute rheumatic fever and RHD with penicillin in South Africa

Irlam J, Mayosi BM, Engel M, Gaziano TA. Primary prevention of acute rheumatic fever and rheumatic heart disease with penicillin in South African children with pharyngitis: a cost-effective analysis. Circulation. Cardiovascular Quality and Outcomes 2013; 6(3):343–51. [61]

3.3.1 Study background

The most common cause of acquired heart disease among children worldwide is RHD [62], which affects 32 million individuals globally and is responsible for over a quarter of a million deaths each year [63]. The global burden of disease study suggests that 18.2 million years are lived with disability worldwide due to RHD; the vast majority of these deaths occur in children, adolescents, and young adults [64,65]. The incidence of acute rheumatic fever has decreased dramatically over the past 50 years in high-income countries. However, this does not eliminate the possibility of RHD outbreaks in the future [66]. Primary prevention strategies against acute rheumatic fever and RHD involve applying penicillin treatment to patients presenting with group A streptococcus infection. However, this primary prevention technique is difficult to implement in LMIC due to numerous barriers including limited access to primary care, the expense of microbiological diagnosis, a dearth of physicians, poor community awareness about group A streptococcus, and the high incidence of acute rheumatic fever without the presence of a sore throat [67,68].

3.3.2 Study aims

Prior to this study there was a paucity of studies assessing the most appropriate diagnostic strategy to apply to those presenting with pharyngitis in high-incidence areas. Also acknowledging the expense of treatment strategies using intramuscular penicillin injection and ancillary resources to apply them [67,69], the aim of the current study was to describe potentially cost-effective diagnostic and treatment strategies for the primary prevention of acute rheumatic fever in urban communities in South Africa.

3.3.3 Study methods

3.3.3.1 The 7-strategy Markov decision analysis cohort model

Whether to treat a pharyngitis patient is a complex decision. Physicians must weigh the benefits of preventing acute rheumatic fever and RHD (and their considerable associated morbidity and mortality) against the potential for significant medication interactions. They must also assess the costs of pharyngitis management against the costs of future treatment for acute rheumatic fever and RHD. A Markov decision analysis cohort model was thus created to assist the decision-making process for evaluating and managing children aged 3 to 13 years presenting without a history of acute rheumatic fever and with pharyngitis in an urban primary care setting in South Africa. As shown in Figure 3.1, this model includes the annual recurrent rates of pharyngitis with the possibility of multiple infections. However, the model excludes the risk of RHD from the first stage of pharyngitis. The model additionally includes the analysis of the development of acute rheumatic fever, penicillin treatment complications, diagnosis of RHD and CHF, and the possibility of group A streptococcus infection and mortality. As South Africa experiences various resource-specific limitations, screening and treatment strategies for possible group A streptococcus infection is based on a clinical

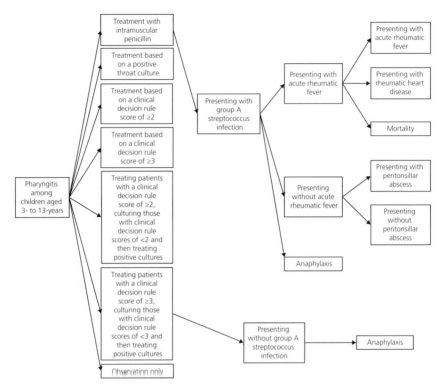

Figure 3.1 The seven-strategy Markov decision analysis cohort model.

decision rule, and/or throat culture results. The clinical decision rule used in this model was adapted from the WHO's recommended rule [70] that considers the presence of enlarged anterior cervical lymph nodes and the absence of rhinitis and/or rash in deciding whether to administer antibiotics. This model has been utilized in a previous study among an Egyptian population with a socioeconomic and health status similar to that of sub-Saharan Africa [71].

3.3.4 Study findings

Table 3.3 displays the costs, cost-effectiveness, and incremental effects associated with the various strategies for primary prevention of acute rheumatic fever and RHD. The most expensive strategy was the treatment based on positive throat culture at US$27.21 per pharyngitis patient, while the least expensive was the treatment of all patients with an intramuscular penicillin injection, at US$11.19 per patient. This cost includes any expenses associated with future pharyngitis events, hospitalizations, or posthospitalization treatments, as well as the initial visit of each patient.

Compared to the strategy of treating all patients with the intramuscular penicillin injection, the strategy of treatment based on a clinical decision rule score of ≥2

Table 3.3 The costs, cost-effectiveness, and incremental effects associated with the various strategies for primary prevention of acute rheumatic fever and RHD.

Strategy	Cost per Patient (US$)	Incremental Cost-Effectiveness Ratio ($/quality-adjusted life year)	Incremental Effect
Treatment based on			
All patients with an intramuscular penicillin injection	$11.19	—	—
Positive throat culture	$27.21	127,600	0.000126
Clinical decision rule score of ≥2	$11.20	136	0.000066
Clinical decision rule score of ≥3	$13.00	(Dominated)	−0.000041
Clinical decision rule score of ≥2, culturing those with clinical decision rule scores of <2 and subsequently treating positive cultures	$16.42	(Dominated)	0.000015
Clinical decision rule score of ≥3, culturing those with clinical decision rule scores of <3 and subsequently treating positive cultures	$23.89	(Dominated)	0.000099
Observation only	$14.39	(Dominated)	−0.000103

Note: *Dominated* equates to both cost savings and better outcomes.

presented an incremental cost-effectiveness ratio of US$136 per quality-adjusted life year and was thus the preferred strategy. The strategy of treatment based on a clinical decision rule score of ≥3 was dominated as it was more expensive and resulted in fewer quality-adjusted life-years than treatment based on a clinical decision rule score of ≥2. The observation-only strategy was eliminated as it was more costly and led to fewer quality-adjusted life-years than the treatment of all patients with an intramuscular penicillin injection.

3.3.4.1 Sensitivity analysis

The overall group A streptococcus infection prevalence rate was approximately 15% but could range from 1.6 to 30% given the variability in the findings. At a group A streptococcus infection prevalence of 1.6 to 2.8%, the most inexpensive strategy would be treatment based on a clinical decision rule score of ≥3; however, the most effective strategy at the same prevalence level would be treatment based on a positive throat culture. The latter strategy presented an incremental cost-effectiveness ratio of US$127,600 per quality-adjusted life year, higher than the WHO's recommended gross domestic product per capita for a cost-effective strategy. If underlying prevalence reached 2.9 to 12.9%, the most inexpensive strategy would become treatment based on a clinical decision rule score of ≥2, with the treatment based on a clinical decision rule score of ≥3 strategy being the most effective, presenting an incremental cost-effectiveness ratio of US$198–US$30,000 per quality-adjusted life year. Finally, with an underlying prevalence of group A streptococcus infection of 12.9 to 30%, the most inexpensive strategy would become the treatment of all patients with an intramuscular penicillin injection. However, the strategy of treatment based on a clinical decision rule score of ≥2 would remain the most preferred strategy at <US$30,000 per quality-adjusted life year. The current analysis varied the probability of patients with untreated group A streptococcus infection developing acute rheumatic fever from 0.1 to 5%. At a probability of 0.1 to 0.29% and a willingness-to-pay of US$30,000 per quality-adjusted life year, the most inexpensive and preferred strategy would be treatment based on a clinical decision rule score of ≥2 (US$10–US$12 per patient). With a probability of 0.30 to 1%, the most inexpensive strategy would become the treatment of all patients with an intramuscular penicillin injection; however, the preferred strategy would become the treatment based on a clinical decision rule score of ≥2, with an incremental cost-effectiveness ratio of US$5–US$29,000 per quality-adjusted life year. Finally, at a probability of >1% the most preferred strategy would be the treatment of all patients with an intramuscular penicillin injection. The cost of throat culture was assumed to involve a return visit to the clinic to receive the penicillin injection, and a US$1 cost was allowed for a follow-up phone call. However, the results were not sensitive to the costs of the intramuscular penicillin injection, the management of acute rheumatic fever, the clinic visit, valve surgery, throat cultures, or the long-term management of subsequent RHD.

3.3.5 Study interpretation

The incidence rates of acute rheumatic fever and RHD in South Africa are relatively high, and are a significant health concern in LMIC [72,73]. The most inexpensive strategy for treating children presenting with pharyngitis at primary care clinics in South Africa was universal treatment with intramuscular penicillin injection. However, the most cost-effective strategy was based on treatment being applied via the application of a clinical decision rule score of ≥2. The remaining strategies resulted in an extremely high incremental cost per quality-adjusted life year gained, or did not result in long-term quality-adjusted life-years gained. Two important variables influencing the cost analyses were the underlying prevalence of group A streptococcus infection and the subsequent probability of developing acute rheumatic fever with group A streptococcus infection. The treatment of those patients presenting with pharyngitis was a low-cost strategy, resulting in $158 per 100,000 children per year aged 3 to 15 years. Additionally, the health benefits of preventing acute rheumatic fever and RHD were demonstrated to outweigh the potential risk of anaphylaxis; this finding is consistent with previous studies [74,75].

3.3.6 Study limitations

As with all studies of this kind, there are numerous assumptions that feed into the modeling of costs and health outcomes, hence the need for robust sensitivity analyses.

3.3.7 Study conclusions

In conclusion, this study determined that the most cost-effective strategy for preventing acute rheumatic fever and RHD is the treatment of all patients presenting with pharyngitis in urban primary care clinics in sub-Saharan Africa with an intramuscular penicillin injection. However, further investigation into the most cost-effective prevention strategies in other settings is required, given that cost-effectiveness is markedly influenced by numerous external factors, including the underlying prevalence of group A streptococcus infection.

3.4 The REMEDY Registry of RHD from an African perspective

Zuhlke L, Engel ME, Karthikeyan G, Rangarajan S, Mackie P, Cupido B, Mauff K, Islam S, Joachim A, Daniels R, Francis V, Ogendo S, Gitura B, Mondo C, Okello E, Lwabi P, Al-Kebsi M, Hugo-Hamman C, Sheta S, Haileamlak A, Daniel W, Goshu D, Abdissa S, Desta A, Shasho BA, Begna DM, ElSayed A, Ibrahim A, Musuku J, Bode-Thomas F, Okeahialam BN, Ige O, Sutton C, Misra R, Fadl A, Kennedy N, Damasceno A, Sani M, Ogah O, Olunuga T, Elhassan H, Mocumbi A, Adeoye AM, Mntla P, Ojji D, Mucumbitsi J, Teo K, Yusuf S, Mayosi BM. Characteristics, complications, and gaps in evidence-based interventions in rheumatic heart disease registry (the REMEDY study). *European Heart Journal* 2015; 36(18):1115–22. [76]

3.4.1 Study background

RHD is a major noncommunicable disease in LMIC and reportedly contributes to 1.4 million deaths per annum [77,78]. There is a known association between RHD, atrial fibrillation (AF), and infective endocarditis and significant complications during pregnancy [79–81]. The World Heart Federation's aim to reduce RHD mortality by 25% by the year 2025 requires an understanding of its characteristics, complications, treatments, and long-term outcomes. However, there is a paucity of research into all such aspects of this major public health issue [82,83]. Fortunately, RHD and its associated morbidity and mortality are highly preventable [84,85], with secondary prophylaxis via long-term penicillin use capable of reducing the recurrence of subsequent episodes of acute rheumatic fever [86]— see Section 3.3. However, previous studies have reported inadequate adherence to secondary prophylaxis and poor control of oral anticoagulant therapy and other evidence-based interventions [87–89].

3.4.2 Study aims

The aim of this study was to document the characteristics and treatment patterns with regard to valvular involvement, the use of key treatments, and the prevalence of adverse cardiac events [90] in patients presenting with RHD and enrolled via the REMEDY study (an international hospital-based registry of patients with RHD).

3.4.3 Study methods
3.4.3.1 Patient enrollment
During the period January 2010 to November 2012, patients were enrolled from 25 settings in 12 African countries, India, and Yemen, where assessment and treatment were recorded for each patient. For the current analysis, countries were grouped into income level. Low-income countries included Malawi, Ethiopia, Rwanda, Kenya, Zambia, and Uganda; lower-middle-income countries included Yemen, India, Egypt, Nigeria, Mozambique, and Sudan; and upper-middle-income countries included South Africa and Namibia [91]. Patients presenting with a primary diagnosis of symptomatic RHD from emergency departments, inpatient facilities, or outpatient clinics were enrolled based on clinical and echocardiogram criteria [92]. Ethical approval and informed patient consent were obtained prior to the study.

3.4.4 Study findings
As shown in Figure 3.2, a total of 3,343 patients with RHD were enrolled in the study. The majority of the patients were enrolled from South Africa (n = 597), followed by Ethiopia (n = 400), Kenya (n = 316), Uganda (n = 311), Yemen (n = 301), India (n = 293), Egypt (n = 286), Namibia (n = 266), Nigeria (n = 199), Sudan (n = 175), Zambia (n = 116), Mozambique (n = 41), Malawi (n = 37), and Rwanda (n = 5).

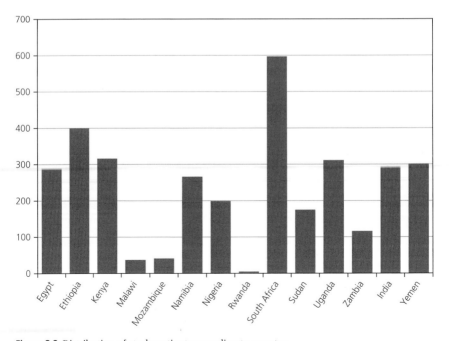

Figure 3.2 Distribution of study patients according to country.

3.4.4.1 Cohort profile

Table 3.4 displays the demographic and clinical characteristics of patients presenting with RHD. Overall, study patients were relatively young (median age of 28 years) and were predominantly women (66.1%; the majority of childbearing age [54.6%]), a large proportion being unemployed (54.3%). Those patients from low-income countries tended to present with more CHF, dilated LV end diastolic dimension in children, and left atrial thrombus. Those from LMIC tended to

Table 3.4 Patients' demographic and clinical characteristics.

	Low-Income Countries (n = 1,110)	Lower-Middle-Income Countries (n = 1,370)	Upper-Middle-Income Countries (n = 863)	All (n = 3,343)
Demographic characteristic				
Age (years)	24 (IQR 15–34)	28 (IQR 18–38)	39 (IQR 22–52)	28 (IQR 18–40)
Unemployed adults	529 (47.7%)	766 (55.9%)	520 (60.3%)	1,815 (54.3%)
Women	728 (65.6%)	867 (63.3%)	616 (71.4%)	2,211 (66.1%)
Women of childbearing age	630 (56.8%)	783 (57.2%)	412 (47.7%)	1,825 (54.6%)
Children	405 (36.5%)	349 (25.5%)	167 (19.4%)	921 (27.6%)
Adults with no formal education	66 (5.9%)	354 (25.8%)	38 (4.4%)	458 (13.7%)
Completed primary level education	246 (22.2%)	278 (20.3%)	204 (23.6%)	728 (21.8%)
Completed secondary level education	373 (33.6%)	372 (27.2%)	436 (50.5%)	1,181 (35.3%)
Completed tertiary level education	13 (1.2%)	10 (0.7%)	11 (1.3%)	34 (1.0%)
Clinical characteristic				
NYHA functional class III and IV	306 (27.6%)	384 (28.0%)	119 (13.8%)	809 (24.2%)
Medical history				
Acute rheumatic fever	247 (22.3%)	593 (43.3%)	500 (59.0%)	1,340 (40.1%)
Congestive HF	476 (42.9%)	285 (20.8%)	349 (57.9%)	1,110 (33.2%)
Infective endocarditis	25 (2.3%)	59 (4.3%)	49 (5.8%)	133 (4.0%)
PH	329 (29.6%)	465 (33.9%)	163 (18.9%)	957 (28.6%)
Stroke	58 (5.2%)	52 (3.8%)	125 (14.5%)	235 (7.0%)
Major bleeding	21 (1.9%)	38 (2.8%)	30 (3.5%)	89 (2.7%)
Peripheral embolism	3 (0.3%)	3 (0.2%)	19 (2.2%)	25 (0.8%)
Cardiovascular complications	96 (8.7%)	137 (10.0%)	191 (22.2%)	424 (12.7%)
AF	163 (14.7%)	241 (17.6%)	182 (21.1%)	586 (17.5%)

present more frequently with a history of acute rheumatic fever, PH, infective endocarditis, major bleeding and AF, dilated LV end diastolic dimension in adults, and decreased LVEF in both adults and children. Alternatively, patients from upper-middle-income countries were more likely to present a history of stroke, peripheral embolism, and cardiovascular complications. The majority of enrolled patients from upper-middle-income countries (71%) were categorized as postintervention or postsurgery.

3.4.4.2 Pattern and severity of native valve disease and the use of secondary prophylaxis

Most of the study patients presenting with mitral stenosis (72.9%), aortic stenosis (61.9%), MR (60.4%), pulmonary stenosis (59.4%), and tricuspid stenosis (54.2%) had moderate to severe disease, while 55.2% of the patients with aortic regurgitation were classified as mild. Overall, 23% of the adult patients and 16.4% of the child patients presenting with native valve disease had a dilated LV; 18.3% and 5.6% of adult and child patients, respectively, also presented with a reduced LVEF. Regarding the use of secondary prophylaxis, 54.8% of the patients were prescribed secondary penicillin prophylaxis, with intramuscular penicillin injections being the most common form of administration (89.5%); the remainder either received oral penicillin treatment or erythromycin in the case of penicillin allergy. Postsurgery patients were less likely to be on secondary prophylaxis compared with the patients awaiting surgery (31.1% versus 61.5%, p <0.001)

3.4.5 Study interpretation

This large, global study yielded a number of important findings. First, RHD patients from LMIC were young, predominantly women, and the majority were unemployed. Second, patients were typically and significantly affected by their disease as demonstrated by associated PH and LV dysfunction and moderate to severe VHD. Third, and of concern, developing countries reported a low use of secondary antibiotic prophylaxis, an important preventive treatment. On the other hand, use of oral anticoagulants was high overall (69.5%), while being low in high-risk mitral stenosis patients (those in sinus rhythm at high risk of stroke). Finally, significant differences were noted with respect to concurrent cardiovascular complications and the application of percutaneous and surgical interventions for RHD in LMIC. All of these factors and issues were evident in the significant number of registry patients enrolled via countries in sub-Saharan Africa.

3.4.6 Study limitations

As with any observational registry, the potential for selection bias and therefore a misrepresentation of the true burden and profile of target cases is ever present. Moreover, any comparisons between participating centers should be treated with caution given likely differences in the geographic distribution of available cases as well as variable issues relating to patient access to these centers.

3.4.7 Study conclusions

In conclusion, these data confirm an important gap between the potential and real-world application of proven surgical and medical interventions to best mitigate the adverse consequences of RHD in younger individuals in LMIC [83,92]. Despite the large contribution of South African data (given availability of surgery in the country), these findings are still relevant to sub-Saharan Africa. As described in Chapter 7, when focusing on the incidence and characteristics of RHD in the adult population, there is a clear imperative to prevent the disease through investment in proven, cost-effective strategies for primary prevention (including penicillin for prophylaxis of secondary streptococcal infections—see Section 3.3) and optimal management (including appropriate applied and monitored oral anticoagulant therapy and noninvasive surgical interventions for valvular dysfunction).

3.5 EMF among patients in Mozambique

Mocumbi AO, Ferreira MB, Sidi D, Yacoub MH. A population study of endomyocardial fibrosis in a rural area of Mozambique. *New England Journal of Medicine* **2008 Jul 3; 359(1):43–9. [93]**

3.5.1 Study background

EMF is the most common restrictive CMO worldwide, with an estimated 10 million people affected [94]. Importantly, EMF disproportionately affects African children. The disease has been reported in specific regions of several African countries, namely Uganda, Nigeria, Ivory Coast, and Mozambique. Sporadic cases have also been reported from Tanzania, Egypt, Congo, South Africa, Ethiopia, Zimbabwe, Senegal, Sudan, Zambia, Ghana, Malawi, and Kenya [95]. The etiology of EMF remains unknown, its prognosis is poor, and to date there is no specific treatment, making it one of the most neglected diseases worldwide.

3.5.2 Study aims

This study was designed using systematic sampling of the community coupled with detailed echocardiographic examination in randomly selected subjects from Inharrime, Mozambique, primarily composed of very-low-income residents. The aim of the study was to determine the prevalence of EMF in Inharrime, a coastal district from which arose most cases detected in referral units. Other objectives were to describe the mode of presentation and severity of EMF in the community, as well as to investigate its possible determinants.

3.5.3 Study methods
3.5.3.1 Patient enrollment

A random sample of 1,063 subjects of all age groups was obtained using an adaptation of the two-stage cluster sampling approach. Thirty-three villages were selected by simple random sampling and their leaders were asked to create a list of all households of each small county. The first household to be studied in each county was then selected by random sampling, and second-stage clustering was completed after arrival to the index household. Households surrounding the index family within the limits of the village were noted; a number was attributed to each and simple random selection of the next household to be visited was performed. This procedure was repeated for the following families until a minimum of 30 patients was reached.

3.5.3.2 Clinical profiling

Standardized questionnaires were used to collect demographic data from every subject of the selected family. Detailed transthoracic echocardiography was performed using a hand-carried echocardiography battery-operated system with M-mode, two-dimensional as well as pulsed, continuous and colour Doppler. Major and minor criteria for the diagnosis were defined based on knowledge of advanced disease and pathology findings of early stages described in postmortem studies. EMF was diagnosed in the presence of two major criteria, or one major criterion associated with two minor criteria (see Table 3.5). EMF was classified according to location of structural lesions: (a) biventricular when lesions involved both ventricles without predominance of one side, (b) right-sided when the lesions affected only or predominantly the RV, and (c) left-sided when the lesions were confined to or affected predominantly the LV. Finally, a severity scoring system was used considering the type and degree of structural and functional changes; according to the scoring system, the severity of EMF was classified as mild (<8), moderate (8–15), or severe (>15). The National Bioethical Committee of Mozambique approved this research protocol.

Table 3.5 Criteria for diagnosis and assessment of the severity of EMF.

Criterion	Score
Major criterion	
Endomyocardial plaques >2 mm in thickness	2
Thin (≤1 mm) endomyocardial patches affecting more than one ventricular wall	3
Obliteration of the RV or LV apex	4
Thrombi or spontaneous contrast without severe ventricular dysfunction	4
Retraction of the RV apex (RV apical notch)	4
Atrioventricular-valve dysfunction due to adhesion of the valvular apparatus to the ventricular wall	1–4
Minor criterion	
Thin endomyocardial patches localized to one ventricular wall	1
Restrictive flow pattern across mitral or tricuspid valves	2
Pulmonary-valve diastolic opening	2
Diffuse thickening of the anterior mitral leaflet	1
Enlarged atrium with normal-size ventricle	2
M-movement of the interventricular septum and flat posterior wall	1
Enhanced density of the moderator or other intraventricular bands	1

3.5.4 Study findings

A prevalence of EMF of 19.8±2.4% was found in this cohort, with highest levels (28.1±5.5%) in those subjects aged 10 to 19 years old. The disease was found to be more prevalent in men (23.0% versus 17.5%, p=0.026). Of the 1,249 patients belonging to the 217 families visited, 186 (14.9%) were not at home and could not be examined. There were no refusals to participate, but echocardiography was not performed for two patients who had psychiatric problems with uncontrolled and aggressive behaviour. Transthoracic echocardiography was performed in 1,063 patients, with a mean age of 22.5±0.7 years; of these, 611 (57.5±3.0%) were women. Overall, 211 patients were found to have EMF. Of these, 163 (77.2%) patients had mild lesions, 39 (18.5%) had moderate lesions, and 9 (4.3%) had severe EMF. Biventricular EMF was the most common EMF diagnosis (n=117, 55.5%), followed by right-sided EMF (n=59, 28%) and left-sided EMF (n=35, 16.6%). Only 48 (22.7%) patients with echocardiographic features of EMF reported being symptomatic. The most frequent lesions in the mild disease category were apical obliteration of the right ventricle, diffuse thickening of the mitral valve, and mild mitral or tricuspid regurgitation. There were differences in prevalence of EMF among the various age groups (p<0.001); the highest percentage being found in the 10 to 19 years old age group was 28.1%. The prevalence of EMF was significantly higher in men (23.0% versus 17.5%, p=0.026), but type of EMF lesion did not differ between the two sexes. Familial occurrence was high in this community. Out of 214 families, 99 (46.3%) had no EMF cases, 63 (29.4%) had one case and 52 (24.3%) had more than one case. There was no correlation between the percentage of subjects with EMF in a family and the observed family size, but the chance of having the disease was higher when other members of the family were affected.

3.5.5 Study interpretation

This study has determined, for the first time, the prevalence of EMF in a rural area using echocardiography screening (the standard technique for its diagnosis). As in a prior hospital-based study [96], EMF prevalence demonstrated bimodal age distribution, the first peak occurring during the second decade of life. Because criteria described in the literature defined only advanced and deforming stages [97,98] and there are no consensual criteria for early diagnosis of EMF, the proposed classification may be very helpful in studies focusing on its natural history. At 19.8%, EMF prevalence was higher than was found in a previous survey (8.9%) that used cardiac auscultation to select individuals for echocardiographic examination [99]. The study corroborated prior reports of clinical-echocardiographic dissociation and identified early stages of EMF, varying from asymptomatic patchy endocardial fibrosis to extensive mural-valvular endocardial fibrosis associated with severe structural and functional changes.

3.5.6 Study limitations

In the absence of major plaques of fibrosis, and considering that the area is also endemic for RHD, the distinction between left-sided EMF and rheumatic MR was not always straightforward; diffuse thickening of the anterior leaflet, hyper-dense papillary muscles, small-sized LV in the presence of severe MR, and disproportionate PH were used to favor left EMF. Familial clustering of this disease emphasizes the need to uncover the role of genetic susceptibility, environmental agents, and nutritional factors in its pathogenesis. Moreover, there is need for prospective studies examining the natural history of mild asymptomatic lesions.

3.5.7 Study conclusions

EMF is common in this rural area of Mozambique when assessed by echocardiography. Echocardiography detected early and asymptomatic stages of the disease, and systematic screening programs should be considered in this context. These findings provide a unique opportunity to study and evolve effective management schemes for the detection and management of EMF in Africa and beyond.

S2.2 The challenge of protecting the heart health of African children

The studies highlighted in this section, regardless of their congenital or acquired heart disease focus, collectively demonstrate the challenges in improving heart health outcomes among African infants and children. Access to appropriate care often comes all too late for the affected child or not at all (although such cases are difficult to quantify and define). When appropriate specialist care is applied in a timely manner, health outcomes are positive. Future investments in regional/national centers of excellence in pediatric management are clearly required to improve typically poor outcomes, particularly among those countries not fortunate to have specialist centers of care. At the same time, the cost analysis of preventive strategies for RHD, beyond a general improvement in living standards and household hygiene, clearly proves once again that prevention is better than cure, particularly in the resource-poor countries of Africa. Finally, the REMEDY registry is a timely reminder of the collaborative efforts being made to better understand the extent and nature of key threats to the heart health of African children (in this case RHD). Such studies are critical to informing public health policy and developing and applying cost-effective health care programs.

References

1 Mocumbi AO. The challenges of cardiac surgery for African children. *Cardiovasc J Afr.* 2012;23(3):165–7.

2 Mocumbi AO, Lameira E, Yaksh A, Paul L, Ferreira MB, Sidi D. Challenges on the management of congenital heart disease in developing countries. *Int J Cardiol.* 2011;148(3):285–8.

3 Hewitson J, Brink J, Zilla P. The challenge of pediatric cardiac services in the developing world. *Semin Thorac Cardiovasc Surg.* 2002;14(4):340–5.

4 Central Intelligence Agency. *The World Factbook: Mozambique.* Washington, DC: Central Intelligence Agency; 2015 [updated August 17 2015; accessed August 2015]. Available from: https://www.cia.gov/library/publications/the-world-factbook/geos/mz.html.

5 The World Bank. World Development Indicators: Urban Population [dataset] 2013. Available from: http://data.worldbank.org/indicator/SP.URB.TOTL.IN.ZS/countries.

6 Central Intelligence Agency. *The World Factbook: Cameroon.* Washington, DC: Central Intelligence Agency; 2011 [updated August 25 2015; accessed September 2015]. Available from: https://www.cia.gov/library/publications/the-world-factbook/geos/cm.html.

7 The World Bank. Cameroon Economic Update. Unlocking the Labor Force: An Economic Update on Cameroon. 2012. Available from: http://siteresources.worldbank.org/INTCAMEROON/Resources/CMR_Economic_update.January.2012.pdf.

8 The World Bank. Cameroon Economic Update. Mitigating Poverty, Vulnerability and Risk: A Special Focus on Social Safety Net. 2013. Available from: http://www-wds.worldbank.org/external/default/WDSContentServer/WDSP/IB/2013/01/23/000356161_20130123142046/Rendered/PDF/NonAsciiFileName0.pdf.

9 The World Bank. Better Access to Health Care for All Cameroonians. Story highlights from the Cameroon Economic Update. 2013. Available from http://www.worldbank.org/en/country/cameroon/publication/better-health-care-access-for-all-cameroonians.

10 Central Intelligence Agency. *The World Factbook: Malawi.* Washington, DC: Central Intelligence Agency; 2015 [updated September 2015; accessed September 2015].

11 Central Intelligence Agency. *The World Factbook: Country Comparison: Total Fertility Rate.* Washington, DC: Central Intelligence Agency [accessed September 2015]. Available from: https://www.cia.gov/library/publications/the-world-factbook/rankorder/2091rank.html#cm.

12 The World Bank. World Development Indicators: Poverty headcount ratio at national poverty lines [dataset]. 2010 [accessed September 2015]. Available from: http://data.worldbank.org/indicator/SI.POV.NAHC/countries.

13 Schmiedeknecht K, Perera M, Schell E, Jere J, Geoffroy E, Rankin S. Predictors of workforce retention among Malawian nurse graduates of a scholarship program: a mixed-methods study. *Global Health: Science and Practice.* 2015;3(1):85–96.

14 Central Intelligence Agency. *The World Factbook: Zimbabwe.* Washington, DC: Central Intelligence Agency; 2015 [updated September 2015; accessed September 2015]. Available from: https://www.cia.gov/library/publications/the-world-factbook/geos/zi.html.

The Heart of Africa: Clinical Profile of an Evolving Burden of Heart Disease in Africa, First Edition.
Edited by Simon Stewart, Karen Sliwa, Ana Mocumbi, Albertino Damasceno, and Mpiko Ntsekhe.
© 2016 John Wiley & Sons, Ltd. Published 2016 by John Wiley & Sons, Ltd.

15 The World Bank. World Development Indicators: Rural poverty headcount ratio at national poverty lines [dataset]. 2011 [accessed September 2015]. Available from: http://data.worldbank.org/indicator/SI.POV.RUHC/countries.

16 Chirwa Y, Witter S, Munjoma M, Mashange W, Ensor T, McPake B, et al. The human resource implications of improving financial risk protection for mothers and newborns in Zimbabwe. *BMC Health Serv Res.* 2013;13:197.

17 The World Bank. World Development Indicators: Mortality rate, infant (per 1,000 live births) [dataset]. 2014 [accessed September 2015]. Available from: http://data.worldbank.org/indicator/SP.DYN.IMRT.IN/countries.

18 World Health Organization. Zimbabwe: WHO statistical profile. 2015. Available from: http://www.who.int/gho/countries/zwe.pdf

19 Awori MN, Ogendo SW, Gitome SW, Ong'uti SK, Obonyo NG. Management pathway for congenital heart disease at Kennyatta National Hospital, Nairobi. *East Afr Med J.* 2007;84(7):312–7.

20 Diop IB, Ba SA, Ba K, Sarr M, Kane A, Fall M, et al. [Congenital cardiopathies: anatomo-clinical, prognostic, and therapeutic features apropos of 103 cases seen at the Cardiology Clinic of the Dakar University Hospital Center]. *Dakar Med.* 1995;40(2):181–6.

21 Okoromah CA, Ekure EN, Ojo OO, Animasahun BA, Bastos MI. Structural heart disease in children in Lagos: profile, problems and prospects. *Niger Postgrad Med J.* 2008;15(2):82–8.

22 Ellis J, Martin R, Wilde P, Tometzki A, Senkungu J, Nansera D. Echocardiographic, chest X-ray and electrocardiogram findings in children presenting with heart failure to a Ugandan paediatric ward. *Trop Doct.* 2007;37(3):149–50.

23 Omokhodion SI, Lagunju IA. Prognostic indices in childhood heart failure. *West Afr J Med.* 2005;24(4):325–8.

24 Marijon E, Tivane A, Voicu S, Vilanculos A, Jani D, Ferreira B, et al. Prevalence of congenital heart disease in schoolchildren of sub-Saharan Africa, Mozambique. *Int J Cardiol.* 2006;113(3):440–1.

25 Sani MU, Mukhtar-Yola M, Karaye KM. Spectrum of congenital heart disease in a tropical environment: an echocardiography study. *J Natl Med Assoc.* 2007;99(6):665–9.

26 Jaiyesimi F, Antia AU. Congenital heart disease in Nigeria: a ten-year experience at UCH, Ibadan. *Ann Trop Paediatr.* 1981;1(2):77–85.

27 Zuhlke L, Mirabel M, Marijon E. Congenital heart disease and rheumatic heart disease in Africa: recent advances and current priorities. *Heart.* 2013;99(21):1554–61.

28 Bernstein D. Congenital heart disease. In: Behrman RE, Kliegman RM, Jenson HB, editors. *Nelson Textbook of Pediatrics* 17th ed., 2004. p. 1501–9.

29 Sulafa KM, Karani Z. Diagnosis, management and outcome of heart disease in Sudanese patients. *East Afr Med J.* 2007;84(9):434–40.

30 Yacoub MH. Establishing pediatric cardiovascular services in the developing world: a wake-up call. *Circulation.* 2007;116(17):1876–8.

31 Tchoumi JCT, Ambassa JC, Chelo D, Djimegne FK, Giamberti A, Cirri S, et al. Pattern and clinical aspects of congenital heart diseases and their management in Cameroon. *Bulletin de la Societe de Pathologie Exotique.* 2011;104(1):25–8.

32 Tchoumi JCT, Ambassa JC, Kingue S, Giamberti A, Cirri S, Frigiola A, et al. Occurrence, aetiology and challenges in the management of congestive heart failure in sub-Saharan Africa: experience of the Cardiac Centre in Shisong, Cameroon. *Pan Afr Med J.* 2011;8:11.

33 Bannerman CH, Mahalu W. Congenital heart disease in Zimbabwean children. *Ann Trop Paediatr.* 1998;18(1):5–12.

34 Ejim EC, Ike SO, Anisiuba BC, Onwubere BJ, Ikeh VO. Ventricular septal defects at the University of Nigeria Teaching Hospital, Enugu: a review of echocardiogram records. *Trans R Soc Trop Med Hyg.* 2009;103(2):159–61.

35 Bassili A, Mokhtar SA, Dabous NI, Zaher SR, Mokhtar MM, Zaki A. Congenital heart disease among school children in Alexandria, Egypt: an overview on prevalence and relative frequencies. *J Trop Pediatr*. 2000;46(6):357–62.

36 Kennedy N, Miller P. The spectrum of paediatric cardiac disease presenting to an outpatient clinic in Malawi. *BMC Res Notes*. 2013;6:53.

37 UNICEF. State of the world's children 2009. New York: United Nations Children's Fund, 2008.

38 Hoosen EG, Cilliers AM, Hugo-Hamman CT, Brown SC, Lawrenson JB, Zuhlke L, et al. Paediatric cardiac services in South Africa. *S Afr Med J*. 2011;101(2):106–7.

39 Daniel E, Abegaz B. Profile of cardiac disease in an out-patient cardiac clinic. *Trop Geogr Med*. 1993;45(3):121–3.

40 el Hag AI. Pattern of congenital heart disease in Sudanese children. *East Afr Med J*. 1994; 71(9):580–6.

41 Marijon E, Ou P, Celermajer DS, Ferreira B, Mocumbi AO, Jani D, et al. Prevalence of rheumatic heart disease detected by echocardiographic screening. *N Engl J Med*. 2007;357(5):470–6.

42 Nkomo VT. Epidemiology and prevention of valvular heart diseases and infective endocarditis in Africa. *Heart*. 2007;93(12):1510–9.

43 Lubega S, Zirembuzi GW, Lwabi P. African Heart disease among children with HIV/AIDS attending the paediatric infectious disease clinic at Mulago Hospital. *Afr Health Sci*. 2005;5:219–26.

44 Miller RF, Kaski JP, Hakim J, Matenga J, Nathoo K, Munyati S, et al. Cardiac disease in adolescents with delayed diagnosis of vertically acquired HIV infection. *Clin Infect Dis*. 2013;56(4):576–82.

45 Joint United Nations Programme on HIV/AIDS. Global report annexes. 2010.

46 Ferrand RA, Bandason T, Musvaire P, Larke N, Nathoo K, Mujuru H, et al. Causes of acute hospitalization in adolescence: burden and spectrum of HIV-related morbidity in a country with an early-onset and severe HIV epidemic: a prospective survey. *PLoS Med*. 2010;7(2):e1000178.

47 Ferrand RA, Desai SR, Hopkins C, Elston CM, Copley SJ, Nathoo K, et al. Chronic lung disease in adolescents with delayed diagnosis of vertically acquired HIV infection. *Clin Infect Dis*. 2012;55(1):145–52.

48 Brown SC, Schoeman CJ, Bester CJ. Cardiac findings in children admitted to a hospital general ward in South Africa: a comparison of HIV-infected and uninfected children. *Cardiovasc J S Afr*. 2005;16(4):206–10.

49 Fisher SD, Easley KA, Orav EJ, Colan SD, Kaplan S, Starc TJ, et al. Mild dilated cardiomyopathy and increased left ventricular mass predict mortality: the prospective P2C2 HIV Multicenter Study. *Am Heart J*. 2005;150(3):439–47.

50 Lipshultz SE, Easley KA, Orav EJ, Kaplan S, Starc TJ, Bricker JT, et al. Left ventricular structure and function in children infected with human immunodeficiency virus: the Prospective P2C2 HIV Multicenter Study. Pediatric Pulmonary and Cardiac Complications of Vertically Transmitted HIV Infection (P2C2 HIV) Study Group. *Circulation*. 1998;97(13):1246–56.

51 Lipshultz SE, Easley KA, Orav EJ, Kaplan S, Starc TJ, Bricker JT, et al. Cardiac dysfunction and mortality in HIV-infected children: the Prospective P2C2 HIV Multicenter Study. Pediatric Pulmonary and Cardiac Complications of Vertically Transmitted HIV Infection (P2C2 HIV) Study Group. *Circulation*. 2000;102(13):1542–8.

52 Okoromah CA, Ojo OO, Ogunkunle OO. Cardiovascular dysfunction in HIV-infected children in a sub-Saharan African country: comparative cross-sectional observational study. *J Trop Pediatr*. 2012;58(1):3–11.

53 Pongprot Y, Sittiwangkul R, Silvilairat S, Sirisanthana V. Cardiac manifestations in HIV-infected Thai children. *Ann Trop Paediatr*. 2004;24(2):153–9.

54 Starc TJ, Lipshultz SE, Easley KA, Kaplan S, Bricker JT, Colan SD, et al. Incidence of cardiac abnormalities in children with human immunodeficiency virus infection: The prospective P2C2 HIV study. *J Pediatr*. 2002;141(3):327–34.

55 Starc TJ, Lipshultz SE, Kaplan S, Easley KA, Bricker JT, Colan SD, et al. Cardiac complications in children with human immunodeficiency virus infection. Pediatric Pulmonary and Cardiac Complications of Vertically Transmitted HIV Infection (P2C2 HIV) Study Group; National Heart, Lung, and Blood Institute. *Pediatrics.* 1999;104(2):e14.

56 Ferrand RA, Luethy R, Bwakura F, Mujuru H, Miller RF, Corbett EL. HIV infection presenting in older children and adolescents: a case series from Harare, Zimbabwe. *Clin Infect Dis.* 2007;44(6):874–8.

57 Bannerman C, Chitsike I. Cor pulmonale in children with human immunodeficiency virus infection. *Ann Trop Paediatr.* 1995;15(2):129–34.

58 Kavanaugh-McHugh A, Ruff A, Rowe S, Holt E, Wilfert C, Modlin JF. Cardiac abnormalities in a multi-center interventional study of children with symptomatic HIV infection. *Pediatr Res.* 1991;29:176A (Abstract).

59 Lubega S, Zirembuzi GW, Lwabi P. Heart diseases among children with HIV/AIDS attending the pediatric infectious disease clinic at Mulago hospital. *Afr Health Sci.* 2005;5:219–26.

60 World Health Organization. *Antiretroviral therapy for HIV infection in infants and children: towards universal access. Recommendations for a public health approach.* Geneva: WHO; 2010.

61 Irlam J, Mayosi BM, Engel M, Gaziano TA. Primary prevention of acute rheumatic fever and rheumatic heart disease with penicillin in South African children with pharyngitis: a cost-effectiveness analysis. *Circ Cardiovasc Qual Outcomes.* 2013;6(3):343–51.

62 Carapetis JR, McDonald M, Wilson NJ. Acute rheumatic fever. *Lancet.* 2005; 366(9480):155–68.

63 Marijon E, Mirabel M, Celermajer DS, Jouven X. Rheumatic heart disease. *Lancet.* 2012; 379(9819):953–64.

64 Global Burden of Disease Study C. Global, regional, and national incidence, prevalence, and years lived with disability for 301 acute and chronic diseases and injuries in 188 countries, 1990-2013: a systematic analysis for the Global Burden of Disease Study 2013. *Lancet.* 2015.

65 Michaud C, Rammohan R, Narula J. Cost-effectiveness analysis of intervention strategies for reduction of the burden of rheumatic heart disease. In: Narula J, Virmani R, Reddy KS, Tandon R, editors. *Rheumatic Fever.* Washington, DC: American Registry of Pathology; 1999. p. 485–97.

66 Pastore S, De Cunto A, Benettoni A, Berton E, Taddio A, Lepore L. The resurgence of rheumatic fever in a developed country area: the role of echocardiography. *Rheumatology (Oxford).* 2011;50(2):396–400.

67 Karthikeyan G, Mayosi BM. Is primary prevention of rheumatic fever the missing link in the control of rheumatic heart disease in Africa? *Circulation.* 2009;120(8):709–13.

68 Milne RJ, Lennon D, Stewart J, Scuffham P, Hoorn SV, Cooke J, et al. *Economic evaluation of a school intervention to reduce the risk of rheumatic fever: a report to the Ministry of Health.* Auckland, NZ: University of Auckland; 2011.

69 Gaziano TA. Economic burden and the cost-effectiveness of treatment of cardiovascular diseases in Africa. *Heart.* 2008;94(2):140–4.

70 Rimoin AW, Hamza HS, Vince A, Kumar R, Walker CF, Chitale RA, et al. Evaluation of the WHO clinical decision rule for streptococcal pharyngitis. *Arch Dis Child.* 2005;90(10): 1066–70.

71 Steinhoff MC, Walker CF, Rimoin AW, Hamza HS. A clinical decision rule for management of streptococcal pharyngitis in low-resource settings. *Acta Paediatr.* 2005;94(8):1038–42.

72 Tibazarwa KB, Volmink JA, Mayosi BM. Incidence of acute rheumatic fever in the world: a systematic review of population-based studies. *Heart.* 2008;94(12):1534–40.

73 World Health Organization, WHO-CHOICE website. Choosing interventions that are cost-effective. Available from: http://www.who.int/choice/en/.

74 Lieu TA, Fleisher GR, Schwartz JS. Cost-effectiveness of rapid latex agglutination testing and throat culture for streptococcal pharyngitis. *Pediatrics.* 1990;85(3):246–56.

75 Webb KH. Does culture confirmation of high-sensitivity rapid streptococcal tests make sense? A medical decision analysis. *Pediatrics.* 1998;101(2):E2.

76 Zuhlke L, Engel ME, Karthikeyan G, Rangarajan S, Mackie P, Cupido B, et al. Characteristics, complications, and gaps in evidence-based interventions in rheumatic heart disease: the Global Rheumatic Heart Disease Registry (the REMEDY study). *Eur Heart J.* 2015;36(18): 1115–22a.

77 Carapetis JR, Steer AC, Mulholland EK, Weber M. The global burden of group A streptococcal diseases. *Lancet Infect Dis.* 2005;5(11):685–94.

78 Paar JA, Berrios NM, Rose JD, Caceres M, Pena R, Perez W, et al. Prevalence of rheumatic heart disease in children and young adults in Nicaragua. *Am J Cardiol.* 2010;105(12):1809–14.

79 Benjamin EJ, Wolf PA, D'Agostino RB, Silbershatz H, Kannel WB, Levy D. Impact of atrial fibrillation on the risk of death: the Framingham Heart Study. *Circulation.* 1998; 98(10):946–52.

80 Diao M, Kane A, Ndiaye MB, Mbaye A, Bodian M, Dia MM, et al. Pregnancy in women with heart disease in sub-Saharan Africa. *Arch Cardiovasc Dis.* 2011;104(6–7):370–4.

81 Koegelenberg CF, Doubell AF, Orth H, Reuter H. Infective endocarditis in the Western Cape Province of South Africa: a three-year prospective study. *QJM.* 2003;96(3):217–25.

82 Carapetis JR. Rheumatic heart disease in Asia. *Circulation.* 2008;118(25):2748–53.

83 Remenyi B, Carapetis J, Wyber R, Taubert K, Mayosi BM, World Heart F. Position statement of the World Heart Federation on the prevention and control of rheumatic heart disease. *Nat Rev Cardiol.* 2013;10(5):284–92.

84 Carapetis JR, Mayosi BM, Kaplan EL. Controlling rheumatic heart disease in developing countries. *Cardiovasc J S Afr.* 2006;17(4):164–5.

85 Lawrence JG, Carapetis JR, Griffiths K, Edwards K, Condon JR. Acute rheumatic fever and rheumatic heart disease: incidence and progression in the Northern Territory of Australia, 1997 to 2010. *Circulation.* 2013;128(5):492–501.

86 Manyemba J, Mayosi BM. Intramuscular penicillin is more effective than oral penicillin in secondary prevention of rheumatic fever: a systematic review. *S Afr Med J.* 2003; 93(3):212–8.

87 Bassili A, Zaher SR, Zaki A, Abdel-Fattah M, Tognoni G. Profile of secondary prophylaxis among children with rheumatic heart disease in Alexandria, Egypt. *East Mediterr Health J.* 2000;6(2–3):437–46.

88 Oldgren J, Healey JS, Ezekowitz M, Commerford P, Avezum A, Pais P, et al. Variations in cause and management of atrial fibrillation in a prospective registry of 15,400 emergency department patients in 46 countries: the RE-LY Atrial Fibrillation Registry. *Circulation.* 2014;129(15):1568–76.

89 Pelajo CF, Lopez-Benitez JM, Torres JM, de Oliveira SK. Adherence to secondary prophylaxis and disease recurrence in 536 Brazilian children with rheumatic fever. *Pediatr Rheumatol Online J.* 2010;8:22.

90 Karthikeyan G, Zuhlke L, Engel M, Rangarajan S, Yusuf S, Teo K, et al. Rationale and design of a Global Rheumatic Heart Disease Registry: the REMEDY study. *Am Heart J.* 2012;163(4): 535–40 e1.

91 Webb R, Wilson NJ, Lennon D. Rheumatic heart disease detected by echocardiographic screening. *N Engl J Med.* 2007;357(20):2088; author reply -9.

92 World Health Organization. *Rheumatic fever and rheumatic heart disease: report of a WHO expert consultation, Geneva, 29 October–1 November 2001.* Geneva: WHO, 2004.

93 Mocumbi AO, Ferreira MB, Sidi D, Yacoub MH. A population study of endomyocardial fibrosis in a rural area of Mozambique. *N Engl J Med.* 2008;359(1):43–9.

94 Mocumbi AO, Yacoub S, Yacoub MH. Neglected tropical cardiomyopathies: II. Endomyocardial fibrosis: myocardial disease. *Heart.* 2008;94(3):384–90.

95 Mocumbi AO. Recent trends in the epidemiology of endomyocardial fibrosis in Africa. *Paediatr Int Child Health.* 2012;32(2):63–4.

96 Rutakingirwa M, Ziegler JL, Newton R, Freers J. Poverty and eosinophilia are risk factors for endomyocardial fibrosis (EMF) in Uganda. *Trop Med Int Health.* 1999;4(3):229–35.

97 Berensztein CS, Pineiro D, Marcotegui M, Brunoldi R, Blanco MV, Lerman J. Usefulness of echocardiography and doppler echocardiography in endomyocardial fibrosis. *J Am Soc Echocardiogr.* 2000;13(5):385–92.

98 Mady C, Salemi VM, Ianni BM, Arteaga E, Fernandes F, Ramires FJ. [Quantitative assessment of left ventricular regional wall motion in endomyocardial fibrosis]. [Article in Portuguese]. *Arq Bras Cardiol.* 2005;84(3):241–4.

99 Ferreira MB. *Endomyocardial fibrosis in Mozambique.* Paris: Paris Descartes University; 2000.

SECTION 3

Spectrum of cardiovascular risk and heart disease in sub-Saharan Africa

Simon Stewart

Australian Catholic University, Melbourne, Victoria, Australia

S3.1 Antecedent risk and heart disease in adult Africans

It is now well established that urban communities in sub-Saharan Africa, unlike rural populations in whom traditional lifestyles are more often preserved, are undergoing various epidemiologic transitions [1–3] with the emergence of non-communicable forms of heart disease (see Chapter 6) [4–6]. As described in Section 4, this has meant a relative decline in communicable forms of heart disease. The central paradox around the phenomenon of epidemiological transition is that despite increasing longevity, there is increased exposure to potentially devastating chronic disease in those who have escaped the traditional killers such as malnutrition and infectious disease; sometimes there is a legacy effect (e.g., late-stage RHD [7]—see Chapter 7) that leaves an individual more prone to develop chronic, noncommunicable disease later in life [8]. Unlike high-income countries in whom aging populations have already been exposed to a high burden of antecedent risk for decades, with peak (age-adjusted) rates of heart disease long passed [9–11], it appears sub-Saharan Africa is only just entering into a new era of non-communicable disease where heart disease will play a major role. However, it would be a mistake to assume that this diverse and populous region will follow the exact same pathway. We already know that younger generations in high-income countries are exposed to different patterns of antecedent risk (i.e., obesity and metabolic disorders including type 2 diabetes [12]) due to changing lifestyles (including sedentary behaviors [13]). We also know that older generations are exposed to a more compressed phase of debilitating chronic disease (including CHF [14,15] and AF [16,17]). Consequently, successful strategies (and even treatments such as the polypill with a strong focus on lipid-lowering therapy [18]) from the

The Heart of Africa: Clinical Profile of an Evolving Burden of Heart Disease in Africa, First Edition.
Edited by Simon Stewart, Karen Sliwa, Ana Mocumbi, Albertino Damasceno, and Mpiko Ntsekhe.
© 2016 John Wiley & Sons, Ltd. Published 2016 by John Wiley & Sons, Ltd.

past and/or applied to high-income populations and patient cohorts to prevent and treat heart disease do not readily apply in the sub-Saharan Africa context.

From a primary prevention perspective, a simple truism holds true—before you develop cost-effective, primary prevention strategies you must understand the prevalence of underlying risk in the target population. This includes understanding the "intensity" of risk not only in terms of numbers affected but the spectrum and complexity of risk values and coexisting risk factors. Beyond a "Westernized" perspective of risk (i.e., the all-encompassing Framingham Study [19]) it is important to accept that different populations may well have different pathways to heart disease; this alternative perspective is never more striking than considering the case of heart disease in Africa [20].

In this section of the *Heart of Africa*, we highlight a number of studies that have, over a relatively short period of time, highlighted the contemporary burden of underlying risk of noncommunicable forms of CVD in the region and the evolving spectrum of disease that has now emerged in a number of representative communities. As noted in the preface, we do not purport to provide the reader of this book with a definitive review of a healthy growth in the African literature (that will perhaps come with future editions of the book), representing an increasing area of research activity. Rather, we highlight key studies that have contributed to our current knowledge in this regard, noting the importance of previous and ongoing studies such as the sub-Saharan Africa Survey of Heart Failure (THESUS-HF) [21], the Sympathetic Activity and Ambulatory Blood Pressure in Africans (SABPA) Study [22–24], the Transition and Health during Urbanisation of South Africans (THUSA) Study [20,25,26], and the Cardiovascular Risk in Black South Africans (CRIBSA) Study [27–29].

In Chapter 4 we summarize risk surveillance data from the community of Soweto in South Africa in addition to Abia State in Nigeria, providing important insights into the likely increase in noncommunicable forms of heart disease throughout sub-Saharan Africa. In Chapter 5, we present the results of one of the most important studies undertaken from a pan-African perspective (the African INTERHEART study), demonstrating common pathways to AMI from a global to African-specific basis. Last, Chapter 6 summarizes the multiple facets of the Heart of Soweto Study based at the Baragwanath Hospital in Soweto, outlining the broad spectrum of communicable versus noncommunicable forms of heart disease now evident in the urban African context.

S3.1.1 Geographical context

Section 3 of this book sees a return to Soweto, South Africa, in Chapters 4 and 6 (see Section 1 for snapshots of South Africa and Soweto). Chapter 4 also familiarizes us with Nigeria, various regions of which will feature again in Section 6. In Chapter 5, eight diverse African countries are represented in the multisite INTERHEART study.

Nigeria, located in West Africa, is the continent's most populous country, with 181,562,056 inhabitants and an annual population growth rate of 2.45% [30].

It is home to more than 250 ethnic groups, the most populous and politically influential being the Hausa, Fulani, Yoruba, and Igbo, which together account for almost 70% of the population [30]. English, Hausa, Yoruba, Igbo, and Fulani are thus the most common languages, with over 500 additional indigenous languages also in use. Urbanization is occurring rapidly in Nigeria, with 47.8% of the population currently identified as urban and a 4.66% rate of change per annum [30]. Although the last official poverty statistics (2010) estimated that 46% of Nigerians live below the poverty line, a recent update by the World Bank suggested that this figure might have improved to 33% [31]. However, individual poverty, shortages of heath personnel, and inadequate pharmaceutical and medical supplies continue to impede access to timely and quality health care despite this economic growth [32]. Life expectancy remains low at 53 years, and Nigeria has the world's tenth-highest rate of infant mortality at almost 74 deaths per 1000 live births [30].

Abia State, the specific Nigerian setting of Chapter 4, is situated in the southeastern portion of Nigeria. Segmented into urban and rural sections, the state has a population of more than 3 million inhabitants, 70% of whom are concentrated in the rural regions [33] and 60% of whom are estimated to live below the poverty line [34]. Difficulties at the system level and a critical lack of resources continue to affect the availability and quality of health services and supplies in Abia State [33].

CHAPTER 4

Cardiovascular risk in urban and rural African settings

Kemi Tibazarwa[1], Karen Sliwa[2], Melinda Jane Carrington[3], Okechukwu Samuel Ogah[4], and Simon Stewart[3]

[1] Muhimbili National Hospital, Dar es Salaam, Tanzania
[2] University of Cape Town, South Africa; University of the Witwatersrand, Johannesburg, South Africa
[3] Australian Catholic University, Melbourne, Victoria, Australia
[4] University College Hospital, Ibadan, Oyo, Nigeria

4.0 Introduction

In this chapter we present three key studies (two are derived from Soweto [35,36] and the other from Nigeria [37]) that offer important insights into the spectrum of risk for heart disease in urban and to a lesser extent rural African communities in sub-Saharan Africa. Importantly, given the enormity of the continent and diverse populations who live there, this represents just the beginning of our understanding of this risk burden, and many more studies are required in the years to come to fully protect both urban and rural African communities from highly preventable forms of heart disease [38].

4.1 A time bomb of risk in an urban African community: "Heart Awareness Days" in Soweto

Tibazarwa K, Ntyintyane L, Sliwa K, Gerntholtz T, Carrington M, Wilkinson D, Stewart S. A time bomb of cardiovascular risk factors in South Africa: results from the Heart of Soweto Study "Heart Awareness Days." *International Journal of Cardiology* **2009; 132(2):233–39. [36]**

4.1.1 Study background

The world-renowned township of Soweto adjacent to Johannesburg in the Republic of South Africa is the quintessential African urban community. Soweto was the epicenter of the apartheid-era struggles and, in just a small corner in the heart of its community, raised two notable luminaries and Nobel Peace Prize

Winners—the late Nelson Mandela (inaugural President of the country) and Archbishop Desmond Tutu (spiritual leader and moral compass for the country). From a public health perspective, at the turn of the 20th century and in the first decade of the 21st century, Soweto was also the epicenter of epidemiological transition in urban African communities across the continent as the benefits of political and economic transformation started to provide even the poorest communities with greater freedom and economic opportunity. At the time of the study described below, there was little attention on heart and CVDs within urban African communities, and this was reflected also in poor awareness of the relative dangers imposed by potentially high levels of antecedent risk for noncommunicable forms of heart disease and stroke. The primary focus of this study therefore, was to undertake initial screening for cardiovascular risk factors in Soweto and to raise community awareness of heart disease in the process via a series of "Heart Awareness Days" conducted on the streets and at key locations within the community.

4.1.2 Study aims

Over and above the broader strategy of raising awareness and visibly engaging the local community to highlight the risks of developing heart disease and other forms of CVD, the primary objective of this study (via a systematic program of voluntary community-based screening) was to determine the likely prevalence of the most common risk factors for communicable forms of heart disease in Soweto.

1.1.3 Study methods

Following ethics approval, the 12-month study was implemented from June 2006 to May 2007 with prescheduled screening days every 4 weeks with a 3-month pause in late 2006 to early 2007. Participation was improved by facilitating a surveillance monitoring stand situated in Soweto's Maponya Mall and the Soweto Taxi Rank. All patients who were screened as well as individuals within a 200-m radius from the monitoring site were educated on the different types and consequences of the risk factors for heart disease.

4.1.3.1 Patient enrollment

With Soweto's total population size of an estimated one million individuals, the predetermined target of the study was 1,800 patients in the first 9 months of active screening. Convenience sampling was used to screen patients who approached the clearly marked "Heart Awareness Days" stands. The same team of health professionals (comprising qualified nurses, a dietician, and supervising cardiologist) conducted each event in a standardized manner. During the screening days, patient consent was obtained followed by structured questions to ascertain each patient's self-reported demographic status and any history of documented CVD, diabetes, or commonly-known related diseases, in the language the patient was most comfortable with. A structured interview investigating patient alcohol intake, smoking habits, and family history of CVD was introduced 5 months after study commencement. All patients then visited a sequence of "stations" where their BP and BMI were measured. Random blood glucose and cholesterol levels were also measured via validated point-of-care machines. All data throughout the study were captured on standardized study forms with unique identifiers for each patient. These were then transferred electronically to a dedicated data management team in Australia (Baker IDI Institute) for analysis and statistical interpretation. At the end of the screening process, all findings were interpreted to patients as well as the distribution of education materials. Dietary counseling and other life-style advice were provided to all patients with identified risk factors.

4.1.4 Study findings

Overall, 1,691 patients (representing 93.9% of the target number) were screened throughout the nine conducted "Heart Awareness Days." In total, 1,540 (91.1%) patients completed the full suite of screening measures. The majority of the patients were of African ancestry (99%), and more than half were women (64.9%). In total, 476 patients (just under one-third) reported a history of CVD or the presence of a closely related risk factor. Of these, 381 (80%) patients reported being hypertensive and 52 (10.9%) having type 2 diabetes (9% self-reporting both). While 938 (55.5%) patients completed the interview in the last half of the study, 197 (21%) of these reported a history of cigarette smoking, 272 (29%) reported regular alcohol intake, and 56 (6%) reported a combination of both alcohol intake and cigarette smoking.

4.1.4.1 Demographic and risk factor characteristics

Strikingly, obesity was by far the most prevalent risk factor for future CVD; not only were 1,184 (70%) patients found to be overweight, but 727 (43%) were considered obese. As shown in Table 4.1, women were more likely to report a history of CVD or type 2 diabetes ($p < 0.001$) and to present with a higher BMI ($p < 0.001$), while men were more likely to report former or current smoking habits ($p < 0.001$). The overall prevalence of obesity was significantly lower in men than in women (23% versus 55%; odds ratio [OR] 0.24; 95% CI 0.19 to 0.30; $p < 0.001$) (see Figure 4.1). Of those with recorded BP levels, 19% had evidence of both systolic and diastolic hypertension with no difference between the sexes in this regard.

As shown in Figure 4.2, one-third of patients had either an elevated systolic or diastolic BP, representing 196 (33%; 95% CI 29 to 37%) of men and 373 (34%; 95% CI 31 to 37%) of women. In contrast, 230 (13.64%; 95% CI 12 to 16%) patients had an elevated (nonfasting) blood cholesterol level with slightly more women presenting this (15% versus 10.9%), and only 54 (3.2%) had an elevated blood glucose level with men presenting slightly higher in this regard (3.5% versus 3%). Smoking was particularly prevalent in 3.0% of men (almost half) but not in women.

4.1.4.2 Pattern of risk for future heart disease

Excluding self-reported history, it was striking that only one in five patients (19%) had no obvious risk factors for the future development of heart disease. Overall, women were significantly more likely to have ≥1 risk factor for heart disease than

Table 4.1 Patients' demographic and risk factor characteristics.

Characteristic	Women (n = 1,097)	Men (n = 594)
Age (years)	47 ± 14	45 ± 15
History of CVD and/or type 2 diabetes	406 (37%)	154 (25.9%)
Former or current cigarette smoker	132 (12%)	244 (41.1%)
BMI (kg/m²)	31.9 ± 7.5	26.4 ± 5.8
Systolic BP (mm Hg)	133 ± 20	133 ± 19
Diastolic BP (mm Hg)	84 ± 14	83 ± 15
Random blood glucose (mmol/L)	4.8 (IQR 4.2–5.7)	5.0 (IQR 4.3–5.8)
Total blood cholesterol (mmol/L)	3.9 (IQR 3.0–4.7)	3.0 (IQR 3.0–4.4)

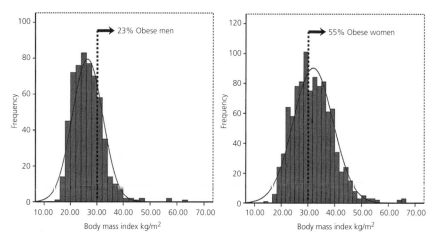

Figure 4.1 Frequency distribution of BMI levels according to sex.

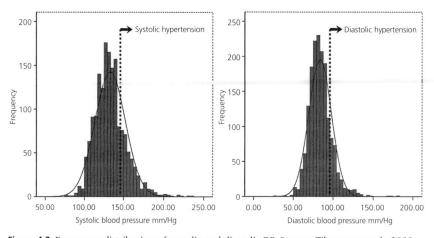

Figure 4.2 Frequency distribution of systolic and diastolic BP. Source: Tibazarwa et al., 2009 [36]. Reproduced with permission of Elsevier.

men (87% versus 68%; p<0.001). Alternatively, there were no sex differences in respect to elevated BP or blood glucose levels. However, women were significantly more likely to have a high serum cholesterol than were men (16% versus 11%, OR 0.67; 95% CI 0.48 to 0.93). As already noted, women were significantly more likely to be overweight than men (82% versus 56%; OR 0.28, 95% CI 0.22 to 0.35; p<0.001). Elevated total cholesterol levels and increasing BMI was associated with the presence of systolic and diastolic hypertension. Among obese men and women, however, there were some differences in respect to concurrent risk factors. For example, obesity in men (but not women) was almost significantly associated with the presence of hyperglycemia ($p=0.06$). Conversely, obesity in women (but not in men) was significantly associated with hypercholesterolemia ($p=0.001$). Consistent with the potential presence of metabolic syndrome in this population overall, an elevated cholesterol was positively correlated with hyperglycemia (OR 2.5, 95% CI 1.3 to 4.8; $p=0.03$).

4.1.5 Study interpretation

This was a "first of a kind" study in the largest township in sub-Saharan Africa and with the greatest concentration of Africans living in an urban setting at the time. Surprisingly, the same highly prevalent risk factors for heart disease in Western societies were also found to be highly prevalent in Soweto. For example, as in countries such as Australia [39] and the United States [40], one-third of adults had elevated BP with 4 in 5 patients demonstrating at least one easily identifiable risk factor for heart disease. Obesity was found to be the most prevalent risk factor overall (one-third of men and one-half of women), but this has to be placed in a cultural and health context of historically high levels of malnutrition and HIV/AIDS-induced body wasting. Not unexpectedly, given the likely presence of high levels of metabolic syndrome [36,41], being overweight was closely associated with hypertension and more importantly with elevated lipid levels. These findings were consistent with equivalent surveys undertaken in other South African provinces (for example, Kwa-Zulu Natal, Limpopo, North West, and northern provinces) [1,20,25,42–44]. As a whole, these data suggest that urban communities in sub-Saharan Africa will become increasingly at risk from epidemiologic transition toward more affluent disease states such as coronary artery disease (CAD) and ischemic stroke, although the relatively low levels of dyslipidemia provide at least some comfort [45–47] when compared to the immediate threat of elevated BP. Sub-Saharan Africa is therefore joining other communities in LMIC in entering a new and potentially devastating phase of noncommunicable disease [2–5]. Given that the urban proportion of South Africa's population (currently at 64% [48]) will continue to grow rapidly, the absolute number of potentially emerging cases of heart disease and other forms of CVD is potentially devastating to the livelihood of the population and its health system. Inequitable provision of health services and the persistence of low indices of suspicion for underlying CVD in health practitioners serving this population would be doubly devastating in this context; hence, the attempt to highlight high-risk levels and raise awareness of an emerging health problem is timely.

4.1.6 Study limitations

Due to resource constraints and the many unknowns about the true demographic structure and profile of Soweto, this was not a purposefully selected cohort designed to be representative of the community. As such, just over half of the study patients were self-selected, which may have led to oversampling of those who would gain the most from this screening program. Even though ushers at the recruitment stands alerted passers-by of the screening process, most recruits presented to the stand without knowledge of its purpose.

4.1.7 Study conclusions

Despite a number of limitations, these data highlighted the enormous potential for noncommunicable forms of heart disease to take hold in Soweto and other urban African communities. The role of obesity, within a historical setting of malnourishment and then the stigma of body-wasting related to HIV/AIDS, provides a challenging backdrop to these findings. At the very least, this study raised awareness of emerging risk factors for noncommunicable forms of heart disease not only in the community of Soweto but in other urban African communities and the wider global health community.

4.2 A time bomb of risk in an urban African community: a primary care perspective in Soweto

Stewart S, Carrington MJ, Pretorius S, Ogah OS, Blauwet L, Antras-Ferry J, Sliwa K. Elevated risk factors but low burden of heart disease in urban African primary care patients: a fundamental role for primary prevention. *International Journal of Cardiology* 2012; 158(2):205–10. [35]

4.2.1 Study background

The results of the "Heart Awareness Days," described in Section 4.1 above, demonstrate potentially high levels of modifiable risk factors for heart disease in the urban African community of Soweto. However, as in other parts of sub-Saharan Africa, it was unclear if apparently high levels of risk factors and advanced forms of heart disease were reflected in the case mix seen in primary care services within that community. It would be fair to say that preventive primary care services (particularly focused on noncommunicable disease) remain underdeveloped across the continent. This reflects a historical reliance and investment in tertiary health services. For example, as described in Chapter 6, only 6.8% of confirmed cases of heart disease were directly referred from local clinics in the Heart of Soweto clinical registry. Primary care research in sub-Saharan Africa remains in its infancy and, even with the best of intentions, this is unlikely to be readily addressed without substantive investment in a skilled workforce; at the time of this study the primary care nurses would be routinely confronted with a caseload in excess of 100 patients per day without substantive medical support. In recognition of the central importance of primary health care to assess cardiovascular risk and in turn implement proactive prevention and treatment programs to tackle an unavoidable rise of noncommunicable forms of disease, the Heart of Soweto research program (see Chapter 6) was extended from the community and hospital setting into the primary care setting.

4.2.2 Study aims

By using the annual number of prevalent and incident cases managed by the Chris Hani Baragwanath Hospital, it was hypothesized that the caseload of heart disease in each of the 12 primary care clinics in Soweto would be ~350 cases per annum, representing a previously undocumented caseload of heart disease in primary care. The study was designed, therefore, to determine the burden and spectrum of risk and established heart disease in primary care clinics servicing the urban African community of Soweto.

4.2.3 Study methods
4.2.3.1 Patient enrollment

Following appropriate ethics approval, the study involved 50 days of prospective screening of primary care patients in target clinics over a 6-month period. Data were systematically collected on consecutive patients attending two selected primary care clinics (Mandela Sissulu Clinic and Pimville Primary Care Clinic) in two diverse locations within Soweto. Both primary care clinics managed more than 300 patients per day with a wide range of health issues. A study team comprising an experienced cardiac nurse, electrocardiogram (ECG) technician, and study coordinator invited consecutive consenting patients aged ≥16 years who presented to the primary care clinic to be screened. All patients were reviewed by a primary health care nurse prior to assessment, and the study had a patient target of 25 consecutive patients per screening day, which would result in a minimum total of 1,000 patients.

4.2.3.2 Advanced cardiac profiling

The study team applied a standardized protocol of sociodemographic (self-report) and clinical profiling using validated point-of-care instruments. All patients suspicious of having possible underlying heart disease or a confirmed diagnosis were investigated further at the Cardiology Unit of the Chris Hani Baragwanath Hospital. The same standardized protocol of classification and assessment, as outlined in the Heart of Soweto Study (see Chapter 6), were applied. All data from the study were recorded on standardized forms before being sent to Australia (Baker IDI Institute) for independent analysis and interpretation.

4.2.4 Study findings
4.2.4.1 Demographic and clinical characteristics

A larger than expected cohort comprising 1,311 primary care patients was studied throughout the program. As shown in Table 4.2, 92.1% patients reside in Soweto, 98.6% were of African ancestry, and just over half (65.8%) were women. It was

Table 4.2 Patients' demographic and clinical characteristics.

	Women (n = 862)	Men (n = 449)	All (n = 1,311)
Demographic characteristics			
Age (years)	41 ± 16	38 ± 14	40 ± 16
African ancestry	853 (99.0%)	439 (97.8%)	1,292 (98.6%)
Reside in Soweto	786 (91.2%)	421 (93.8%)	1,207 (92.1%)
Years residing in Soweto	30 ± 20	26 ± 18	29 ± 19
<6 years education	193 (22.4%)	89 (19.8%)	282 (21.5%)
Unemployed	613 (71.1%)	131 (29.2%)	744 (56.8%)
Risk profile			
Family history of CVD	455 (52.8%)	185 (41.2%)	640 (48.8%)
History of cigarette smoking	124 (14.4%)	210 (46.8%)	334 (25.5%)
Dyslipidaemia	12 (1.4%)	4 (0.9%)	16 (1.2%)
BMI (kg/m^2)	29.9 ± 9.2	24.8 ± 8.3	28.2 ± 9
Waist circumference (cm)	93 ± 19	85 ± 15	90 ± 18
No regular exercise	787 (91.3%)	385 (85.8%)	1,172 (89.4%)
Preexisting CVD			
Diabetes	32 (3.7%)	13 (2.9%)	45 (3.4%)
Hypertension	333 (38.6%)	97 (21.6%)	430 (32.8%)
Stroke	6 (0.7%)	6 (1.3%)	12 (0.9%)
Any CVD	42 (4.9%)	23 (5.1%)	65 (5.0%)
Clinical characteristics			
NYHA Class II or III	154 (17.8%)	61 (13.6%)	215 (16.4%)
Palpitations	144 (16.7%)	56 (12.5%)	200 (15.3%)
Chest pain on exertion	143 (16.6%)	77 (17.2%)	220 (16.8%)
Syncopal episodes	160 (18.6%)	58 (12.9%)	218 (16.6%)
Peripheral edema	30 (3.5%)	10 (2.2%)	40 (3.1%)
Heart rate (beats/min)	73 ± 12	72 ± 12	72 ± 12
Systolic BP (mmHg)	132 ± 22	131 ± 20	132 ± 22
Diastolic BP (mmHg)	85 ± 16	84 ± 16	84 ± 157
Blood glucose level (mmol/L)	5.5 ± 2.0	5.3 ± 2.0	5.5 ± 2.0

found that women were more likely to be older (p < 0.001), unemployed (p < 0.0001), and reside in Soweto for longer (p < 0.001).

As shown in Figure 4.3, patients sought primary care management for a wide range of conditions. Most notably (from a cardiovascular perspective), 4.9% of patients were found to have preexisting CVD, and around one-third overall (comprising 39% women and 22% men; OR 1.79, 95% CI 1.47–2.17) presented with hypertension. Predictably, cases of stroke (0.9%) and CAD (0.2%) were scarce, while 3.4% had been diagnosed with type 2 diabetes. Other than hypertension, the most common conditions seen were respiratory disease, gastrointestinal disorders, musculoskeletal disorders, skin disorders, systemic infectious disease, and neurological disorders.

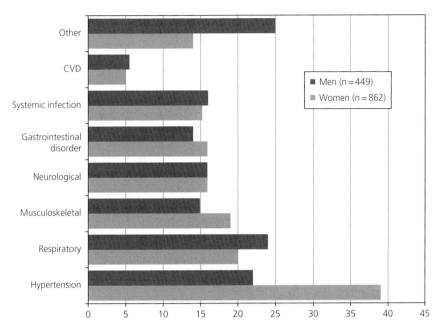

Figure 4.3 Diagnostic profile of primary care patients according to sex. Source: Tibazarwa et al., 2009 [36]. Reproduced with permission of Elsevier.

4.2.4.2 Cardiovascular risk profile

In addition to presenting with more hypertension, more women than men reported a family history of any form of heart condition (OR 1.28, 95% CI 1.16–1.46) and were more likely found to be obese (42% versus 14%; OR 4.54, 95% CI 3.33–5.88). They also reported more symptoms suggestive of underlying heart disease (including exercise intolerance, palpitations, chest pain on exertion, and syncope). Men on the other hand were far more likely to smoke cigarettes (OR 5.23, 95% CI 4.01–6.82) and men with hypertension had higher BP than their female counterparts (151 ± 22/97 ± 16 versus 146 ± 22/92 ± 15 mm Hg; p < 0.05 for both comparisons). Sedentary behaviors were common in both sexes (nearly all patients); this was counteracted with around one in five patients reporting physically active employment. Figure 4.4 shows the relationship between BP levels, heart rate, blood glucose levels, and body fatness levels in nonobese (top panels) and obese (bottom panels) patients on an age-specific basis. Overall, there was a consistent age gradient in all parameters. Significantly, the largest gradients were found in obese women, particularly in respect to systolic BP and blood glucose levels, the latter rising from 4.5 ± 1.0 to 6.8 ± 3.2 mmol/L in the youngest versus oldest age group. On an adjusted basis, obese women were twofold more likely to record a blood glucose level of >7.0 mmol/L (p = 0.01) and a systolic BP >140 mm Hg (p = 0.007), respectively, than obese men, reinforcing a higher latent risk for early onset diabetes and premature heart disease in obese women.

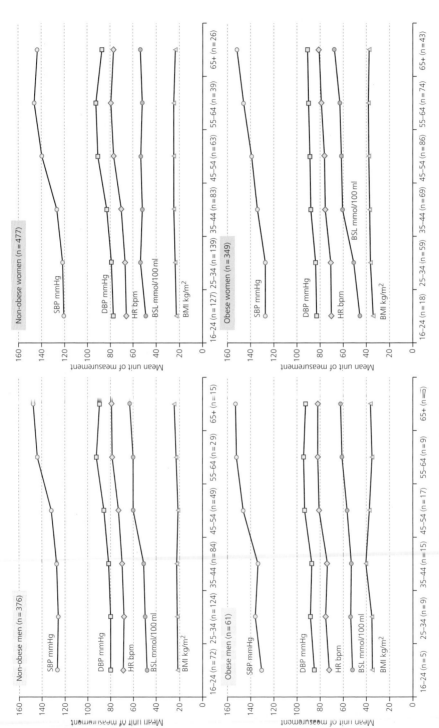

Figure 4.4 Differential risk profiles according to age and obese status in men and women.

4.2.4.3 Advanced cardiac assessment

Overall, 63 (7.3%) women (aged 40 ± 16 years) and 36 (8%) men (aged 37 ± 14 years), were referred for more advanced cardiologic assessment via the Cardiology Clinic of the Baragwanath Hospital due to hypertension. Beyond those with preexisting heart disease, 31 (2.4%) patients were reviewed. Subsequently, 17 (1.3%) patients were found to have LV systolic dysfunction and 12 (0.9%) had evidence of diastolic dysfunction. Ultimately, these referrals for more extensive investigation revealed an additional 15 (1.1%) de novo cases of hypertensive HF, 3 (0.2%) cases of CAD, 3 (0.2%) cases of degenerative valve disease (a total of 28 patients having some form of valvular dysfunction but none with RHD), 3 (0.2%) cases with a serious tachyarrhythmia (two cases of AF plus one Wolf-Parkinson-White Syndrome), 2 (0.2%) cases of idiopathic CMO, 2 (0.2%) cases of acute myocarditis (postviral infection), and 1 (0.1%) case of PPCMO (see Chapter 1). Notably, 8 of these patients had no history of CVD or cardiovascular risk factors.

4.2.5 Study interpretation

As with the "Heart Awareness Days" [36], this represented a first-of-its-kind study, reflecting a systematic attempt to quantify the contribution of clinically overt and subclinical heart disease in primary care clinics servicing an urban African community in sub-Saharan Africa. Consistent with relevant reports outlining the broad spectrum of disease in the region [4], infectious disease predominated, both in the form of systemic infection such as HIV/AIDS and localized manifestations such as TB. Respiratory disease and musculoskeletal disorders were also common reasons for a primary care presentation. Although the contribution of established heart disease to the clinical case mix was relatively small (1–3 cases per 100 presentations depending on the level of scrutiny and investigation), consistent with community surveillance data, cardiovascular risk factors were disturbingly high with around one-third (but with more women than men affected) being hypertensive. This is consistent with previous estimates of this highly modifiable cardiovascular risk factor [49] and resembles BP levels often seen in high-income countries [39]. The disproportionate contribution of obese women was important in this regard, particularly when one considers the higher, age-adjusted gradients in BP levels in obese women.

4.2.6 Study limitations

There were a number of study limitations that require comment. First, this study was unable to provide accurate estimates of the proportion of cases captured due to the volume of cases managed by the participating primary care clinics and the nature of their medical record system. Secondly, study personnel were unable to verify each and every diagnosis as there was a combination of self-report and primary care clinic records. Finally, it is worth noting that more individuals with subclinical or undiagnosed heart disease would have been identified if all patients were subject to the same level of screening.

4.2.7 Study conclusions

Despite a number of limitations, these data provide a fascinating and important insight into the case-mix of primary care presentations in Soweto, noting immediately the expectation that many factors would affect the distribution and nature of cases over time. Overall, study findings were consistent with initial estimates that around 1 in 100 primary care patients in Soweto have an established form of heart disease [50]. However, this number increased to 3 in 100 cases when greater scrutiny (in the form of referral to more extensive cardiologic investigation) was applied. Such a "return for effort" needs to be carefully evaluated, particularly in association with other potentially more sophisticated strategies (e.g., cardiac biomarkers [51] and handheld imaging [52]). Moreover, more basic methods such as well-defined clinical assessments for heart disease (e.g., auscultating for cardiac murmurs) and screening with 12-lead ECG should be considered, the latter being tempered by the finding that a significant proportion of urban Africans without heart disease demonstrate some form of ECG "abnormality" [53]. Regardless of the exact methods that might be applied, these data reinforce the call for strengthening primary care services and preventive strategies in the sub-Saharan Africa context [54]. These are essential to combat an expected rise in noncommunicable forms of heart disease, noting the particularly elevated risk levels in obese African women.

4.3 A time bomb of hypertension in urban and rural African communities in Nigeria

Okpechi IG, Chukwuonye, II, Tiffin N, Madukwe OO, Onyeonoro UU, Umeizudike TI, et al. Blood pressure gradients and cardiovascular risk factors in urban and rural populations in Abia State South Eastern Nigeria using the WHO STEPwise approach. *PLoS One* 2013; 8(9):e73403. [37]

4.3.1 Study background

As revealed by surveillance data derived from the urban, African community of Soweto, hypertension represents a particular challenge to the wider sub-Saharan African community, but quantifying the risk imposed by hypertension and the necessary response in terms of primary prevention is particularly problematic for the diverse peoples of the African continent and, specifically, those living in sub-Saharan Africa. This requires a greater diversity of surveillance studies to determine the underlying prevalence and contribution of hypertension to CVD in the region, particularly as the pattern of risk and the demographic profile of African populations evolve. For example, in what can be described a landmark systematic review of 25 surveillance studies (>400 patients in each and conducted between 1987 and 2004), data from 10 sub-Saharan African countries provided clear evidence of the diversity of risk in the pattern of hypertension [49]. Across the

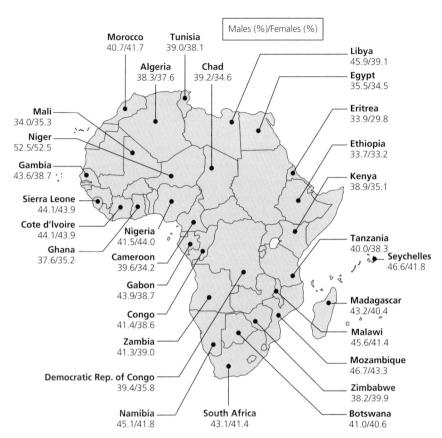

Figure 4.5 Estimated prevalence of hypertension in African men and women. Source: Stewart et al., 2012. Reproduced with permission of Elsevier.

continent the estimated prevalence of hypertension ranged from 13% to 48%, with markedly lower prevalence evident in rural versus urban communities (with gradients linked to epidemiologic transition) and a large burden among women of African ancestry [49]. This latter sex-specific bias toward greater hypertension among African women is emphasized by WHO estimates of the prevalence of hypertension across the African continent according to sex (see Figure 4.5). Population prevalence estimates for the region range from 33.9% in Eritrea to 52.5% in Niger [55].

4.3.2 Study aims

Despite these seemingly impressive data, there is a paucity of studies assessing the relationship between the frequency of cardiovascular risk factors and gradients of hypertension derived from large population studies in the region. This study focused on the pattern of hypertension relative to other risk factors in one of the most populous countries in sub-Saharan African (Nigeria) and, specifically, Abia State. Unlike the data from Soweto described earlier, it focused on both urban- and rural-dwelling adults. Given the paucity of data, the aim of this study was to examine the relationship between hypertension and other common risk factors for heart disease in urban and rural adults residing in Abia State, South East Nigeria.

4.3.3 Study methods
4.3.3.1 Patient enrollment
A cross-sectional design (applying the WHO STEPwise approach [56]) to determine the risk factor profiles of men and women aged ≥18 years in the region was applied. During the period August 2011 to March 2012, study patients were enrolled from the 24 Enumeration Areas and the 6 local government areas by using a multistage stratified cluster sampling technique. In each broad area, four local areas were randomly selected for inclusion. The selection was such that not more than two eligible patients of either sex were selected from each household. Overall, 2,999 patients were enrolled in the study, with complete data available for 2,983 patients. The WHO STEPwise approach surveillance questionnaire was used for data collection and was administered by a team of trained health workers comprising six supervisors and interviewers. Information collected included sociodemographic parameters such as age, sex, cigarette smoking, alcohol intake, and dietary information on consumption of fruits and vegetables.

4.3.3.2 Anthropometry and BP measurement
Weight and height were recorded in order to determine each patient's BMI and then categorized using standard cut-off values for overweight and obese patients. BP measurements were performed with a battery-powered Omron Digital BP machine and were measured with patients sitting with their legs uncrossed and after resting for 5 minutes.

4.3.4 Study findings
4.3.4.1 Demographic and clinical characteristics
Overall, there were more women patients (52.1%) and a slightly higher sampling of patients in rural areas (53.2%). Just under half of the patients were aged 20 to 39 years (mean overall age 42 years), two-thirds were actively employed (67.4%), and 10.7% had no formal education. As shown in Figure 4.6, other than hypertension, there were high overall levels of alcohol intake contrasted by inadequate consumption of fruits and vegetables as well as low physical activity. Alcohol intake was higher in men, while a larger proportion of women were overweight or obese. Despite high antecedent levels of risk, overall only 3.6% of patients had type 2 diabetes. In contrast, hypertension affected approximately one-third of the cohort, with more men than women affected. Specifically, more men were classified as prehypertensive than women in both urban and rural areas. Alternatively, stage 2 and 3 hypertension was observed in similar proportions of men and women.

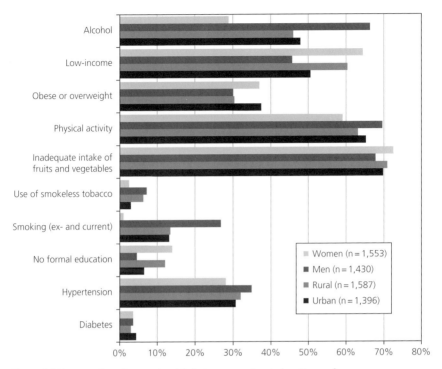

Figure 4.6 Pattern of cardiovascular risk factors according to location and sex.

4.3.4.2 Correlates of hypertension

Overall, strong correlations between elevated BP and sex (more elevated in men), increasing age, lower level of education, being obese or overweight, lower annual income, and use of smokeless tobacco were observed. On an adjusted basis, the most important determinants of hypertension were increasing age, being male, and being overweight or obese.

4.3.5 Study interpretation

When combined with other reports from sub-Saharan Africa, including those described above in respect to Soweto in South Africa, these data corroborate real concerns that high underlying risk factors (in particular hypertension) will contribute to the future burden of noncommunicable forms of heart disease in the continent. Importantly, these data highlight key sociodemographic and cultural factors, such as poverty, level of education, and the use of smokeless tobacco, that influence BP levels. At a regional level, these data confirm other reports from Nigeria that, unlike the broad trends reported elsewhere, the prevalence of hypertension is high in rural Nigerian communities (around 20% [57]). At the same time, they confirm that low-income earners (just over 40%) in Nigeria are most likely to present as hypertensive [58] with low overall awareness of the presence of elevated BP levels. The latter observation not only mirrors the trigger for "Heart Awareness Days" in Soweto but reaffirms data from Cameroon published by Dzudie and colleagues [59].

4.3.6 Study limitations

The discordant findings in this study in respect to relatively high BP levels in rural Nigerian communities not only defy the findings of a previous systematic review of BP levels in sub-Saharan Africa overall [49], but more specifically the International Collaborative Study of Hypertension in those of African ancestry conducted in several populations of West Africa [60]. In the current study, 31%–32% of urban- and rural-dwelling adults were found to have hypertension; other than the potential for different pathways to these relatively high levels, a major reason for this observation may well reflect the similarity in diets between rural- and urban-dwelling patients. It is not inconceivable that in this part of Nigeria, therefore, healthy behaviours previously common to rural communities have been replaced by the equally unhealthy diets and lifestyles adopted by urban communities as part of the phenomenon of epidemiological transition. Such a possibility is concerning given the assumption that African rural communities have been largely spared the future risk of developing noncommunicable forms of heart disease.

4.3.7 Study conclusions

These data demonstrated that, as in other parts of sub-Saharan Africa, the prevalence of hypertension is high in both urban and rural communities of Abia State, Nigeria. Important differentials in the pattern of hypertension (and other common risk factors for CVD), according to sociodemographic and cultural factors, reinforce the need to consider both broad and regional-specific strategies to prevent an increasing burden of noncommunicable forms of heart disease from a continent to region-specific perspective [61–63].

CHAPTER 5

The African INTERHEART study

Krisela Steyn[1] and Karen Sliwa[2]

[1] Medical Research Council, Tygerberg, South Africa
[2] University of Cape Town, South Africa; University of the Witwatersrand, Johannesburg, South Africa

5.0 Introduction

With the African continent so large and diverse, from industrialized cities where Westernized lifestyles have become the norm to more remote rural regions where traditional lifestyles still predominate, there are inherent disadvantages on focusing on specific communities and regions. As already suggested by potentially discordant data from South Africa and Nigeria, relative to each other and to historical reports, the phenomenon of epidemiological transition towards noncommunicable forms of heart disease is far from uniform. Indeed, it is subject to the vagaries of geography, culture, and economic development across the continent. Large-scale registries or observational studies that collect less detailed but uniform data across a range of populations play an important role in understanding both the common and unique factors driving any particular disease state from a national to global perspective. It was on this premise that the Global INTERHEART Study (an observational case-control study) examined the pattern of risk in cases of AMI across 52 countries (including representative data from Africa) [64]. Predictably, perhaps, the study demonstrated that regardless of the population, the same risk factors (see Figure 5.1) feature heavily in this common manifestation of CAD.

5.1 The African INTERHEART study

Steyn K, Sliwa K, Hawken S, Commerford P, Onen C, Damasceno A, Ounpuu S, Yusuf S. Risk factors associated with myocardial infarction in Africa: the INTERHEART Africa Study. *Circulation* **2005; 112(23):3554–61. [64]**

5.1.1 Study aims

Following the release of the major findings from the global INTERHEART study, a more detailed analysis of the study data from Africa was published. The African INTERHEART study investigated the pattern of AMI and risk within the African population. Specifically, it examined the differences in the risk profiles of three

The Heart of Africa: Clinical Profile of an Evolving Burden of Heart Disease in Africa, First Edition.
Edited by Simon Stewart, Karen Sliwa, Ana Mocumbi, Albertino Damasceno, and Mpiko Ntsekhe.
© 2016 John Wiley & Sons, Ltd. Published 2016 by John Wiley & Sons, Ltd.

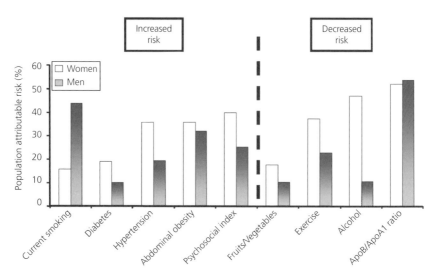

Figure 5.1 Pattern of risk factors for AMI according to sex.

distinct ethnic/cultural African groups to identify any key differences in epidemiological transition between groups. The three target groups (as labeled) were those of African ancestry, colored Africans, and European/other Africans.

5.1.2 Study methods

5.1.2.1 Patient enrollment and data collection

From 1999 to 2003, the African INTERHEART study investigators collected data on 578 de novo cases of AMI and 785 age- and sex-matched controls from nine sub-Saharan African countries (Benin, Botswana, Cameroon, Kenya, Mozambique, Nigeria, Seychelles, South Africa, and Zimbabwe). Cases of AMI were derived from systematic screening of patients in the medical wards or coronary care units of participating centers (with relevant data collected within 24 hours). Case controls were derived from visitors to the participating centers. Trained staff collected profiling data from the participating sites in a standardized manner: sociodemographic profile, family cardiovascular history, lifestyle behaviors (including smoking habits and physical activity), and clinical history (including a history of hypertension and/or type 2 diabetes) were included. Active measurements of anthropometric profile, mental health status, and lipid profile (available for 76% of the patients) were also obtained.

5.1.3 Study findings

5.1.3.1 Cohort profile

Overall, 81.2% of the patients were from South Africa (this represents an important caveat when interpreting study data), and the overall ethnic groups comprised 46.9% colored Africans, 36.4% of African ancestry, and 17% European/other Africans (see Figure 5.2). Nearly 66% were men. Once again, this profile provides an important caveat in any interpretation of study findings.

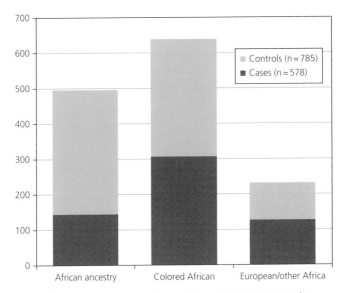

Figure 5.2 Cases and controls by ethnicity in the African INTERHEART Study.

5.1.3.2 Overall pattern of risk associated with a de novo AMI

Consistent with the overall pattern and natural history of AMI [9,65,66], in both the global INTERHEART study and the African INTERHEART study, there were more men than women cases (p<0.0001), with men presenting younger than women (mean age of 53 ± 12 years versus 56 ± 11 years; p=0.0014) (see Table 5.1). Across the three ethnic groups, the age of a de novo AMI was similar (mean age of 54 years), and overall, those of African ancestry were around 4 years younger than their international counterparts. The major risk factors linked to AMI and other forms of CVD around the globe were just as predominant in those of African ancestry, with a history of hypertension and diabetes representing the strongest risk factors in this regard. Consistent with the findings presented in Chapter 4 suggesting a greater role for hypertensive-related diseases, compared to case controls, hypertension was significantly more likely to occur in African ancestry cases than overall (OR of concurrent hypertension 3.4 versus 2.5; p<0.01). Along with hypertension, abdominal obesity and apolipoprotein B (apoB)/apolipoprotein A-1 (apoA1) ratio were also more likely to present in AMI de novo patients of African ancestry (compared to controls). Overall, however, current and former cigarette smoking and stress were found to be the strongest risk factors in the African INTERHEART patients.

5.1.3.3 Ethnic differences

Some important differences in the risk profiles of cases and controls were evident according to ethnicity. Consistent with community surveillance and the Heart of Soweto registry data, the lipid profile of African ancestry controls was more benign and less likely to lead to atherogenesis than those of the other ethnic groups. This included lower levels of low-density lipoprotein (LDL) cholesterol,

Table 5.1 Patients' risk factor profiles according to the African INTERHEART Study and the Global INTERHEART Study.

	African INTERHEART Study		Global INTERHEART Study	
	Controls (n = 14,637)	Cases (n = 12,461)	Controls (n = 785)	Cases (n = 578)
Men	10,846 (74.1%)	9,458 (75.9%)	507 (64.6%)	385 (66.6%)
Mean Age	52.21±11.53	54.3±11.29	56.9±12.2	58.1±12.2
Hypertension	3,206 (21.9%)	4,860 (39%)	148 (18.8%)	244 (42.3%)
Diabetes	1,098 (7.5%)	2,305 (18.5%)	60 (7.6%)	136 (23.6%)
Current cigarette smoking	3,923 (26.8%)	5,632 (45.2%)	299 (38.1%)	302 (52.3%)
Former smoker	7,040 (48.1%)	65.2 (65.2%)	442 (56.3%)	418 (72.3%)
Exercise	2,825 (19.3%)	1,782 (14.3%)	133 (16.9%)	87 (15.1%)
Alcohol intake	3,586 (24.5%)	2,991 (24%)	210 (26.8%)	128 (22.2%)
Daily fruits and vegetables intake	6,206 (42.4%)	4,461 (35.8%)	309 (39.4%)	216 (37.4%)
Depression	2,561 (17.5%)	2,991 (24%)	175 (22.3%)	184 (31.8%)
Stress	629 (4.3%)	959 (7.7%)	35 (4.5%)	55 (9.6%)

total cholesterol, apoB/apoA1 ratio, and apoB (adjusted for differences in smoking status, sex, and age). In the African ancestry group, relative to those with less than 8 years of schooling, those with tertiary education had an elevated risk for AMI. The direction of this observed association between education level and de novo AMI was reversed in the European/other African group. In the latter group, less education was associated with an increased risk of presenting with an AMI. This same pattern was observed when the relationship between AMI and income was examined. Relative to those with the lowest income, those of African ancestry with the highest income were more likely to present with a de novo AMI (OR 2.75; 95% CI 1.53–4.94). Alternatively, in the European/other African group, higher income was associated with less AMI cases ($p < 0.001$ for income-ethnicity interactions).

5.1.3.4 Population-attributable risks

A population-attributable risk perspective (reflecting the prevalence of any one risk factor combined with the strength of the risk it poses) seeks to determine the relative contribution of an observed risk to actual events. Classically, a highly "virulent" risk factor affecting a relatively small number of cases can cause fewer cases when compared to a highly prevalent factor with only marginal risk for converting that risk into an actual event, the latter having a higher population attributable risk for an event. This was indeed observed from a U.S. analysis of the population impact of marginally elevated BP levels derived from the National Health and Nutrition Examination Survey Study [67]. It provides a population target and potential solution (e.g., salt reduction in the food supply chain [68]) beyond the individual level. In this instance, a history of hypertension (30% of AMI cases) was markedly more important than in the global cohort (41.9% versus 23.4%) as a target for preventing de novo AMI. Likewise, abdominal obesity (58.4% versus

33.7%) and less favorable apoB/apoA1 ratios (61.8% versus 46.2%) were also more important contributors to AMI in the African cohort.

5.1.3.5 Cumulative effects of risk factors

Taking into account the cumulative impact of multiple risk factors in the African cohort, a history of diabetes, smoking, and/or hypertension was associated with a population-attributable risk of just under two-thirds of cases (64.5%), with a 17-fold increased risk of presenting as an AMI case compared to controls. When apoB/apoA1 was considered, these values rose to 80.6% and 29-fold, respectively, increasing once again to 89.2% and 49-fold when waist-to-height ratio was additionally considered. Overall, the population-attributable risks for the African cohort were higher than the overall global cohort when all five of these risk factors were assessed. When all nine risk factors of interest were combined (including irregular consumption of fruits/vegetables, no alcohol intake, physical inactivity, and psychosocial stressors) the overall population-attributable risk for de novo AMI in the African cohort related to these factors was 97.4% (i.e., almost all observed cases).

5.1.4 Study interpretation

Beyond aforementioned caveats relating to the geographic location and composition of the study cohort, the African INTERHEART study's findings strongly suggest that only five risk factors account for almost 9 in 10 de novo presentations of AMI (regardless of ethnicity). As will be discussed in Chapters 6 and 10, while AMI remains relatively rare in those of African ancestry (representing the major portion of the population at risk of future cardiac events) in comparison to high-income countries [9,65,69], the signs are ominous when considering the findings from this research and that outlined in the previous chapter. The INTERHEART investigators concluded that five highly modifiable risk factors indicative of potentially unhealthy lifestyles drove the majority of the AMI patients documented in the global and African-specific component of this landmark study. The major contribution of hypertension to AMI patients is of concern (particularly when considering that CAD and AMI are not the main consequences of undiagnosed/untreated high BP in the African context), as is diabetes.

Key differences according to education and income among the three ethnic groups studied clearly demonstrates that the phenomenon known as epidemiological transition [1–3] is in play. Those of European origin displayed similar patterns of risk according to socioeconomic status as high-income countries [64]. In contrast, it is those of African ancestry who can now "afford" (due to their increased wealth) an unhealthy Westernized diet who appear to be most at risk of AMI. Potential differences in the epidemiological transition of population are also reflected in the pattern of cardiovascular-related case-fatalities. Burden of disease estimates suggest that in South Africa in the year 2000, those of African ancestry had stroke (including hemorrhagic events) and IHD rates of 143/100,000 and 70/100,000, respectively, compared with 72/100,000 and 230/100,000 in those of European origin.

Significantly, there was a clear differential in the median age of the African INTERHEART cohort when compared to the global cohort. Applying to both sexes, the median age of African cases was 4 to 5 years younger overall. Consistent with the overall pattern of noncommunicable forms of heart disease (see Chapter 6), this critical finding suggests that the African population is at particular risk of premature AMI. This may well reflect a pervasive lack of awareness, early detection, effective management, and prevention measures targeting cardiovascular risk factors in vulnerable African communities, noting the relative wealth and resources of South Africa when compared to the remainder of the continent.

Data from the European/other African group reflects an advanced stage of the epidemiological transition as there was found to be a high prevalence rates of cigarette smoking, abdominal obesity, and dyslipidemia, whereas lower prevalence rates of diabetes and hypertension were found. The risk of an elevated apoB/apoA1 ratio was significantly higher in the European/other African group than that found in the global INTERHEART study. Additionally, the most educated and wealthiest segment of the European/other African group had the lowest risk of AMI. This pattern corresponds, for example, to the lower IHD risk factor rates and levels found in the wealthier sector of the population in the UK [70,71]. Their risk profile is also corresponding with the mortality pattern reported above. It is worth noting that the median age of cases in this particular cohort was 54 years, whereas the median age of patients for the global INTERHEART study was 62 years; residually high rates of smoking and dyslipidemia (relative to population changes elsewhere in the world [69]) may well play a significant role in this finding.

The colored African group mainly consisted of individuals from mixed ethnicity ancestry and was predominantly recruited from South Africa. The adoption of Westernization, industrialization, and urbanization among this group is also associated with the epidemiological transition. The recruitment took place at the public sector health services that provided assistance for the poor working class. The risk profile of the controls in this ethnic group nicely illustrates the dangers of adopting potentially hazardous Westernized/industrialized lifestyles. Both men and women were found to have high cigarette smoking habits in addition to often being overweight or obese with parallel increases in the prevalence of hypertension and diabetes in particular. Such a differential in risk is reflected in the estimated rates of CAD and stroke in this ethnic group—higher than those of African ancestry and with much higher rates of stroke than for Europeans.

Overall, the African INTERHEART study's findings contradicted the prevailing theory (see Chapter 10) that people of African ancestry are essentially "immune" to developing AMI, even when exposed to the type of risk factors [19,72] that drive cases of AMI in the rest of the world. As noted in Chapter 4, reports from various African countries document a changing spectrum and pattern of cardiovascular risk factors (predominantly in urban areas). This must be understood in the context of lifetime exposure to unhealthy lifestyles before these well-known risk factors have a sufficient impact and subjects present with established forms of

CVD, particularly relating to atherosclerotic events and noting competing risks for premature mortality in the African context. Supporting this position is the fact that two to three decades ago, African Americans had lower rates of CVD than Caucasian North Americans. However, over time and with extended exposure to risk factors, this has changed, with African Americans demonstrating higher risk of cardiovascular events in the United States [73]. In this context, the risk profile of the Indigenous African group in the African INTERHEART study demonstrates an early stage of epidemiological transition. The study found that there was a relatively small number of AMI cases found among those of African ancestry. However, this may well change given an evolving pattern of risk outlined in Chapter 4. From a more optimistic perspective, these data suggest that AMI in the less-developed areas of sub-Saharan Africa is relatively rare, and in other African countries, the population may be at an even earlier epidemiological transition stage than, for example, South Africa. However, the incremental risk posed by hypertension within those of African ancestry when compared to the global INTERHEART study cohort is of particular concern. As will be highlighted in Chapter 6 and Chapter 13, the impact of highly prevalent hypertension will not only influence de novo cases of AMI but also a broad spectrum of other forms of noncommunicable heart disease without special efforts to control this particular risk factor in those of African ancestry.

5.1.5 Study limitations

As part of the global INTERHEART study, the African-specific findings, outlined above, have the same potential limitations as those reported previously. These include possible confounding if there is differential ascertainment of risk factors between cases and controls, such as possible recall bias when cases of AMI are influenced more because of stress than in controls. The inclusion of patients with first AMI reduces the possibility that individuals with previous CVDs may have altered their lifestyles and risk factor patterns. To minimize bias in the selection of controls, individuals in whom the risk factors of interest in this study were implicated as being protective or harmful were excluded.

5.1.6 Study conclusions

Despite these limitations, it is reasonable to conclude that the African INTERHEART study data revealed that a key set of common risk factors for CVDs accounted for ~90% of case presentations of de novo AMI. As such, the association of five major risk factors for AMI in the African population is consistent with that found in the global INTERHEART study cohort. Fortunately, these data also confirm that those of African ancestry are in early epidemiological transition toward noncommunicable forms of heart disease and specifically AMI. There is still time, therefore, to invest in lifestyle modification, primary prevention, early diagnosis, rapid-access treatment options, and secondary prevention strategies, adapted to the African context, in order to prevent a future epidemic of AMI and to minimize its potentially devastating consequences if a primary event should occur.

CHAPTER 6

The spectrum of heart disease in urban Africans: The Heart of Soweto Study

Melinda Jane Carrington[1], Karen Sliwa[2], and Simon Stewart[1]

[1] *Australian Catholic University, Melbourne, Victoria, Australia*
[2] *University of Cape Town, South Africa; University of the Witwatersrand, Johannesburg, South Africa*

6.0 Introduction

This chapter provides an overview of the Heart of Soweto Study [74], now regarded as a landmark study in our attempts to understand the evolving burden of heart disease in sub-Saharan Africa. However, given its limited scope and lack of prospective follow-up data, this study is only the beginning in this regard. The Heart of Soweto Study was built on the premise that while the burden of CVD has stabilized in most high-income countries (with age-adjusted rates of acute and chronic heart disease events continuing to fall [9–11]), in LMIC there was clear evidence it was beginning to rise [75]. In a setting of scarce health care resources, these countries are ill-equipped to cope with the rise of the noncommunicable diseases [38]; particularly when the traditional killers of malnourishment and infection remain prevalent [76]. As discussed in the original reports, there is little scope to tackle new prototypes of heart disease arising from changing risk behaviours due to epidemiologic transition [3]. As also described in Chapter 4, there is clear evidence that urban communities (including Soweto) contain a rising burden of antecedent risk that will fuel a rising burden of non-communicable forms of heart disease. This begged an important question: How does this emerging threat compete and interact with the historically dominant, communicable forms of heart disease (see Section 4) in sub-Saharan Africa? As shown in Figure 6.1, the Heart of Soweto Study generated a series of reports describing various aspects of the spectrum of heart disease in the world-renowned community of Soweto. Many of these were "first of a kind" reports within the African context. The two most encompassing reports from this study (in chronological order) are initially summarized before a review of the

The Heart of Africa: Clinical Profile of an Evolving Burden of Heart Disease in Africa, First Edition.
Edited by Simon Stewart, Karen Sliwa, Ana Mocumbi, Albertino Damasceno, and Mpiko Ntsekhe.
© 2016 John Wiley & Sons, Ltd. Published 2016 by John Wiley & Sons, Ltd.

Increasing evidence of epidemiological transition towards noncommunicable disease in urban African communities—spectrum & burden of heart disease unknown

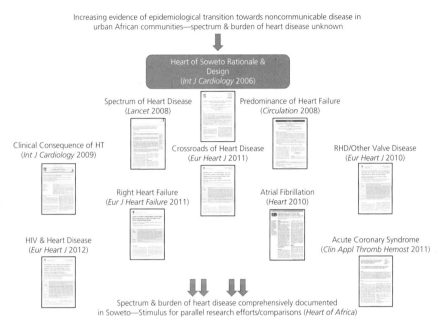

Figure 6.1 A family tree of key research reports from the Heart of Soweto Study.

specific diagnoses (from AF to pulmonary arterial hypertension (PAH)/RHF—see Chapter 15) subject to more intensive analysis and interpretation are presented.

6.1 Initial findings of the Heart of Soweto Study

Sliwa K, Wilkinson D, Hansen C, Ntyintyane L, Tibazarwa K, Becker A, Stewart S. Spectrum of heart disease and risk factors in a black urban population in South Africa (the Heart of Soweto Study): a cohort study. *The Lancet* **2008; 371:915–22. [50]**

As described in the initial report of the rationale and design of the Heart of Soweto Study, this was a prospective clinical registry of all heart disease presentations to the Cardiology Unit of the Chris Hani Baragwanath Hospital in Soweto, South Africa (see Chapter 4). Specifically, all individuals presenting with suspected or confirmed CVD to the hospital were recorded on a prospectively designed registry. The registry was compiled and maintained via a dedicated team of staff and facilities using standardized case report forms (with each patient provided with a unique identifier). A key component of the study was the presence of expert cardiologic review, echocardiography, and 12-lead ECGs for each and every patient attending the purposely built Heart of Soweto clinic that formed the basis for the registry.

6.1.1 Study methods

Wherever possible, the study adhered to the STROBE guidelines for collecting and interpreting observational data [77]. Critically, at the time of the study the hospital provided almost exclusive cardiac services to the community, with many patients bypassing the overstretched primary care services to go straight to the hospital for treatment. The Chris Hani Baragwanath Hospital, therefore, did and still does represent an important barometer (if not complete given a number of caveats) of the heart health of Soweto and, by implication, the heart health of urban communities in sub-Saharan Africa in epidemiological transition.

6.1.1.1 Patient profiling

The Heart of Soweto registry captured basic sociodemographic (including self-reported years of education, origin, and history of any preexisting CVD) in addition to any advanced clinical profiling (described in detail in study reports [50,78,79]) according to clinical need. As noted above, a critical component of the study was the capture of echocardiography (performed and reviewed according to gold-standard criteria [80]), and 12-lead ECG (subject to detailed and blinded Minnesota coding [81]) in each and every presentation to the clinic to facilitate profiling. This reflected the typical lack of "clinical workup" of those presenting de novo with often complex conditions in advance stages of illness. Those of African ancestry were typically of Zulu or Xhosa origin and migrants to Soweto were defined as those not self-reporting to be born in Soweto.

6.1.1.2 Diagnostic classifications

An enormous amount of clinical data from many patients with complex disease states were generated from the registry. Using predominantly European Society of Cardiology guidelines [79] relevant to the time of analyses, these data were independently reviewed and adjudicated (consensus approach) by the principal investigators. Table 6.1 summarizes the broad classification of clinical cases according to communicable versus noncommunicable heart disease, noting that in the case of valvular disease and dysfunction, a new system of classification was devised [7]. Study data were documented on standardized forms and entered into a preliminary database at the Soweto Cardiovascular Research Unit based at the Chris Hani Baragwanath Hospital before being transferred and entered into the definitive trial registry by an Australian team based at the Baker IDI Heart and Diabetes Institute in Melbourne. These data were then used to derive the final classification of cases according to broad classes.

6.1.1.3 Study timeline

The initial phase of the Heart of Soweto Study took place from January 1, 2006 to December 31, 2006. During that period, 129,633 inpatients were managed by the hospital's internal medicine specialists. The estimated case load for the cardiology unit during the same period was 5,000 patients, generating 21,000 patient contacts overall, all with access to gold-standard cardiologic review and advanced diagnostic investigations.

Table 6.1 General classification of Heart of Soweto case presentations.

Study Classification	Primary Diagnoses	General Characteristics
Hypertension and/or type 2 diabetes	Hypertension and type 2 diabetes	These are increasingly prevalent risk factors in urban communities and are strongly associated with lifestyle risk factors. It is considered a primary diagnosis only when no evidence of cardiac dysfunction is found.
Historically prevalent heart disease	RHD, nonischemic CMO, pericardial disease, and pulmonary heart disease (10)	These are the main contributors to heart disease in sub-Saharan Africa arising from infectious diseases such as TB, streptococcal infection, and HIV-infection.
Noncommunicable heart disease	Hypertensive HF and CAD	These are strongly associated with lifestyle risk factors.
CHD	Congenital heart defects and cardiac trauma	Fairly rare
Other heart disease	Miscellaneous diagnoses, including cardiac trauma or cases without a definitive diagnosis	Fairly rare
Other CVD	Peripheral arterial and cerebrovascular disease	These are almost exclusively linked to lifestyle risk factors.

6.1.2 Study findings

As shown in Figure 6.2, 4,506 patients were assessed and entered into the Heart of Soweto Registry in 2006. Of these, 344 (7.6%), who were on average a decade younger and had a similar sex profile, were found not to have underlying CVD and were excluded from further analyses. Therefore, the study population consisted of 4,162 confirmed cases of heart disease. Of these, 1,593 (38.3%) were newly diagnosed patients and 2,569 (61.7%) patients had been previously diagnosed with one or more forms of heart disease. On average, patients with preexisting heart disease were 1.7 years older than the de novo cases.

6.1.2.1 Cohort profile

As expected, most (n = 1,359; 85.3%) patients were of African ancestry. The study cohort mainly consisted of women (n = 939; 59.0%), and those of African ancestry reported the lowest education levels compared to other ethnic groups. Consistent with an overall picture of premature heart disease, 862 (54.1%) patients were younger than 55 years, and 399 (25.1%) were younger than 40 years. With more than half the patients residing in Soweto (n = 842; 52.9%), only 42 (5.0%) reported residing there for <5 years.

6.1.2.2 Spectrum of risk and disease

A broad spectrum of CVD and risk factors were identified within the study cohort; the most common diagnoses were HF, hypertension, CAD, and VHD (see the following sections). Patients diagnosed with VHD were on average more than a decade

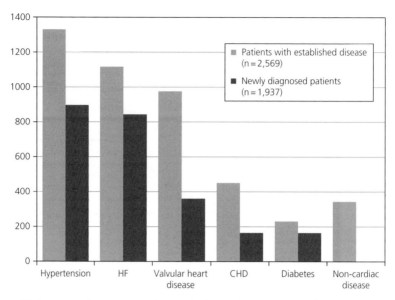

Figure 6.2 Spectrum of case presentations in the Heart of Soweto 2006 cohort.

younger than those with hypertension or HF. Renal disease, anemia, and concurrent diabetes was also diagnosed in some of the patients in the study (n = 115/1,182 [9.7%]; n = 156/1,185 [13.2%]; and n = 165 [10.4%] respectively), and 74 (4.7%) tested HIV positive. In 146 (9.3%) patients, the most common diagnosis was pericardial effusion as a complication due to HIV/AIDS, TB, or a combination of both (n = 80; 54.8%). Overall, 639 (40.1%) of the newly diagnosed patients had rheumatic (valvular) heart disease, tuberculous pericardial effusion, or CMOs. Although stroke diagnosis was rare, 145 (9.1%) patients reported a family history of stroke and 64 (4%) were diagnosed with an acute stroke. Those patients of African ancestry were more likely to be diagnosed with HF than the rest of the cohort (739 [54%] versus 105 [45%]; OR 1·46, 95% CI 1·11−1·94; p = 0·009). On the other hand, they were far less likely to be diagnosed with CAD than any other ethnic group (77 [6%] versus 88 [38%]; OR 0·10, 0·07−0·14; p < 0·0001). Although the total proportions of men and women diagnosed with diabetes and hypertension were very similar, proportionately more women than men were diagnosed with VHD (240 [26%] versus 120 [18%]; OR 1·30, 1·11−1·52; p = 0·001). Commonly presenting symptoms across all diagnostic groups were angina pectoris/chest pain (n = 451; 28.3%), dyspnoea (NYHA Class III/IV), and peripheral oedema (n = 494; 31%). Echocardiographic and ECG profiling demonstrated that 487 (34%) patients presented with underlying cardiac dysfunction, structural disease, and/or tachycardia. Of the 844 patients with HF, 332 (39.3%) had concurrent valvular dysfunction, 203 (24.1%) had a mixed underlying etiology, and 67 (7.9%) had a primary diagnosis of valve disease. The dilated CMOs (OR 35%; 95% CI 32−38), which include HF secondary to hypertensive heart disease (OR 33%; 30−36), RHF (OR 27%; 24−30), and PPCMO, were the three most common forms of HF.

6.1.3 Study limitations

A critical but understandable limitation of this and other African studies high-lighted in this book is the risk of selection bias—in this case predominantly due to the fact that the study's reliance on presentations to the cardiology unit at the hospital. This meant that milder forms of heart disease, fatal events in the community, and even stroke cases directed toward neurology services would be underreported and influence findings if known. Fortunately, the hospital services the community of Soweto almost exclusively and thus serves as a broad, if not specific, barometer of health and disease in the community. Although systematic ECG and echocardio-graphic investigations were applied, beyond basic clinical profiling, patients in the study were profiled according to clinical need.

6.1.4 Study conclusions

The initial publications arising from the Heart of Soweto Study generated more questions than answers, providing tantalizing glimpses (via the broad data generated) of important aspects on the specific changes that were/are driving a transition from predominant communicable heart disease toward a mixture of the old and new, the new being noncommunicable heart disease. These data confirmed at least the hypothesis that epidemiological transition was driving Soweto (and other parts of Africa) toward profound changes, not only from a socioeconomic perspective but in health and health outcomes. As previously shown in Figure 6.1, a number of research reports focused on key contributors to the spectrum of heart disease in Soweto; more detailed descriptions of the spectrum of HF (Chapter 13), HIV infection of the heart (Chapter 9), ACS (Chapter 10), RHD (Chapter 7), and RHF associated with PAH (Chapter 15) are described later in the book. The following sections highlight some of the other key findings from the study, noting the same strengths and weaknesses/limitations that applied throughout.

6.2 Nexus between communicable and noncommunicable forms of heart disease in Soweto

Stewart S, Carrington MJ, Pretorius S, Methusi P, Sliwa K. **Standing at the crossroads between new and historically prevalent heart disease: effects of migration and socio-economic factors in the Heart of Soweto cohort study.** *European Heart Journal* **2011; 32(4):492–9.**

6.2.1 Study background

The initial phase of data derived from the Heart of Soweto Study as outlined above [74] immediately suggested that epidemiologic transition was broadening the spectrum of advanced forms of heart disease in that community. It was immediately apparent that a high burden of complex cases in young individuals and women (a pattern rarely seen in high-income countries) required further investigation [50]. In this context, the intrinsic balance between historically prevalent and emergent forms of heart disease in sub-Saharan Africa was unknown. As noted in the original report [74], with high levels of rural migration and extreme poverty counterbalanced by sufficient consumer demand for new, state-of-the-art shopping precincts, Soweto represented an ideal community to study epidemiologic transition via the Heart of Soweto Study. Collectively, the investigators postulated that the balance between largely communicable versus noncommunicable forms of heart disease [82] had irrevocably changed, and this would be observed in this study cohort, particularly when examining de novo presentation of heart disease at the Cardiology Unit of the Chris Hani Baragwanath Hospital. Specifically, it was hypothesized that in addition to finding an equitable balance between new and historically prevalent forms of heart disease in the study cohort, sociodemographic gradients in the pattern of case presentations as well as a significant role for lifestyle risk factors in contributing to more advanced presentations in those with historically prevalent heart disease would be evident, with the latter representing the confluence of communicable and noncommunicable heart disease.

6.2.2 Study methods

6.2.2.1 Patient enrollment

During the extended period 2006 to 2008, data were subsequently captured on 6,006 de novo presentations at the Cardiology Unit of the Chris Hani Baragwanath Hospital. Of these, 678 cases (11.2%) were found not to have any form of CVD or major risk factors. Of the 5,328 remaining cases, 401 (7.5%) were derived from the emergency case presentations, 367 (7.1%) from external referrals from local primary care clinics, 1,992 (37.4%) from internal referrals as a hospital inpatient, and 2,568 (48.2%) from referrals from other outpatient departments.

6.2.3 Study findings

Overall, 4,626 (86.8%) patients were of African ancestry, with a predominance of women in this group (see Table 6.2).

Figure 6.3 highlights the spectrum of 5,328 de novo cases according to sex and ethnicity; the pattern of presentation was also determined by level of education and migrant status. Historically prevalent heart disease was diagnosed in 2,092 (39.3%) patients (comprising 60% women and 93% Africans). Newer, noncommunicable forms of heart disease were found in 35% of the patients (comprising 56% women and 79% Africans; $p < 0.001$ for both comparisons). A similar proportion of men and women were diagnosed with any other form of CVD (including 87 (60.4%) patients with stroke/cerebrovascular disease and 57 (39.6%) with peripheral arterial disease. An additional 999 (18.8%) patients (almost all with hypertension) presented with a high risk of developing heart disease but with no evidence of the same at that time.

6.2.3.1 Soweto at the crossroads

Significantly, the proportion of historically prevalent communicable versus newer noncommunicable forms of heart disease was evenly poised (1.8 ± 0.9 versus 2.4 ± 0.8). Adjusting for sociodemographic profile, communicable cases of heart disease were more likely to be younger, of African ancestry, and men. The influence of sex, age,

Table 6.2 Patients' demographic and clinical characteristics.

	Women (n = 3,168)	Men (n = 2,160)	African (n = 4,626)	Other (n = 702)
Demographic characteristics				
Age (years)	51.5 ± 17.9	52.8 ± 16.5	51.5 ± 17.7	56.7 ± 14.1
African ancestry	2,863 (90.4%)	1,763 (81.6%)	4,626 (100%)	—
Women	3,168 (100%)	—	2,863 (61.9%)	305 (43.5%)
<6-years education	1,331 (42%)	933 (43.2%)	2,018 (43.6%)	246 (35%)
Soweto originated	1,756 (55.4%)	1,079 (50%)	2,807 (60.7%)	28 (4%)
Residing in Soweto (years)	39.2 ± 18.1	38.2 ± 17.7	38.8 ± 18.0	38.6 ± 15.8
Risk factors				
Family history	1,430 (45.1%)	727 (33.7%)	1,800 (39%)	357 (50.9%)
Total cholesterol (mmol/L)	4.4 ± 1.3	4.1 ± 1.3	4.2 ± 1.3	4.8 ± 1.3
History of cigarette smoking	971 (30.7%)	1,454 (67.3%)	200 (4.3%)	425 (60.5%)
BMI (kg/m²)	29.8 ± 7.6	25.7 ± 6.0	28.2 ± 7.2	28.0 ± 7.5
Clinical characteristics				
NYHA II, III, or IV	2,274 (71.8%)	1,371 (63.5%)	3,214 (69.5%)	431 (61.4%)
Systolic BP (mm Hg)	133 ± 27	132 ± 28	133 ± 27	132 ± 26
Diastolic BP (mm Hg)	75 ± 16	76 ± 16	76 ± 15	74 ± 14
Chest pain/angina pectoris	385 (12.2%)	241 (11.2%)	505 (10.9%)	121 (17.2%)
Peripheral oedema	1,054 (33.3%)	648 (30%)	1,579 (34.1%)	123 (17.5%)
Mean LVEF (%)	56.3 ± 15.8	51.7 ± 16.7	54.2 ± 16.5	55.8 ± 14.7
LV systolic dysfunction	597 (18.9%)	592 (27.4%)	1,074 (23.2%)	115 (16.4%)
Diastolic dysfunction	469 (14.8%)	290 (13.4%)	676 (14.6%)	83 (11.8%)
Primary diagnosis				
Hypertensive HF	732 (23.1%)	414 (19.2%)	1,050 (22.7%)	96 (13.7%)
Hypertension	645 (20.4%)	343 (15.9%)	854 (18.3%)	134 (19.1%)
Valve disease	491 (15.5%)	233 (10.8%)	660 (14.3%)	64 (9.1%)
CAD	239 (7.5%)	342 (15.8%)	271 (5.9%)	310 (44.2%)
Idiopathic dilated CMO	234 (7.4%)	268 (12.4%)	470 (10.2%)	32 (4.6%)
RHF/PH	185 (5.8%)	160 (7.4%)	311 (6.7%)	34 (4.8%)
HIV-related heart disease	321 (10.1%)	197 (9.1%)	500 (10.8%)	18 (2.6%)

and urban transition with uptake of lifestyles was more likely to lead to noncommunicable forms of heart disease, but less exposure to some forms of communicable disease was evident in the pattern of heart disease in the cohort. Overall, there were more cases of historically prevalent than new heart disease up to the age of 49 years for women and 59 years for men, before this pattern reversed in older age groups. For Sowetan women, new heart disease case presentations continuously increased across all age groups compared to historically prevalent cases, which peaked in those aged 30 to 39 years before declining slowly thereafter. Alternatively, for Sowetan men, new forms of heart disease cases peaked in the age bracket 60 to 69 years and decreased thereafter, while historically prevalent cases peaked in the 50- to-59-year age group before decreasing thereafter. This pattern was very similar for migrant African men. For female migrants however, new heart disease case presentations

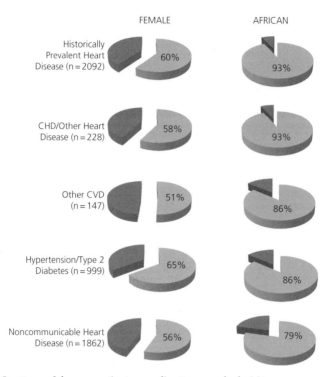

Figure 6.3 Spectrum of de novo patients according to sex and ethnicity

peaked in those aged 50 to 59 years before declining compared to historically prevalent cases; which decreased across all age groups. Although there was no interaction between age, sex, and presentation in "migrants," there was a borderline association in native Sowetans (p=0.059); the probability of a woman aged 20 to 29 years presenting with historically prevalent heart disease was 1.25-fold greater, but this probability was 0.67-fold less in the >70 years age group relative to age-matched men.

6.3 Hypertension and hypertensive heart disease in Soweto

Stewart S, Libhaber E, Carrington MJ, Damasceno A, Abbasi H, Hansen C, Wilkinson D, Sliwa K. The clinical consequences and challenges of hypertension in urban-dwelling black Africans: insights from the Heart of Soweto Study. *International Journal of Cardiology* **2011; 146(1):22–27.**

As outlined in Chapter 4 and Chapter 5, it is highly probable that, for the foreseeable future, hypertension represents the single greatest threat to the development of noncommunicable forms of heart disease in sub-Saharan Africa. As part of the original cohort studied, 761 (84.8%) cases of hypertension among those of African ancestry (comprising 63.3% women) were subject to further scrutiny. On presentation, chest pain, palpitations, and/or dizziness were common. Hypertension was the primary diagnosis in only 35% (n=266); with a presentation of concurrent non-IHD (54%), concurrent LVH (39%), renal dysfunction (24%), anaemia (11%), and CAD (6.2%). Overall, therefore, 494 (64.9%) patients presented with an advanced form of CVD. An additional 98 (12.9%) patients had a valvular abnormality detected by echocardiography with more men than women presenting with impaired LV systolic function. The majority of the valvular cases (n=58; 59.2%) were due to underlying structural valve disease, mainly comprising rheumatic valve disease (n=47; 81%) and degenerative valve disease (n=9; 15.5%). Although women presented with more clinical symptoms, proportionately, they were less likely to be diagnosed HF and renal disease. The study concluded that more women than men were affected with advanced forms of hypertensive heart disease in the Heart of Soweto cohort. Overall, these data reinforce the potential for untreated and undetected hypertension to ultimately lead to advanced forms of heart disease in many individuals within sub-Saharan Africa. As such, the development and application of sex-specific community-based screening and prevention programs adapted to the African context are urgently required to truncate an almost inevitable rise in the burden of hypertensive heart disease in vulnerable communities in the region.

6.4 A predominance of HF in Soweto

Stewart S, Wilkinson D, Hansen C, et al. Predominance of heart failure in the Heart of Soweto Study cohort: emerging challenges for urban African communities. *Circulation* **2008; 118(23):2360–7. [79]**

The syndrome HF represents a common pathway for most forms of CVD when associated cardiac damage and ventricular dysfunction is left untreated and/or poorly managed. Even in the setting of optimal prevention and management, progressive cardiac dysfunction is inevitable as the body ages. At the time of the Heart of Soweto Study, the single largest HF study had been conducted in Africa in the early 1960s and too few data from previous studies were derived from echocardiography presentations. As part of a more detailed examination of the original 2006 cohort, data from 1,960 HF patients and related CMO's were analyzed to bridge this critical gap in the African literature (see Section 6) however, demographic and clinical data was collected from all 844 (43.1%) de novo presentations. Overall, 739 (87.6%) patients were of African ancestry, 479 (56.8%) were women, and the mean age (in stark contrast to that seen in high-income countries) was 55 ± 16 years. A complex picture of HF and comorbidity was noted, with the most common diagnoses being hypertensive (n=281; 33.3%), idiopathic dilated CMO (n=237; 28.1%), tricuspid regurgitation (n=234; 27.7%), RHF (n=225; 26.7%), isolated diastolic dysfunction (n=180; 21.3%), and concurrent renal dysfunction (n=172; 20.4%). Figure 6.4 highlights the ethnic differences in HF presentation. Not unexpectedly, given the paucity of CAD overall (see Chapter 5), only 41 (5.6%) patients of African ancestry presented with ischemic CMO compared to 36 (34.3%) in the rest of the cohort (p<0.0001). Alternatively,

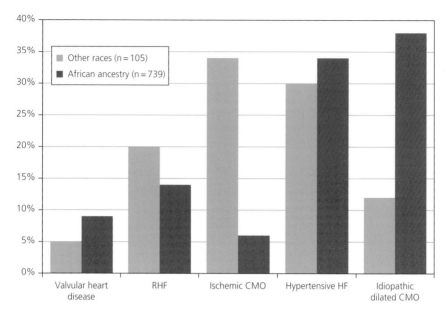

Figure 6.4 Etiology of heart failure according to ethnicity.

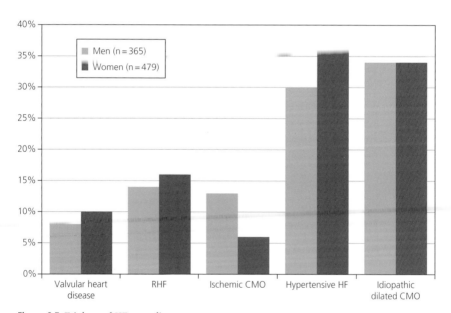

Figure 6.5 Etiology of HF according to sex.

285 (38.6%) patients of African ancestry presented with an idiopathic dilated CMO compared to 13 (12.4%) for the rest (p<0.0001).

Similarly, Figure 6.5 compares the etiology of HF according to sex in those of African ancestry. While there were almost double the number of ischemic CMO cases in men compared to women (13.4% versus 5.9%), the latter were more likely to present with valvular HF, RHF, and hypertensive HF.

6.5 RHF—A not so rare form of HF in Soweto

Stewart S, Mocumbi AO, Carrington MJ, Pretorius S, Burton R, Sliwa K. A not-so-rare form of heart failure in urban black Africans: pathways to right heart failure in the Heart of Soweto Study cohort. *European Journal of Heart Failure.* **2011; 13(10):1070–77. [83]**

In the first year of conducting the Heart of Soweto Study, it was soon clear that one in every five cases of HF involved a component of RV dysfunction/RHF, an otherwise rare form of HF reported in cohorts derived from high-income countries. Consistent with these figures, of the 5,328 heart disease patients presenting during the period 2006 to 2008, 2,505 (47%) patients had any form of HF and 697 (27.8%) of these were diagnosed with a component of RHF (642 [92.1%] patients were of African ancestry). Figure 6.6 shows the diagnostic profile of these RHF patients according to sex. An important component (given the number of presentations overall) of RHF cases was PAH. As such, Figure 6.7 shows the diagnostic profile of these cases according to sex. The most common forms of PAH found in women were idiopathic (n=32; 34.4%), HIV-related (n=31; 33.3%), and connective tissue disease-related (n=25; 26.9%). Among men,

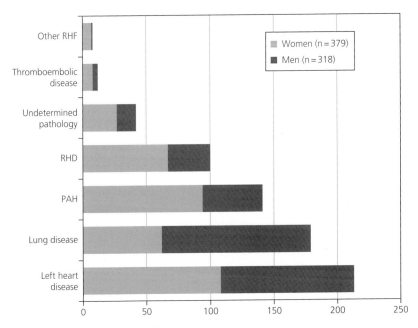

Figure 6.6 Diagnostic profile of RHF according to sex.

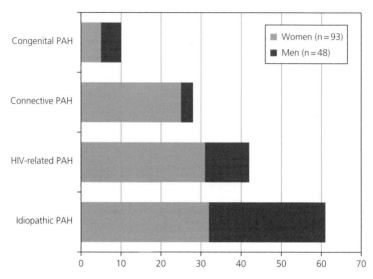

Figure 6.7 PAH diagnostic characteristics according to sex.

idiopathic PAH (n = 29; 60.4%) and HIV-related PAH (n = 11; 22.9%) were predominant. These findings are more fully explored in Chapter 15.

6.6 Pathways to AF in Soweto

Sliwa K, Carrington M, Klug E, Opie L, Lee G, Ball J, Stewart S. Predisposing factors and incidence of atrial fibrillation/flutter in an urban African community: insights from the Heart of Soweto Study. *Heart* **2010; 96:1878–82. [84]**

At the time of the Heart of Soweto Study, there was a paucity of data on the epidemiology of AF in sub-Saharan Africa. Given the twin epidemics of HF and AF in the aging populations of high-income countries [85], an emerging threat in LMIC elsewhere in the world [86], and the predominance of hypertension and HF in the cohort, a close analysis of 12-lead ECG data was logical. During the period 2006 to 2008, 246 (4.6%) of the 5,328 de novo heart disease patients presented with AF. In contrast to typical presentations of AF in high-income countries, the mean age was 59 ± 18 years. Both those of African ancestry (n = 211; 85.8%) and women (n = 150; 61%) predominated. Perhaps not surprisingly, the most common concurrent diagnosis was any form of HF (n = 138; 56.1%) followed by primary valve disease and/or valvular dysfunction (n = 106; 43.1%). A primary diagnosis of valve disease was made in 71 (28.9%) patients, comprising 51 (20.7%) patients with RHD and 20 (8.1%) patients with degenerative valve disease. Overall, 106 (43.1%) patients presented with clinically significant valve disease/dysfunction. Other diagnoses comprised CAD (n=16; 6.5%), Type 2 diabetes (n=9; 3.7%), stroke (n=6; 2.4%) and PPCMO (n=3; 1.2%). Table 6.3 compares

Table 6.3 AF patients' demographic and clinical characteristics according to sex.

	Women (n = 150)	Men (n = 96)	All (n = 246)
Demographic characteristics			
Mean age (years)	60.5 ± 18.5	56.2 ± 17.4	58.8 ± 18.2
African ancestry	135 (90%)	76 (79.2%)	211 (85.8%)
Median (IQR) years in Soweto	45.5 (37.3–55.0)	46.0 (30.0–56.5)	46.0 (35.0–55.0)
Risk factor profile			
History of smoking	46 (30.7%)	70 (72.9%)	116 (47.2%)
Hypertension	96 (64.0%)	52 (54.2%)	148 (60.2%)
BMI (kg/m²)	29.4 ± 6.7	24.6 ± 5.0	27.7 ± 6.5
Serum cholesterol (mmol/L)	4.0 ± 1.2	3.9 ± 1.3	4.0 ± 1.2
Multiple cardiovascular risk factors	69 (46%)	37 (38.5%)	106 (43.1%)
History of alcohol intake	48 (32%)	71 (74%)	119 (48.8%)
Clinical presentation			
NYHA Class II or III	109 (72.7%)	62 (64.6%)	171 (69.5%)
Dizziness	93 (62%)	43 (44.8%)	136 (55.3%)
Palpitations	96 (64%)	49 (51%)	145 (58.9%)
Heart rate (beats/min)	83 ± 20	81 ± 21	82 ± 21
Systolic BP (mm Hg)	130 ± 24	125 ± 26	127 ± 25
Diastolic BP (mm Hg)	75 ± 13	72 ± 15	74 ± 15
eGFR	76 ± 29	85 ± 34	80 ± 31
Probable aetiology of AF			
Lone AF	16 (10.7%)	6 (6.3%)	22 (8.9%)
Valvular AF	65 (43%)	42 (43.8%)	107 (43.5%)
Concurrent disease			
Hypertensive HF	37 (24.7%)	10 (10.4%)	47 (19.1%)
Idiopathic dilated CMO	15 (10%)	23 (24%)	38 (15.9%)
Any type of HF	87 (58%)	51 (53.1%)	138 (56.1%)
RHD	33 (22%)	18 (18.8%)	51 (20.7%)
CAD	6 (4%)	10 (10.4%)	16 (6.5%)
Echocardiography			
LVEF (%)	53 ± 16	48 ± 16	51 ± 16
LV systolic dysfunction (LVEF < 45%)	35 (23.3%)	41 (42.7%)	76 (30.9%)
LVEDD (mm)	45 ± 11	51 ± 8	48 ± 10
LVESD (mm)	34 ± 11	38 ± 10	35 ± 11
RVSP > 35 mm Hg	22 (14.7%)	20 (20.8%)	42 (17.1%)

the demographic and clinical characteristics of those presenting in AF according to sex, noting important differences in this regard. Overall, African women were older (average of 4 years) and far more likely to present as obese (73% versus 40%; OR 1.80, 95% CI 1.28–2.52; p<0.001) and with hypertensive HF (24.7% versus 10.4%; OR 2.37, 95% CI 1.24–4.54; p=0.006). Alternatively, men were more likely to have a smoking history (OR 2.88, 95% CI 1.92–4.04) and to drink

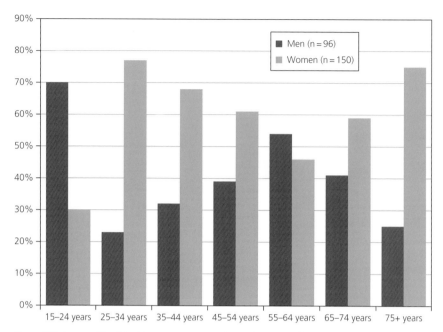

Figure 6.8 Age profile of incident case presentations of AF according to sex.

alcohol (OR 2.61, 95% CI 1.83–3.73). Women were less likely to present with a dilated CMO (OR 0.12, 95% CI 0.23–0.76) or CAD (OR 0.38, 95% CI 0.14–1.02).

Figure 6.8 shows the age profile of incident case presentations of AF in the Heart of Soweto Study cohort. As expected, there was a sharp rise in case presentations with age. There was <1 case per 100,000 for those aged 15 to 24 years compared with 49.6 cases per 100,000 for those aged ≥75 years. After the age of 25 years, significantly more women presented with AF compared with men (ranging from 46% to 77% in each age group), with the peak incidence rate for men occurring in the 55-to-64–year age group.

S3.2 Responding to an evolving spectrum of heart disease in Africa

There are many ways to interpret the studies outlined in this section given their profound implications. In particular, the Heart of Soweto Study and the community data supporting it, given its particular and detailed focus on an African urban community in epidemiological transition, requires careful interpretation. Overall, it joins such notable studies as the SABPA Study [22–24], the THUSA Study [20,25,26], and the CRIBSA Study [27–29] in providing critical data to understand the evolving burden of heart disease in sub-Saharan Africa. Notably, the Heart of Soweto represented (and still does) the most comprehensive cohort study of advanced forms of heart disease from sub-Saharan African [87], representing a key barometer for a region in epidemiological transition [36,87]. Dynamic forces such as economic development, erosion of traditional lifestyles, and rural migration are powerful influences among vulnerable communities, and these were evident in the data presented around a "crossroads" between communicable and noncommunicable heart disease in Soweto. Contrary to contemporary expectations [88], the single most prevalent form of heart disease was hypertensive HF. In combination with CAD, the ratio of these "new" communicable forms of heart disease versus historically prevalent forms of the same was almost equal. As noted in the original report [8], these ominous data suggest that if South Africa and other countries in the region continue to experience positive socioeconomic changes with a residual background of infectious disease (including the HIV epidemic—see Chapter 9), there will be a paradoxical increase in the number of relative older individuals (particularly women, but still of working age) who will develop noncommunicable forms of heart disease that will soon surpass the number of relatively younger individuals affected by communicable forms of heart disease. The former will include hypertensive heart disease, CAD, and AF. The latter may well include a latent population of adults who survived the peak epidemic of RHD (noting its close correlation to social deprivation and vulnerability to streptococcal infection) but with residual valve disease and dysfunction in their later years.

The value of these novel data (along with INTERHEART findings) cannot be overstated when compared to the strengths and weaknesses of previously published, population-based studies across the spectrum of CVD [89]. Within the context of a predominant focus on communicable disease and its impact on the burden of disease in sub-Saharan Africa [90] (most notably the impact of HIV infection and HAART [91]), these data highlight the greatest threat will emanate from a complex set of socioeconomic circumstances and the rise of noncommunicable heart disease. Strikingly, unlike high-income countries, those affected by noncommunicable heart disease were relatively young (i.e., working age) and mostly comprised women. A complex interplay between clinical risk and socioeconomic profile (including migrant status) predicates that the pattern and balance of communicable and noncommunicable forms of heart disease will continue to evolve in Soweto and other urban African communities.

Key surveillance studies from two populous (but geographically and culturally) diverse regions of sub-Saharan Africa, confirmed two key factors that will likely drive the future rise of noncommunicable forms of heart disease on the African continent. First, despite the potential threat to their health, African communities remain poorly informed and unaware of cardiovascular risk factors and the threat they pose to their heart health. Second, the potential threat of epidemiological transition toward less healthy lifestyles has already reached many urban communities and now rural communities in the region.

In summary, complex forces are shaping an important transition from communicable to noncommunicable forms of heart disease in Soweto and other urban African communities. Paradoxically, economic development and the control of infectious diseases will still leave a vulnerable portion of the community (notably obese women) at high risk of developing early and aggressive forms of non-communicable heart disease. Beyond early target organ damage (consistent with previous studies; in an earlier Nigerian study 64%, 41%, and 37% of de novo hypertensive adults demonstrated retinopathy, nephropathy, and LVH, respectively [63]), findings from the Heart of Soweto Study [8,64] support increasing evidence that hypertensive heart disease will emerge as the predominant form of heart disease on the continent. Overall, these data support calls to invest in cost-effective primary and secondary prevention programs/strategies in sub-Saharan Africa [92], with early disease detection and chronic disease programs being an obvious priority [38]. At the same time, there is a need to better understand the underlying dynamics and drivers of epidemiologic transition in different communities across the entire continent.

References

1 van Rooyen JM, Kruger HS, Huisman HW, Wissing MP, Margetts BM, Venter CS, et al. An epidemiological study of hypertension and its determinants in a population in transition: the THUSA study. *J Hum Hypertens.* 2000;14(12):779–87.

2 Yusuf S, Reddy S, Ounpuu S, Anand S. Global burden of cardiovascular diseases: Part II. Variations in cardiovascular disease by specific ethnic groups and geographic regions and prevention strategies. *Circulation.* 2001;104(23):2855–64.

3 Yusuf S, Reddy S, Ounpuu S, Anand S. Global burden of cardiovascular diseases: Part I. General considerations, the epidemiologic transition, risk factors, and impact of urbanization. *Circulation.* 2001;104(22):2746–53.

4 Global Burden of Disease Study Collaborators. Global, regional, and national incidence, prevalence, and years lived with disability for 301 acute and chronic diseases and injuries in 188 countries, 1990–2013: a systematic analysis for the Global Burden of Disease Study 2013. *Lancet.* 2015.

5 Mensah GA, Roth GA, Sampson UK, Moran AE, Feigin VL, Forouzanfar MH, et al. Mortality from cardiovascular diseases in sub-Saharan Africa, 1990–2013: a systematic analysis of data from the Global Burden of Disease Study 2013. *Cardiovasc J Afr.* 2015;26(2 Suppl 1):S6–S10.

6 Tollman SM, Kahn K, Sartorius B, Collinson MA, Clark SJ, Garenne ML. Implications of mortality transition for primary health care in rural South Africa: a population-based surveillance study. *Lancet.* 2008;372(9642):893–901.

7 Sliwa K, Carrington M, Mayosi BM, Zigiriadis E, Mvungi R, Stewart S. Incidence and characteristics of newly diagnosed rheumatic heart disease in urban African adults: insights from the heart of Soweto study. *Eur Heart J.* 2010;31(6):719–27.

8 Stewart S, Carrington M, Pretorius S, Methusi P, Sliwa K. Standing at the crossroads between new and historically prevalent heart disease: effects of migration and socioeconomic factors in the Heart of Soweto cohort study. *Eur Heart J.* 2011;32(4):492–9.

9 Dudas K, Lappas G, Stewart S, Rosengren A. Trends in out-of-hospital deaths due to coronary heart disease in Sweden (1991 to 2006). *Circulation.* 2011;123(1):46–52.

10 Hung J, Teng TH, Finn J, Knuiman M, Briffa T, Stewart S, et al. Trends from 1996 to 2007 in incidence and mortality outcomes of heart failure after acute myocardial infarction: a population-based study of 20,812 patients with first acute myocardial infarction in Western Australia. *J Am Heart Assoc.* 2013;2(5):e000172.

11 Teng TH, Hung J, Knuiman M, Stewart S, Arnolda L, Jacobs I, et al. Trends in long-term cardiovascular mortality and morbidity in men and women with heart failure of ischemic versus non-ischemic aetiology in Western Australia between 1990 and 2005. *Int J Cardiol.* 2012;158(3):405–10.

12 Zimmet PZ, Magliano DJ, Herman WH, Shaw JE. Diabetes: a 21st century challenge. *Lancet Diabetes Endocrinol.* 2014;2(1):56–64.

13 Owen N, Healy GN, Matthews CE, Dunstan DW. Too much sitting: the population health science of sedentary behavior. *Exerc Sport Sci Rev.* 2010;38(3):105–13.

14 Jhund PS, Macintyre K, Simpson CR, Lewsey JD, Stewart S, Redpath A, et al. Long-term trends in first hospitalization for heart failure and subsequent survival between 1986 and 2003: a population study of 5.1 million people. *Circulation.* 2009;119(4):515–23.

15 Stewart S, Ekman I, Ekman T, Oden A, Rosengren A. Population impact of heart failure and the most common forms of cancer: a study of 1 162 309 hospital cases in Sweden (1988 to 2004). *Circ Cardiovasc Qual Outcomes.* 2010;3(6):573–80.

16 Olsson LG, Swedberg K, Lappas G, Stewart S, Rosengren A. Trends in mortality after first hospitalization with atrial fibrillation diagnosis in Sweden 1987 to 2006. *Int J Cardiol.* 2013; 170(1):75–80.

17 Olsson LG, Swedberg K, Lappas G, Stewart S, Rosengren A. Trends in stroke incidence after hospitalization for atrial fibrillation in Sweden 1987 to 2006. *Int J Cardiol.* 2013;167(3):733–8.

18 Lonn E, Bosch J, Teo KK, Pais P, Xavier D, Yusuf S. The polypill in the prevention of cardiovascular diseases: key concepts, current status, challenges, and future directions. *Circulation.* 2010;122(20):2078–88.

19 Sytkowski PA, Kannel WB, D'Agostino RB. Changes in risk factors and the decline in mortality from cardiovascular disease: the Framingham Heart Study. *N Engl J Med.* 1990; 322(23):1635–41.

20 Oosthuizen W, Vorster HH, Kruger A, Venter CS, Kruger HS, de Ridder JH. Impact of urbanisation on serum lipid profiles: the THUSA survey. *S Afr Med J.* 2002;92(9):723–8.

21 Damasceno A, Mayosi BM, Sani M, Ogah OS, Mondo C, Ojji D, et al. The causes, treatment, and outcome of acute heart failure in 1006 Africans from 9 countries. *Arch Intern Med.* 2012;172(18):1386–94.

22 Hamer M, von Kanel R, Reimann M, Malan NT, Schutte AE, Huisman HW, et al. Progression of cardiovascular risk factors in black Africans: 3 year follow up of the SABPA cohort study. *Atherosclerosis.* 2015;238(1):52–4.

23 Huisman HW, Schutte AE, Schutte R, van Rooyen JM, Fourie CM, Mels CM, et al. Exploring the link between cardiovascular reactivity and end-organ damage in African and Caucasian men: the SABPA study. *Am J Hypertens.* 2013;26(1):68–75.

24 Meyburgh D, Malan L, Van Rooyen JM, Potgieter JC. Cardiovascular, cortisol and coping responses in urban Africans: the SAPBA study. *Cardiovasc J Afr.* 2012;23(1):28–33.

25 Kruger HS, Venter CS, Vorster HH, Study T. Physical inactivity as a risk factor for cardiovascular disease in communities undergoing rural to urban transition: the THUSA study. *Cardiovasc J S Afr.* 2003;14(1):16–23.

26 Malan L, Malan NT, Wissing MP, Seedat YK. Coping with urbanization: a cardiometabolic risk? The THUSA study. *Biol Psychol.* 2008;79(3):323–8.

27 Peer N, Lombard C, Steyn K, Levitt N. High prevalence of metabolic syndrome in the Black population of Cape Town: the Cardiovascular Risk in Black South Africans (CRIBSA) study. *Eur J Prev Cardiol.* 2015;22(8):1036–42.

28 Peer N, Steyn K, Lombard C, Gwebushe N, Levitt N. A high burden of hypertension in the urban black population of Cape Town: the Cardiovascular Risk in Black South Africans (CRIBSA) study. *PLoS One.* 2013;8(11):e78567.

29 Peer N, Steyn K, Lombard C, Gaziano T, Levitt N. Alarming rise in prevalence of atherogenic dyslipidaemia in the black population of Cape Town: the Cardiovascular Risk in Black South Africans (CRIBSA) study. *Eur J Prev Cardiol.* 2014;21(12):1549–56.

30 Central Intelligence Agency. *The World Factbook: Nigeria.* Washington, DC: Central Intelligence Agency, 2015 [updated September 2015; accessed September 2015]. Available from: https://www.cia.gov/library/publications/the-world-factbook/geos/ni.html.

31 The World Bank. *Nigeria Economic Report, No. 2.* Washington, DC: World Bank Group, 2014.

32 Adedini SA, Odimegwu C, Bamiwuye O, Fadeyibi O, De Wet N. Barriers to accessing health care in Nigeria: implications for child survival. *Glob Health Action.* 2014;7:23499.

33 Danawi H, Ogbonna F. Impact of socioeconomic status and household structure on infant mortality rate in Abia State of Nigeria. *Int J Childbirth Educ.* 2014;29(4).

34 Umeh CA, Onyi SC. Case based rubella surveillance in Abia State, South East Nigeria, 2007–2011. *PeerJ.* 2014;2:e580.

35 Stewart S, Carrington MJ, Pretorius S, Ogah OS, Blauwet L, Antras-Ferry J, et al. Elevated risk factors but low burden of heart disease in urban African primary care patients: a fundamental role for primary prevention. *Int J Cardiol.* 2012;158(2):205–10.

36 Tibazarwa K, Ntyintyane L, Sliwa K, Gerntholtz T, Carrington M, Wilkinson D, et al. A time bomb of cardiovascular risk factors in South Africa: results from the Heart of Soweto Study "Heart Awareness Days." *Int J Cardiol.* 2009;132(2):233–9.

37 Okpechi IG, Chukwuonye, II, Tiffin N, Madukwe OO, Onyeonoro UU, Umeizudike TI, et al. Blood pressure gradients and cardiovascular risk factors in urban and rural populations in Abia State South Eastern Nigeria using the WHO STEPwise approach. *PLoS One.* 2013;8(9):e73403.

38 Stewart S, Sliwa K. Preventing CVD in resource-poor areas: perspectives from the 'real-world'. *Nat Rev Cardiol.* 2009;6(7):489–92.

39 Carrington MJ, Jennings GL, Stewart S. Pattern of blood pressure in Australian adults: results from a national blood pressure screening day of 13,825 adults. *Int J Cardiol.* 2010;145(3):461–7.

40 Burt VL, Whelton P, Roccella EJ, Brown C, Cutler JA, Higgins M, et al. Prevalence of hypertension in the US adult population. Results from the Third National Health and Nutrition Examination Survey, 1988–1991. *Hypertension.* 1995;25(3):305–13.

41 Cameron AJ, Magliano DJ, Zimmet PZ, Welborn T, Shaw JE. The metabolic syndrome in Australia: prevalence using four definitions. *Diabetes Res Clin Pract.* 2007;77(3):471–8.

42 Alberts M, Urdal P, Steyn K, Stensvold I, Tverdal A, Nel JH, et al. Prevalence of cardiovascular diseases and associated risk factors in a rural black population of South Africa. *Eur J Cardiovasc Prev Rehabil.* 2005;12(4):347–54.

43 Peltzer K. Health behaviour among Black and White South Africans. *J R Soc Promo Health.* 2002;122(3):187–93.

44 Seedat YK, Mayet FGH, Latiff GH, Joubert G. Study of Risk-Factors Leading to Coronary Heart-Disease in Urban Zulus. *J Human Hypertension.* 1993;7(6):529–32.

45 Lyons JG, Sliwa K, Carrington MJ, Raal F, Pretorius S, Thienemann F, et al. Lower levels of high-density lipoprotein cholesterol in urban Africans presenting with communicable versus non-communicable forms of heart disease: the 'Heart of Soweto' hospital registry study. *BMJ Open.* 2014;4(7):e005069.

46 Lyons JG, Stewart S. Prevention: Convergent communicable and noncommunicable heart disease. *Nat Rev Cardiol.* 2012;9(1):12–4.

47 Sliwa K, Lyons JG, Carrington MJ, Lecour S, Marais AD, Raal FJ, et al. Different lipid profiles according to ethnicity in the Heart of Soweto study cohort of de novo presentations of heart disease. *Cardiovasc J Afr.* 2012;23(7):389–95.

48 The World Bank. World Development Indicators: Urban Population [dataset] 2013. Available from: http://data.worldbank.org/indicator/SP.URB.TOTL.IN.ZS/countries.

49 Addo J, Smeeth L, Leon DA. Hypertension in sub-saharan Africa: a systematic review. *Hypertension.* 2007;50(6):1012–8.

50 Sliwa K, Wilkinson D, Hansen C, Ntyintyane L, Tibazarwa K, Becker A, et al. Spectrum of heart disease and risk factors in a black urban population in South Africa (the Heart of Soweto Study): a cohort study. *Lancet.* 2008;371(9616):915–22.

51 Xanthakis V, Larson MG, Wollert KC, Aragam J, Cheng S, Ho J, et al. Association of novel biomarkers of cardiovascular stress with left ventricular hypertrophy and dysfunction: implications for screening. *J Am Heart Assoc.* 2013;2(6):e000399.

52 Stoica R, Heller EN, Bella JN. Point-of-care screening for left ventricular hypertrophy and concentric geometry using hand-held cardiac ultrasound in hypertensive patients. *Am J Cardiovasc Dis.* 2011;1(2):119–25.

53 Sliwa K, Lee GA, Carrington MJ, Obel P, Okreglicki A, Stewart S. Redefining the ECG in urban South Africans: electrocardiographic findings in heart disease-free Africans. *Int J Cardiol.* 2013;167(5):2204–9.

54 World Health Organization. *2008–2013 Action Plan for the Global Strategy for the Prevention and Control of Noncommunicable Diseases.* Geneva: WHO, 2008.

55 World Health Organization. Noncommunicable disease country specific profiles. 2011.

56 World Health Organization. Non-communicable Diseases and Mental Health Cluster. *WHO STEPS Surveillance Manual: The WHO STEPwise Approach to Chronic Disease Risk Factor Surveillance.* Geneva: WHO, 2005.

57 Oladapo OO, Salako L, Sodiq OS, K., Adedapo K, Falase AO. A prevalence of cardiometabolic risk factors among a rural Yoruba south-western Nigerian population: a population-based survey. *Cardiovasc J Afr* 2010;21:26–31.

58 Ulasi, II, Ijoma CK, Onwubere BJ, Arodiwe E, Onodugo O, Okafor C. High prevalence and low awareness of hypertension in a market population in Enugu, Nigeria. *Int J Hypertens.* 2011;2011:869675.

59 Dzudie A, Kengne AP, Muna WF, Ba H, Menanga A, Kouam Kouam C, et al. Prevalence, awareness, treatment and control of hypertension in a self-selected sub-Saharan African urban population: a cross-sectional study. *BMJ Open.* 2012;2(4).

60 Cooper R, Rotimi C, Ataman S, McGee D, Osotimehin B, Kadiri S, et al. The prevalence of hypertension in seven populations of west African origin. *Am J Public Health.* 1997;87(2):160–8.

61 Alwan A, Maclean DR, Riley LM, d'Espaignet ET, Mathers CD, Stevens GA, et al. Monitoring and surveillance of chronic non-communicable diseases: progress and capacity in high-burden countries. *Lancet.* 2010;376(9755):1861–8.

62 Boutayeb A, Boutayeb S. The burden of non communicable diseases in developing countries. *Int J Equity Health.* 2005;4(1):2.

63 Reddy KS. Cardiovascular diseases in the developing countries: dimensions, determinants, dynamics and directions for public health action. *Public Health Nutr.* 2002;5(1A):231–7.

64 Steyn K, Sliwa K, Hawken S, Commerford P, Onen C, Damasceno A, et al. Risk factors associated with myocardial infarction in Africa: the INTERHEART Africa study. *Circulation.* 2005;112(23):3554–61.

65 Tunstall-Pedoe H, Kuulasmaa K, Mahonen M, Tolonen H, Ruokokoski E, Amouyel P. Contribution of trends in survival and coronary-event rates to changes in coronary heart disease mortality: 10-year results from 37 WHO MONICA project populations. Monitoring trends and determinants in cardiovascular disease. *Lancet.* 1999;353(9164):1547–57.

66 Yeh RW, Sidney S, Chandra M, Sorel M, Selby JV, Go AS. Population trends in the incidence and outcomes of acute myocardial infarction. *N Engl J Med.* 2010;362(23):2155–65.

67 Wang Y, Wang QJ. The prevalence of prehypertension and hypertension among US adults according to the new joint national committee guidelines: new challenges of the old problem. *Arch Intern Med.* 2004;164(19):2126–34.

68 Bibbins-Domingo K, Chertow GM, Coxson PG, Moran A, Lightwood JM, Pletcher MJ, et al. Projected effect of dietary salt reductions on future cardiovascular disease. *N Engl J Med.* 2010;362(7):590–9.

69 Kuulasmaa K, Tunstall-Pedoe H, Dobson A, Fortmann S, Sans S, Tolonen H, et al. Estimation of contribution of changes in classic risk factors to trends in coronary-event rates across the WHO MONICA Project populations. *Lancet.* 2000;355(9205):675–87

70 Capewell S, MacIntyre K, Stewart S, Chalmers JW, Boyd J, Finlayson A, et al. Age, sex, and social trends in out-of-hospital cardiac deaths in Scotland 1986–95: a retrospective cohort study. *Lancet*. 2001;358(9289):1213–7.

71 Macintyre K, Stewart S, Chalmers J, Pell J, Finlayson A, Boyd J, et al. Relation between socioeconomic deprivation and death from a first myocardial infarction in Scotland: population based analysis. *BMJ*. 2001;322(7295):1152–3.

72 Mahmood SS, Levy D, Vasan RS, Wang TJ. The Framingham Heart Study and the epidemiology of cardiovascular disease: a historical perspective. *Lancet*. 2014;383(9921):999–1008.

73 Gillum RF. The epidemiology of cardiovascular disease in black Americans. *N Engl J Med*. 1996;335(21):1597–9.

74 Stewart S, Wilkinson D, Becker A, Askew D, Ntyintyane L, McMurray JJ, et al. Mapping the emergence of heart disease in a black, urban population in Africa: the Heart of Soweto Study. *Int J Cardiol*. 2006;108(1):101–8.

75 Abegunde DO, Mathers CD, Adam T, Ortegon M, Strong K. The burden and costs of chronic diseases in low-income and middle-income countries. *Lancet*. 2007;370(9603):1929–38.

76 Essop MR, Wisenbaugh T, Sareli P. Evidence against a myocardial factor as the cause of left ventricular dilation in active rheumatic carditis. *J Am Coll Cardiol*. 1993;22(3):826–9.

77 von Elm E, Altman DG, Egger M, Pocock SJ, Gotzsche PC, Vandenbroucke JP. The Strengthening the Reporting of Observational Studies in Epidemiology (STROBE) statement: guidelines for reporting observational studies. *Lancet*. 2007;370(9596):1453–7.

78 Sliwa K, Carrington M, Mayosi BM, Zigiriadis E, Mvungi R, Stewart S. Incidence and characteristics of newly diagnosed rheumatic heart disease in urban African adults: insights from the heart of Soweto study. *Eur Heart J*. 2010;31(6):719–27.

79 Stewart S, Wilkinson D, Hansen C, Vaghela V, Mvungi R, McMurray J, et al. Predominance of heart failure in the Heart of Soweto Study cohort: emerging challenges for urban African communities. *Circulation*. 2008;118(23):2360–7.

80 Sahn DJ, DeMaria A, Kisslo J, Weyman A. Recommendations regarding quantitation in M-mode echocardiography: results of a survey of echocardiographic measurements. *Circulation*. 1978;58(6):1072–83.

81 Prineas RJ, Crow RS, Blackburn H. *The Minnesota Code Manual of Electrocardiographic Findings: Standards and Procedures for Measurement and Classification*. Boston, Massachusetts: John Wright, 1982.

82 Setel PW, Saker L, Unwin NC, Hemed Y, Whiting DR, Kitange H. Is it time to reassess the categorization of disease burdens in low–income countries? *Am J Public Health*. 2004; 94(3):384–8.

83 Stewart S, Mocumbi AO, Carrington MJ, Pretorius S, Burton R, Sliwa K. A not-so-rare form of heart failure in urban black Africans: pathways to right heart failure in the Heart of Soweto Study cohort. *Eur J Heart Fail*. 2011;13(10):1070–7.

84 Sliwa K, Carrington MJ, Klug E, Opie L, Lee G, Ball J, et al. Predisposing factors and incidence of newly diagnosed atrial fibrillation in an urban African community: insights from the Heart of Soweto Study. *Heart*. 2010;96(23):1878–82.

85 Ball J, Carrington MJ, McMurray JJ, Stewart S. Atrial fibrillation: profile and burden of an evolving epidemic in the 21st century. *Int J Cardiol*. 2013;167(5):1807–24.

86 Lip GY, Brechin CM, Lane DA. The global burden of atrial fibrillation and stroke: a systematic review of the epidemiology of atrial fibrillation in regions outside North America and Europe. *Chest*. 2012;142(6):1489–98.

87 Albert MA. Heart failure in the urban African enclave of Soweto: a case study of contemporary epidemiological transition in the developing world. *Circulation*. 2008; 118(23):2323–5.

88 Brink AJ, Aalbers J. Strategies for heart disease in sub-Saharan Africa. *Heart*. 2009; 95(19):1559–60.

89 Kruger R, Kruger HS, Macintyre UE. The determinants of overweight and obesity among 10- to 15-year-old schoolchildren in the North West Province, South Africa: the THUSA BANA (Transition and Health during Urbanisation of South Africans; BANA, children) study. *Public Health Nutr.* 2006;9(3):351–8.

90 Sridhar D, Batniji R. Misfinancing global health: a case for transparency in disbursements and decision making. *Lancet.* 2008;372(9644):1185–91.

91 World Health Organization. *Sub-Saharan Africa AIDS Epidemic Update Regional Summary.* Geneva, Switzerland: WHO, 2008.

92 Gaziano TA. Cardiovascular disease in the developing world and its cost-effective management. *Circulation.* 2005;112(23):3547–53.

SECTION 4

Infectious heart disease

Mpiko Ntsekhe

University of Cape Town/Groote Schuur Hospital, Cape Town, South Africa

S4.1 The historical and contemporary burden of infectious forms of heart disease in Africa

This section of the book aims to provide a broad overview and current under-standing of infectious heart diseases as experienced by adults living in sub-Saharan Africa. By highlighting three key research areas, it explores aspects of the epide-miology, pathogenesis, clinical manifestations, and potential prevention and man-agement strategies for the main causes of infectious heart disease in African adults. This is achieved by providing simple but concise analyses of the available information from major contemporary observational studies and randomized tri-als conducted on the African continent. Data from around the world suggest that HIV predisposes to heart muscle and pericardial disease, causing PH and large vessel aneurysms. It also increases the risk of acute coronary syndrome (ACS) (in the absence of significant atherosclerosis) and may accelerate progression of chronic coronary atherosclerosis in those with traditional risk factors who are receiving HAART (see Chapter 10). The extent to which this holds true in the African setting, where the HIV burden is highest and the profile of people with HIV differs significantly from most of the rest of the world, is not clear. Chapter 9 helps to unpack some of these issues by providing an analysis of data from the Heart of Soweto Study that sets out to (a) explore the clinical presentation and cardiac disease profile of HIV-infected patients presenting to one of the largest referral hospitals in Africa and (b) quantify the burden of HIV-related cardiac disease relative to other forms of CVD in a community known to have a high background prevalence of HIV infection. TB remains endemic in most of sub-Saharan Africa and can affect all organs of the body, including the heart. In immune-competent hosts, the spread of TB to the heart occurs predominantly via the multiple major lymph glands that surround the heart (mediastinal,

The Heart of Africa: Clinical Profile of an Evolving Burden of Heart Disease in Africa, First Edition.
Edited by Simon Stewart, Karen Sliwa, Ana Mocumbi, Albertino Damasceno, and Mpiko Ntsekhe.
© 2016 John Wiley & Sons, Ltd. Published 2016 by John Wiley & Sons, Ltd.

peritracheal, and peribronchial). Alternatively, in those who are immunocompromised, the spread of TB is predominantly via the hematogenous route. Cardiac involvement is localized to the pericardium in the majority of people with TB-related heart disease, where it presents as sub-acute effusive pericarditis with or without cardiac tamponade or constrictive pericarditis with or without HF. Although not common, TB can also involve the myocardium and endocardium. In this context, Chapter 8 provides an update and summary of recent randomized controlled outcome data designed to explore the potential efficacy of adjunctive immunotherapy for the treatment of effusive TB pericarditis in those with and without HIV.

Finally, in the setting of overcrowding and poverty, both of which are highly prevalent across the African continent, the immune response to Group B Streptococcus pharyngitis can lead to both acute and chronic RHD with devastating effects. The pathogenic interrelationship between poverty, overcrowding, genetic predisposition, and the immune response in this condition is yet to be elucidated, although promising research, which will be crucial to seeing the disease eventually eradicated, is underway. Sadly, rates of cardiovascular morbidity and premature mortality related to rheumatic valvular disease across the continent have been underestimated for decades, with more recent observational data revealing that the burden remains unacceptably high. In Africa, RHD remains an important contributor to the high levels of cardiac-related maternal morbidity and mortality, accounts for a significant proportion of AF and stroke, and is the major predisposing cardiac risk factor for infective endocarditis and its devastating outcomes. The absence of the ability to provide cardiac surgery in most of sub-Saharan Africa is an important consideration that adds to the impetus and calls to implement aggressive primary and secondary preventive strategies such as wider use of empiric penicillin for pharyngitis in susceptible populations. Chapter 7 provides fairly robust data from the Heart of Soweto Study that challenges the previously held myths of RHD as a vanishing disease of bygone eras that affected mainly children and contributed little to the burden of HF in adults.

In summary, sub-Saharan Africa is currently in the midst of a quadruple burden of disease that is characterized by high levels of trauma, a growing epidemic of chronic diseases of lifestyle (see Section 3), poor maternal and child health (see Sections 1 and 2, respectively), and a persistently high burden of communicable disease. In this section we focus on the latter by examining the interrelationship between infectious diseases and CVD in Africa and exploring their contribution to the high burden of structural heart disease. Three organisms and their sequelae account for the vast majority of the cardiac disease that is attributable to infections in sub-Saharan Africa—HIV, TB, and group B streptococcus. Accordingly, it is these infectious pathways to heart disease that feature heavily in the three chapters that compose this section of the book.

S4.1.1 Geographical context

In Section 4, the urban area of Soweto in South Africa provides the setting for Chapters 7 and 9 (see Section 1 for profiles of Soweto and South Africa). Chapter 8 offers a contrasting geographical backdrop, featuring a multicenter trial representing eight African countries across diverse regions of the continent.

CHAPTER 7

Rheumatic heart disease

Simon Stewart[1], Melinda Jane Carrington[1], and Karen Sliwa[2]

[1] *Australian Catholic University, Melbourne, Victoria, Australia*

[2] *University of Cape Town, South Africa; University of the Witwatersrand, Johannesburg, South Africa*

7.0 Introduction

As outlined in more detail in Section 2, RHD with its close link to childhood poverty and heavy exposure to communicable diseases (in this case acute rheumatic fever) represents one of the truly reliable barometers of the socioeconomic wealth of a population and country, particularly in the setting of limited access to even basic preventive health care measures. The poorer the country, the higher the rate of childhood cases of RHD, with often deadly consequences. Beyond clearly identifiable index childhood cases, however, there is undoubtedly a "legacy effect" of acute rheumatic fever (estimated to affect millions of people across the globe)—the subsequent development of subclinical RHD that may well reveal itself in adulthood as increasingly significant valve disease/dysfunction. Certainly, this is most probably the case even in high-income countries among individuals who were exposed to childhood poverty but survived to a very advanced age. Derived from the main results of the Heart of Soweto Study (see Chapter 6), it was postulated that the adult population in Soweto would be particularly vulnerable to this otherwise poorly researched and reported clinical phenomenon.

7.1 A legacy effect of RHD from childhood to adulthood in an urban African community

Sliwa K, Carrington M, Mayosi B, Zigriades E, Mvungi R, Stewart S. Incidence and characteristics of newly diagnosed rheumatic heart disease in urban African adults: insights from the Heart of Soweto Study. *European Heart Journal* **2010; 31(6):719–27. [3]**

7.1.1 Study background

Worldwide it is estimated that almost 16 million people per annum are affected by RHD as a consequence of streptococcal infection with subsequent acute rheumatic fever and involvement of the cardiac valves as part of a systemic inflammatory response/process [1,2]. Consequently, it has been estimated that approximately 200,000 deaths per annum among those living in low-income countries are attributable to RHD [3]. As with most forms of communicable disease, the peoples of sub-Saharan Africa are particularly vulnerable to RHD. However, as these (global) figures largely relate to children and young adults, they are likely to underestimate the true burden of RHD as reflected in the adult population (via the legacy effect described above). As described in Chapter 6, the Heart of Soweto Study cohort provided a perfect opportunity to explore the balance between communicable and noncommunicable forms of heart disease in a population in epidemiological transition.

7.1.2 Study aims

Using systematic clinical profiling of the Heart of Soweto Study cohort to investigate de novo presentations of heart disease, with a careful examination and classification of all cases of valvular disease and dysfunction via echocardiography, this study focused on the probable incidence and clinical characteristics of RHD in the Sowetan community.

7.1.3 Study methods

Overall, 960 patients presenting with valvular abnormalities to the Cardiology Unit at the Chris Hani Baragwanath Hospital during the period 2006 to 2007 and enrolled in the Heart of Soweto Study (see Chapter 6 for detailed study methods and the spectrum of disease presentation) were subject to further clinical investigation and scrutiny as part of this study report. As described in the original report, classifying inherently complex cases of valve disease and dysfunction in this cohort was both challenging and problematic. However, this resulted in the most comprehensive report of the clinical spectrum of valve disease in sub-Saharan Africa (at least from an adult perspective) to that point.

As described in the original report, RHD was diagnosed from a history of acute rheumatic fever and/or a cardiac murmur plus standard echocardiographic criteria [4]; the latter included detection of typical bowing or doming of the mitral valve leaflets in diastole. Similarly, mitral stenosis was diagnosed on the basis of thickening or calcification of the leaflets (typically the posterior leaflet with subvalvular region involvement). Isolated or concomitant MR was diagnosed by any definitive evidence of regurgitation seen in two planes by Doppler evaluation using semiquantitative measures, while severe MR was detected from additional systolic flow reversal in the pulmonary veins.

7.1.4 Study findings
7.1.4.1 Newly diagnosed VHD

Of 4,005 de novo presentations to the Cardiology Unit of the Chris Hani Baragwanath Hospital during the study period, 960 (24.0%) had a valvular abnormality. Affected patients were predominantly of African ancestry (n = 868 [90.4%]), women (n = 570 [59.4%]), and long-term residents of Soweto (n = 512 [53.3%]). Overall, there was an equal balance between structural VHD (n = 481 [50.1%]), and functional VHD (n = 439 [45.7%]). As shown in Table 7.1, the most common structural valve disease presented was RHD, found in 344 (71.5%) patients. Other structural abnormalities included CHD (n = 20; 55.6%), mitral valve prolapse (n = 5; 13.9%), myxomatous mitral valve (n = 3; 8.3%), submitral aneurysm (n = 2; 5.6%), Marfan syndrome (n = 1; 2.8%), subaortic aneurysm (n = 12.8%), hypertrophic CMO (n = 1; 2.8%), and unclassified (n = 3; 8.3%).

Figure 7.1 shows the pattern of structural valve disease abnormalities in this cohort according to sex with roughly similar patterns of presentation on this basis. Similarly, Figure 7.2 shows the pattern of disease associated with functional valve dysfunction according to sex. From this perspective, women were more likely to present with valvular dysfunction associated with hypertensive heart disease (OR 1.70, 95% CI 1.03–2.81; p = 0.042) and dilated CMO (OR 1.52, 95% CI 1.07–2.18; p = 0.026). Alternatively, men were more likely to present with RHF/cor pulmonale (OR 2.11, 95% CI 1.54–2.90; p < 0.0001) and concurrent ischemic CMO (OR 3.56, 95% CI 1.62–7.88; p = 0.026).

7.1.4.2 Newly diagnosed RHD patients

Overall, the patients presenting with newly diagnosed RHD were predominantly women of African ancestry (n = 234; 68.0%), and the prevalence pattern appeared to increase in the economically productive age group before declining again (i.e., age groups 14 to 19 years [3%], 20 to 29 years [16%], 30 to 39 years [24%], 40 to 49 years [17%], 50 to 59 years [19%], 60 to 69 years [12%], and >70 years [8%]). Men were more likely to present in NYHA Class III/IV (20.9% versus 16.2%) when compared to women. Alternatively, women were more likely to present with dyspnea (68.0% versus 60.9%) and peripheral edema (29.5% versus 22.7%). Women also presented with higher heart rates (86 ± 18 versus 81 ± 16) while having similar BP profiles (see Table 7.2).

Table 7.1 Abnormal presentations of structural valve disease according to sex.

Structural Valve Disease Abnormality	Women (n = 325)	Men (n = 156)	All (n = 481)
Degenerative	65 (20.0%)	36 (23.1%)	101 (21.0%)
RHD	234 (72.0%)	110 (70.5%)	344 (71.5%)
Other structural abnormalities	26 (8.0%)	10 (6.4%)	36 (7.5%)
CHD	15 (57.7%)	5 (50.0%)	20 (55.6%)
Hypertrophic CMO	0 (0%)	1 (10.0%)	1 (2.8%)
Marfan syndrome	1 (3.8%)	0 (0%)	1 (2.8%)
Mitral valve prolapse	3 (11.5%)	2 (20.0%)	5 (13.9%)
Myxomatous mitral valve	3 (11.5%)	0 (0%)	3 (8.3%)
Subaortic aneurysm	1 (3.8%)	0 (0%)	1 (2.8%)
Submitral aneurysm	1 (3.8%)	1 (10.0%)	2 (5.6%)
Unclassified	2 (7.7%)	1 (10.0%)	3 (8.3%)

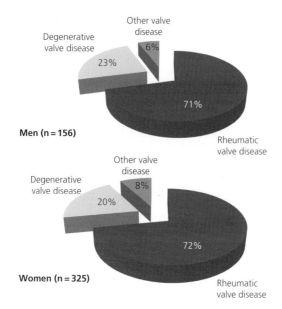

Figure 7.1 The structural valve disease pattern according to sex.

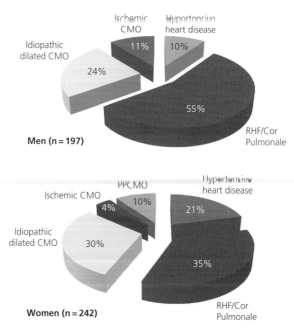

Figure 7.2 Functional valve dysfunction according to sex.

Table 7.2 Patients' demographic and clinical characteristics and clinical presentation.

	Women (n = 234)	Men (n = 110)	All (n = 344)
Demographic characteristics			
African ancestry	220 (94.0%)	94 (85.5%)	314 (91.3%)
Median age in years	41 (30–55)	42 (31–55)	43 (32–56)
Median years in Soweto	35 (20–49)	37 (20–50)	36 (20–50)
Standard education, 0–10 years	213 (91.0%)	101 (91.8%)	314 (91.3%)
Women	234 (100%)	0 (0%)	234 (68.0%)
Clinical characteristics			
Anemia	23 (9.8%)	4 (3.6%)	27 (7.9%)
AF	20 (8.6%)	14 (12.7%)	34 (9.9%)
Renal dysfunction	28 (12.0%)	29 (26.4%)	57 (16.7%)
Clinical presentation			
Heart rate, beats/min	86 ± 18	81 + 16	84 + 17
Systolic BP, mm Hg	122 ± 24	121 + 24	122 + 24
Diastolic BP, mm Hg	69 ± 21	67 ± 18	69 ± 20
Dyspnea on presentation	159 (67.9%)	67 (60.9%)	226 (65.7%)
Palpitations/chest pain	156 (66.7%)	71 (64.6%)	227 (65.9%)
Peripheral edema	69 (29.5%)	25 (22.7%)	94 (27.3%)
Raised jugular venous pressure	12 (5.1%)	7 (6.4%)	19 (5.5%)
NYHA III/IV	38 (16.2%)	23 (20.9%)	61 (17.7%)

As shown in Table 7.3, MR was revealed as the most common valvular lesion (affecting 59% of the patients) and was commonly associated with left and right heart abnormalities. Alternatively, aortic stenosis was the least common valvular lesion (9% of cases).

7.1.4.3 Outcomes

Overall, 90 (26.2%) patients with RHD were admitted to hospital for suspected bacterial endocarditis ≤30 months after diagnosis. Additionally, 75 (21.8%) patients were referred for aortic and mitral valve replacement (22 [29.3%] patients and 32 [42.7%] patients, respectively) and 21 (28%) patients for double valve replacement.

7.1.4.4 Estimated incidence of RHD

These hospital data permitted some estimates of the incidence of RHD in those aged 14 years or more living in the surrounding area of Soweto (on age and sex-specific basis). Overall, it was estimated that, annually, there are ~24 new cases of RHD per 100,000 in Soweto. However, a j-shaped distribution of incident cases was highly evident with incidence rates rising from 15 to 53 cases per 100,000 per annum in those aged between 19 and 60 years (the highest point being in older cases) following an initial (high) rate of 30 cases per 100,000 per annum among those aged 15 to 19 years.

Table 7.3 Patients' RHD echocardiographic presentations according to predominant valvular lesion, and prescribed medication.

	Aortic Regurgitation (n = 126)	Aortic Stenosis (n = 31)	Mitral Regurgitation (n = 204)	Mitral Stenosis (n = 103)	All (n = 344)
Systolic function					
LV diameter systole (mm)	37 ± 14	31 ± 14	38 ± 31	33 ± 13	36 ± 21
LV diameter systole >45 mm	22 (17.5%)	3 (9.7%)	27 (13.2%)	8 (7.8%)	55 (16.0%)
LV diameter diastole (mm)	51 ± 14	49 ± 14	51 ± 11	44 ± 10	49 ± 12
LV diameter diastole >55 mm	40 (31.8%)	6 (9.4%)	49 (24.0%)	7 (6.8%)	86 (25.0%)
LVEF (%)	56 ± 14	60 ± 13	58 ± 13	59 ± 11	58 ± 13
LV systolic dysfunction	23 (18.3%)	7 (2.6%)	28 (13.7%)	11 (10.7%)	50 (14.5%)
Valvular regurgitation (mild-moderate-severe)					
Aortic valve	45-37-18	35-32-13	12-8-3.4	12-6.8-0	126 (36.6%)
Mitral valve	22-8.7-7.1	19-5-3.2	43-40-17	20-17-4.9	103 (29.9%)
Tricuspid valve	9.5-9.5-6.4	13-3.2-3.2	13-9.3-7.4	8.7-14-11	89 (25.9%)
Other abnormalities					
RV systolic pressure >35 mm Hg	19 (15.1%)	3 (9.7%)	40 (19.6%)	26 (25.3%)	62 (18.0%)
Prescribed medication					
Loop diuretics	76 (60.3%)	22 (71.0%)	116 (56.9%)	69 (67.0%)	208 (60.5)
Antiplatelet therapy	50 (39.7%)	12 (38.7%)	67 (32.8%)	45 (43.7%)	130 (37.8%)
ACE-inhibitor	45 (35.7%)	10 (32.3%)	53 (26.0%)	26 (25.2%)	94 (27.3%)
Calcium antagonist	28 (22.2%)	6 (19.3%)	16 (7.8%)	6 (5.8%)	39 (11.3%)
Beta-blocker	24 (19.1%)	9 (29.0%)	44 (21.6%)	42 (40.8%)	89 (25.9%)
Aldosterone inhibitor	20 (18.9%)	6 (19.3%)	28 (13.7%)	13 (12.6%)	47 (13.7%)
Digoxin	16 (12.7%)	3 (9.7%)	24 (11.8%)	14 (13.6%)	43 (12.5%)

7.1.5 **Study interpretation**

As originally reported, this was the first study to examine the incidence of RHD among those of African ancestry aged >14 years [5]. Overall, these data revealed that RHD remains common among the studied adult population, challenging the long-held assumption that RHD predominantly affects children (particularly in populations in epidemiologic transition) [6]. Significantly, these data suggest that RHD principally affects individuals in economically productive age groups in Soweto (particularly those aged 30–39 years). Furthermore, primary VHD plays a vital role in the development of HF in the sub-Saharan African context. Early detection of valvular disease and dysfunction is clearly crucial in this context. However, the challenge of assessing patients with cardiac murmurs in LMIC remains. In total, 960 out of 4,005 de novo patients presented to the cardiac unit with a valvular abnormality (more than half of cases presenting with functional VHD). In developed countries, VHD is not considered a concern and is often over-looked in terms of morbidity and mortality [7]. Numerous reports on the investigation of functional MR in ischemic and nonischemic CMOs have been published, as well as their contribution to the burden of HF [8,9].

7.1.6 **Study limitations**

A number of limitations were noted throughout this study. First, the study sample included only individuals who were privileged enough to seek professional medical care, and these patients usually presented with advanced forms of valvular heart disease. Therefore, this hospital-based study likely underrepresented the true portion of the population of Soweto affected by the full spectrum of valve disease and dysfunction. Unfortunately, given the nature and context of the study population, follow-up of study patients was limited and the long-term impact and natural history of RHD and other forms of valve disease and dysfunction in this and other sub-Saharan African patient populations remains largely unknown.

7.1.7 **Study conclusions**

As noted in the original report, this complex clinical picture of valvular disease and dysfunction required careful interpretation, including a new standard for classifying cases. Quite apart from a unique report on late-stage RHD, this pivotal study uncovered a significant component of valve disease and dysfunction as part of late presentations of heart disease in Soweto. Given the volume of cases derived from the systematic application of echocardiography, there is a clear mandate to explore novel and cost-effective methods (e.g., handheld echocardiography and automated heart sound interpretation) to discover otherwise undiagnosed valve disease/dysfunction and implement preventive treatments.

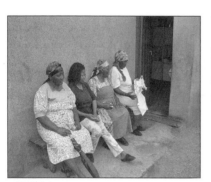 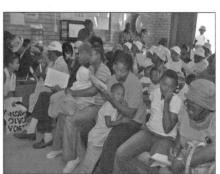

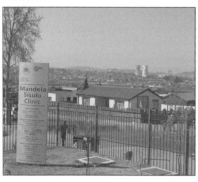 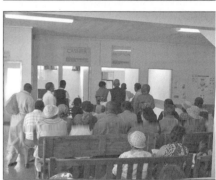

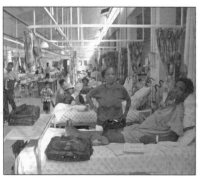 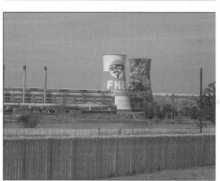

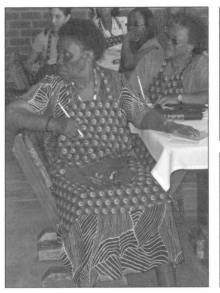
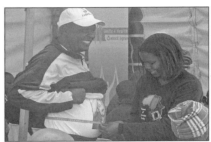
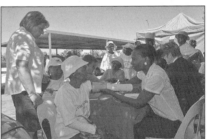
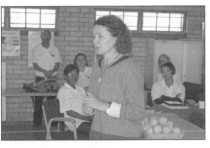
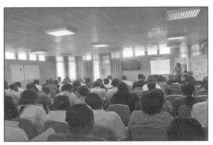
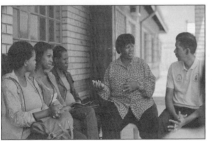
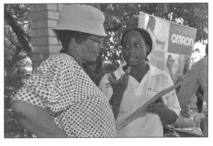

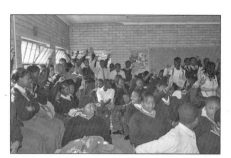

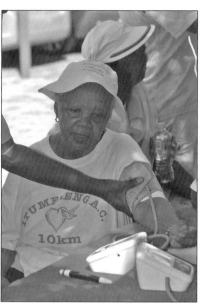

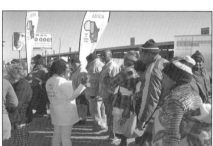

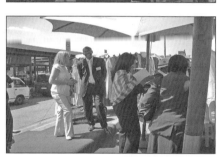

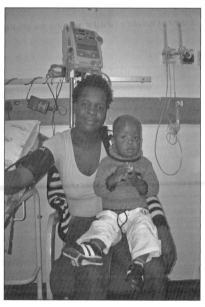

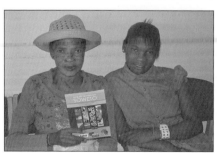

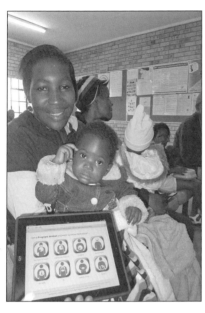

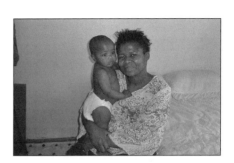

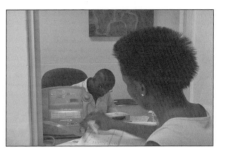

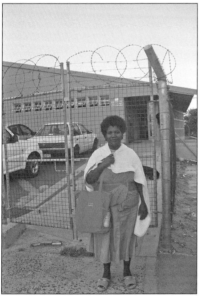

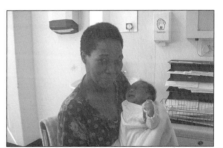

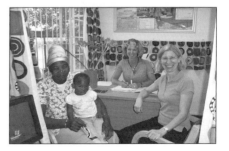

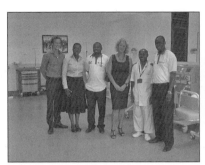
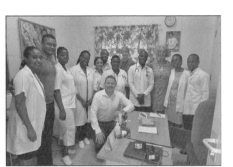
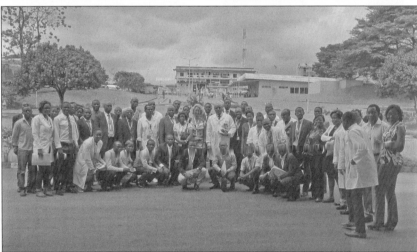
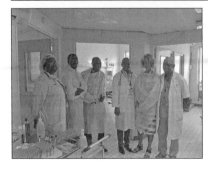
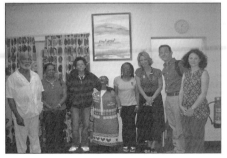

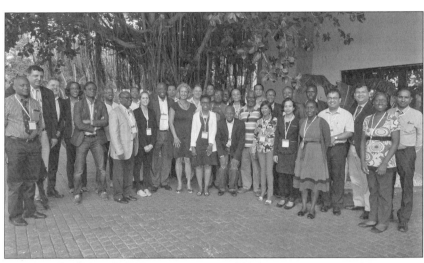

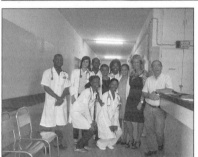

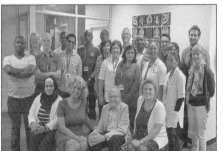

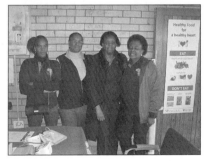

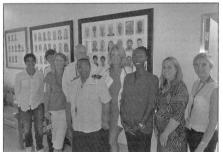

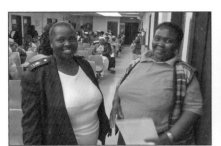

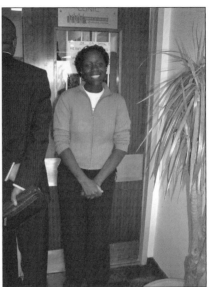

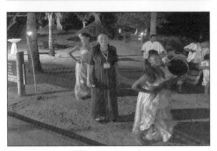

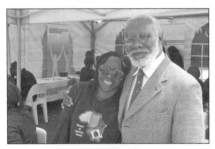

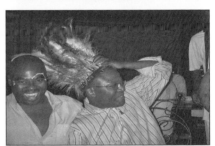

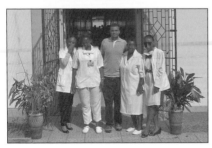

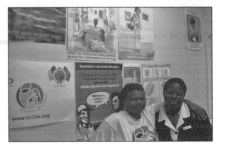

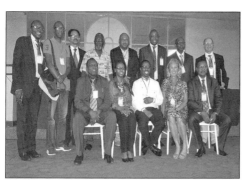
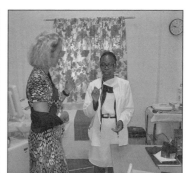
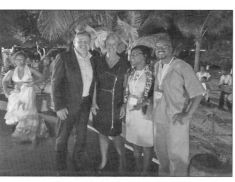
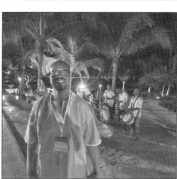
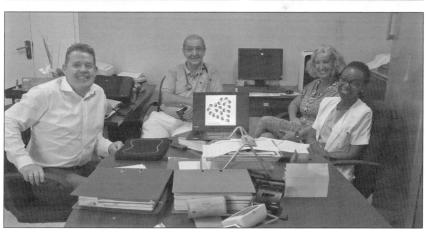

CHAPTER 8

Pericardial disease

Mpiko Ntsekhe

University of Cape Town/Groote Schuur Hospital, Cape Town, South Africa

8.0 Introduction

Inflammation, infection, and other noxious insults to the thin-layered membrane surrounding the heart are capable of triggering a range of responses within the pericardium, which often culminate in clinically evident disease of the pericardium. Traditionally, pericardial diseases are classified by mode of clinical presentation into the following: (a) acute pericarditis with or without pericardial effusion, (b) effusive pericarditis with or without tamponade (c) effusive constrictive pericarditis, and (d) constrictive pericarditis [10]. Pericardial disease is a relatively common cause of cardiac morbidity and mortality in sub-Saharan Africa [11]. In THESUS-HF, pericardial disease was as common a cause of HF as IHD (both approximately 7%) [12] (see Section 5). These results were similar to findings from the large Heart of Soweto Study, which was designed to ascertain the spectrum of heart disease among a prospective cohort of patients referred to one of Africa's largest hospitals for cardiac evaluation [13]. The predominant clinical presentations of pericardial disease in parts of Asia and in sub-Saharan Africa, where TB is endemic and coinfection with HIV is common, are effusive pericarditis with or without tamponade and constrictive pericarditis [14]. Tuberculous pericarditis results in high morbidity and mortality rates despite anti-TB therapy, pericardial drainage, or pericardiectomy [15–17]. Evidence from early studies of patients with tuberculous pericarditis showed that glucocorticoid therapy may improve outcomes and decrease mortality by reducing pericardial constriction and cardiac tamponade. A meta analysis comprising two randomized controlled trials examining glucocorticoid therapy for tuberculous pericarditis reported a nonsignificant reduction in mortality rates [18,19]. However, these studies were limited by small sample sizes and number of events recorded [18–20]. Preliminary data from a number of sources provide a potential mechanism via which adjunctive immunotherapy may improve outcomes in tuberculous pericarditis.

The Heart of Africa: Clinical Profile of an Evolving Burden of Heart Disease in Africa, First Edition.
Edited by Simon Stewart, Karen Sliwa, Ana Mocumbi, Albertino Damasceno, and Mpiko Ntsekhe.
© 2016 John Wiley & Sons, Ltd. Published 2016 by John Wiley & Sons, Ltd.

This evidence indicates that inflammation associated with TB may be reduced by corticosteroids while repeated doses of intradermal heat-killed *Mycobacterium indicus pranii* may increase CD4+ T-cell counts in HIV-positive patients and alter phenotype of the immune response within the pericardium [21–23]. However, a limitation of therapy is data suggesting the potential for an increased risk of cancer in HIV-infected patients [24,25]. It was on this basis that Mayosi and colleagues conducted the Investigation of the Management of Pericarditis (IMPI) randomized controlled trial of the efficacy and safety of adjunctive immunotherapy for patients with tuberculous pericarditis [26].

8.1 Prednisolone and *Mycobacterium indicus pranii* in tuberculous pericarditis

Mayosi BM, Ntsekhe M, Bosch J, Pandie S, Jung H, Gumedze F, Pogue J, Thabane L, Smieja M, Francis V, Joldersma L, Thomas KM, Thomas B, Awotedu AA, Magula NP, Naidoo DP, Damasceno A, Banda AC, Brown B, Manga P, Kirenga B, Mondo C, Mntla P, Tsitsi JM, Peters F, Essop MR, Russell JBW, Hakim J, Matenga J, Barasa AF, Sani MU, Olunuga T, Ogah O, Ansa V, Aje A, Danbauchi S, Ojji D, Yusuf S. Prednisolone and *Mycobacterium indicus pranii* in tuberculous pericarditis. *New England Journal of Medicine* 2014; 371(12):1121–30.

8.1.1 Study aims
This study evaluated the efficacy and safety of adjunctive prednisolone and *Mycobacterium indicus pranii* in African patients who had tuberculous pericarditis with or without concurrent HIV. It was hypothesized that adjunctive prednisolone (by suppressing intrapericardial inflammation), or intradermal *Mycobacterium indicus pranii* (by altering the cellular phenotype of the local immune response) would be of overall benefit with regard to major adverse pericardial disease events. A two-by-two factorial design was conducted to measure intradermal *Mycobacterium indicus pranii* and prednisolone for the treatment of tuberculous pericarditis compared with placebo. The study drugs used were donated and distributed to the research sites by Cadila Pharmaceuticals. The protocol was reviewed by the Canadian Institutes of Health Research and the South African Medical Research Council. Ethics approval was obtained at each participating site along with informed consent from all patients.

8.1.2 Study methods
8.1.2.1 Patient enrollment
Patients included in the study had pericardial effusion confirmed by echocardiography, had probable or definite tuberculous pericarditis, had been receiving anti-TB treatment for less than one week before enrollment, and were >18 years of age. Patients were excluded from the study if they had used glucocorticoids within the last 30 days, if they were pregnant, allergic, or hypersensitive to *Mycobacterium indicus pranii* preparation, or if another cause of pericardial disease was identified.

8.1.2.2 Study procedures

Patients were randomized into either prednisolone or *Mycobacterium indicus pranii* groups and both were compared with two independent placebo groups. With regard to the prednisolone comparison, placebo and prednisolone were given to the different comparison groups for 6 weeks. A dose of 120 mg was administered daily in the first week, 90 mg daily in the second week, 60 mg daily for the third week, 30 mg daily for the fourth week, 15 mg daily for the fifth week, and 5 mg daily for the last week. With regard to the *Mycobacterium indicus pranii* comparison, the placebo and the *Mycobacterium indicus pranii* were administered to both groups in five doses of 0.1 mL. The first dose was administered at baseline by a single injection into the deltoid muscle region of the upper arm, three successive injections were administered at the same site at 2 week intervals, and the remaining fifth dose administered at 3 months. HAART for HIV and antimicrobial treatment for TB was given to the trial patients according to the WHO guidelines [29–32]. No routine testing for drug resistance of either *Mycobacterium* TB isolates or HIV isolates was performed before or during treatment. Follow-up data collection comprised assessments of study outcomes (details in section below), recording of adverse events, and treatment adherence. These data were collected at the time of hospital discharge; at 2, 4, and 6 weeks; at 6 months; and then every 6 months for 2 years and every 12 months thereafter over the 5-year study period. Site monitoring throughout the study was performed through the project coordinating office according to a standard operating procedure.

8.1.2.3 Outcomes and statistical analysis

The primary efficacy outcome in the study was the composite of death, the first occurrence of cardiac tamponade requiring pericardiocentesis, or the development of constrictive pericarditis. The secondary efficacy outcomes were hospitalization as well as the individual components of the primary outcome. Cancer, opportunistic infections, CD4+ T-lymphocyte cell count, and the incidence of immune reconstitution inflammatory syndrome (in those with HIV) comprised the safety outcomes. The sample size calculation was based on the following assumptions: that the event rate among patients receiving placebos for both interventions would be 35% at a mean follow-up of 2 years, the rate of loss to follow-up would be 6%, and approximately 50% of the patients in each intervention's placebo group would receive an effective intervention that would result in 30% relative risk reduction in the event rate. Based on this, a sample size of 1,400 patients would result in 90% power to detect a 22.9% reduction in the hazard ratio, with use of a log-rank test and a two-sided type I error rate of 5%.

8.1.3 Study findings
8.1.3.1 Study population

The trial was conducted during the period January 2009 to February 2014. Patients were recruited from 19 hospitals in 8 African countries (South Africa, Mozambique, Malawi, Uganda, Zimbabwe, Sierra Leone, Kenya, and Nigeria). Overall, a total of 1,400 patients were recruited. These patients were randomized into either the placebo (n = 694; 49.6%) or the prednisolone (n = 706; 50.4%) group for 6 weeks (see Figure 8.1). Median follow-up period was 637 days. Primary outcome status was known for 1,371 (97.9%) of these patients. An additional 1,250 patients were randomized into either the placebo (n = 625; 50%) or the *Mycobacterium indicus pranii* (n = 625; 50%) group (Figure 8.1). Median follow-up period was 721 days. Primary outcome status was known for 1,223 (97.8%) of these patients.

Baseline characteristics of all those who participated in the study are presented in Table 8.1 with a similar profile evident according to group assignment. Both groups had more male than female patients. Approximately two-thirds had a large pericardial effusion, and pericardiocentesis was performed in over 60% of the patients. The diagnosis of tuberculous pericarditis was confirmed in 17.1% of patients, and over two-thirds were found to be HIV positive.

8.1.3.2 Treatment regimens and adherence

With regard to the comparison of placebo with prednisolone, 88.7% of the patients in the placebo group and 88.5% of those in the prednisolone group adhered to the regimen for the full study treatment of 6 weeks. A total of 44 (3.1%) patients received nonstudy glucocorticoids during the trial, and this rate was similar in the placebo and prednisolone groups. Adherence was slightly lower in the *Mycobacterium indicus pranii* and associated placebo group. A total of

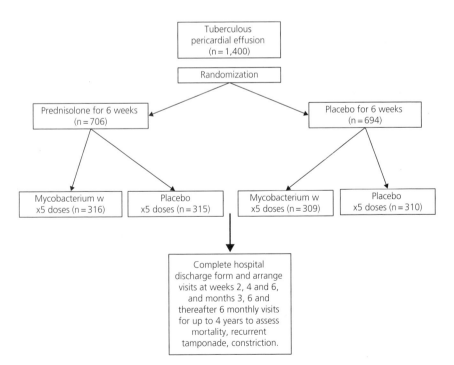

Figure 8.1 Trial study design.

81.4% of the patients in the placebo group and 75.9% of those in the *Mycobacterium indicus pranii* group adhered to the regimen for the full study treatment of 3 months. Of the 1,400 Prednisolone comparison patients enrolled in the trial, 14.5% were receiving HAART and 76.6% were receiving anti-TB treatment at the time of randomization. The growing use of HAART during the course of the trial is attributed to revised WHO guidelines recommending early HAART initiation in HIV-positive patients presenting with TB.

Table 8.1 Patients' baseline, 3-month follow-up, and outcome characteristics.

	Mycobacterium indicus pranii Group (n = 625)	Placebo Group (n = 625)	Prednisolone Group (n = 706)	Placebo Group (n = 694)
Age (years)	37.7 ± 12.5	39.3 ± 14.1	38.8 ± 13.5	38.5 ± 13.3
Men	333 (53.3%)	362 (57.9%)	389 (55.1%)	395 (56.9%)
Weight (kg)	58.6 ± 12.2	59.6 ± 12.0	59.6 ± 12.3	59.2 ± 12.1
Diagnosis at 3-Months				
Definite Tuberculous Pericarditis	100 (16.0%)	105 (16.8%)	116 (16.4%)	122 (17.6%)
Probable Tuberculous Pericarditis				
TB Proven Elsewhere	67 (10.7%)	53 (8.5%)	73 (10.3%)	63 (9.1%)
TB Not Proven Elsewhere	450 (72.0%)	462 (73.9%)	506 (71.7%)	506 (72.9%)
Non-tuberculous cause	8 (1.3%)	5 (0.8%)	11 (1.6%)	3 (0.4%)
HIV-status				
Positive	437 (69.9%)	403 (64.5%)	474 (67.1%)	465 (67.0%)
Negative	175 (28.0%)	209 (33.4%)	218 (30.9%)	213 (30.7%)
Unknown	13 (2.1%)	13 (2.1%)	14 (2.0%)	16 (2.3%)
Pericardiocentesis				
Performed	372 (59.5%)	381 (61.0%)	428 (60.6%)	419 (60.4%)
Not performed	253 (40.5%)	244 (39.0%)	278 (39.4%)	275 (39.6%)
Size of Pericardial Effusion				
Small, < 1 cm	58 (9.3%)	40 (6.4%)	51 (7.2%)	56 (8.1%)
Moderate, 1-2 cm	154 (24.6%)	140 (22.4%)	172 (24.4%)	159 (22.9%)
Large, > 2 cm	391 (62.6%)	428 (68.5%)	462 (65.4%)	460 (66.3%)
Not Measured	22 (3.5%)	17 (2.7%)	21 (3.0%)	19 (2.7%)
HAART	88 (14.1%)	84 (13.4%)	99 (14.0%)	104 (15.0%)
Anti-TB Therapy	460 (73.6%)	462 (73.9%)	541 (76.6%)	531 (76.5%)
Primary Composite Outcomes	156 (25.0%)	152 (24.3%)	168 (23.8%)	170 (24.5%)
Secondary Outcomes				
Cardiac Tamponade	22 (3.5%)	22 (3.5%)	22 (3.1%)	28 (4.0%)
Constrictive Pericarditis	36 (5.8%)	37 (5.9%)	31 (4.4%)	54 (7.8%)
Death From Any Cause	119 (19.0%)	111 (17.8%)	133 (18.8%)	115 (16.6%)
Hospitalisation	152 (24.3%)	141 (22.6%)	146 (20.7%)	175 (25.2%)

8.1.3.3 Prednisolone comparison

The rate of the primary composite outcome (cardiac tamponade requiring pericardiocentesis, constrictive pericarditis, or death) was 14.3 events per 100 person-years of follow-up in the prednisolone group and 14.8 per 100 person-years in the placebo group. When considered individually, there were no significant differences between groups in the rate of cardiac tamponade requiring pericardiocentesis or in the rate of death. The main causes of death were determined to be disseminated TB (18.6%), HIV infection (7.3%), pericarditis (23.8%), and other cardiovascular causes (5.7%). The placebo group had more hospitalizations and a higher rate of constrictive pericarditis than the prednisolone group. Table 8.2 shows the effects of prednisolone and *Mycobacterium indicus pranii* immunotherapy on safety outcomes. The incidence of opportunistic infection was 6.89 cases per 100 patient-years in the prednisolone group as compared with 5.91 per 100 patient-years in the placebo group. The proportion of patients with candidiasis, cancer, and HIV-related cancer was significantly higher in the prednisolone group when compared to the placebo group. Prednisolone was associated with an increased incidence of cancer relative to placebo. This increase was due to a higher incidence of HIV-related cancers in the prednisolone group. A list of the causes of cancer is provided in Table 8.3.

8.1.3.4 *Mycobacterium indicus pranii* comparison

The primary composite outcome rates and components, as well as the rates of opportunistic infection and hospitalization, did not differ significantly between the *Mycobacterium indicus pranii* group and the placebo group. However, as compared with placebo, *Mycobacterium indicus pranii* was significantly associated with an increased cancer incidence (0.92 versus 0.24 cases per 100 person-years; $p=0.03$), which was mainly due to an increase in HIV-related cancer (shown in Tables 8.2 and 8.3). There was a similar nonsignificant difference in the increase in CD4+ T-cell counts, HIV-related cancer, and one immune reconstitution inflammatory syndrome case in both groups. For obvious reasons, patients in the placebo group had fewer injection-site reactions than those in the *Mycobacterium indicus pranii* group. While the majority of these reactions were characterized by inflammation signs and minor symptoms, there was a significantly greater proportion of patients with abscess formation (15% versus 1%, $p<0.001$) in the *Mycobacterium indicus pranii* group than in the placebo group. These injection-site side effects negatively affected adherence to the treatment (21% nonadherence) in the *Mycobacterium indicus pranii* group.

8.1.3.5 Prednisolone and *Mycobacterium indicus pranii* interaction and subgroup analysis

There was no significant interaction between the effects of prednisolone and *Mycobacterium indicus pranii* on the primary efficacy and safety outcomes ($p>0.30$), except for injection-site reactions ($p=0.004$). However, 9 of the 13 cancer cases in the prednisolone group occurred in patients who also received *Mycobacterium*

Table 8.2 Effects of prednisolone and *Mycobacterium indicus pranii* immunotherapy on safety outcome.

Outcome	Prednisolone (n = 706)		Placebo (n = 694)		Mycobacterium indicus pranii (n = 625)		Placebo (n = 625)	
	No. of patients	No. of events/ 100 person-yr	No. of patients	No. of events/ 100 person-yr	No. of patients	No. of events/ 100 person-yr	No. of patients	No. of events/ 100 person-yr
Cancer	13 (1.8%)	1.05	4 (0.6%)	0.22	11 (1.8%)	0.92	3 (0.5%)	0.24
Candida infection	54 (7.6%)	4.68	36 (5.2%)	3.01	47 (7.5%)	4.17	37 (5.9%)	3.20
HIV-related cancer	9 (1.3%)	0.73	1 (0.1%)	0.08	7 (1.1%)	0.58	2 (0.3%)	0.16
Immune reconstitution disease	2 (0.3%)	0.16	1 (0.1%)	0.08	1 (0.2%)	0.08	1 (0.2%)	0.08
Opportunistic infection	78 (11%)	6.89	68 (9.8%)	5.11	75 (12%)	6.86	61 (9.8%)	5.45

Table 8.3 The causes of malignancy according to the prednisolone comparison.

	Prednisolone (n = 706)	Placebo (n = 649)
All malignancies	13 (1.8%)	4 (0.6%)
Gastric/colon cancer	1 (0.1%)	0 (0%)
Kaposi	7 (1%)	1 (0.1%)
Non-Hodgkin's lymphoma	2 (0.3%)	0 (0%)
Progression of preexisting malignancy	1 (0.1%)	1 (0.1%)
Other	2 (0.3%)	2 (0.3%)

indicus pranii. The number of cases is small, although a clinical interaction of the two interventions on cancer cannot be ruled out. As identified by forest plots, the effects of *Mycobacterium indicus pranii* immunotherapy and prednisolone therapy on the primary composite efficacy outcome were similar across the key subgroups (prespecified above).

8.1.4 Study interpretation

Overall, neither *Mycobacterium indicus pranii* immunotherapy nor prednisolone therapy had a significant effect on reducing the primary composite outcome of constrictive pericarditis, cardiac tamponade requiring pericardiocentesis, or mortality. Adjunctive prednisolone therapy decreased the incidence of hospitalization and constrictive pericarditis. However, both interventions increased the incidence of HIV-related cancer among trial patients. The trial had a number of strengths. First, a large cohort of 1,400 patients, 940 of whom were HIV positive, were recruited into the trial, providing a robust platform for testing the study hypotheses. Second, beyond examining treatment efficacy, treatment adherence and adverse events were carefully monitored and analyzed. Previous trials of adjunctive glucocorticoid therapy in those with tuberculous pericarditis were relatively small, included few HIV-infected patients, and provided little detail on potential adverse events. Most important, this was the first study to examine *Mycobacterium indicus pranii* immunotherapy in this patient population. A number of additional aspects to this study require comment. A dose of 120 mg per day of prednisolone was administered at baseline, which is identified to have a therapeutic effect when administered in combination with rifampin, an enzyme inducer that increases the metabolism of glucocorticoids. Throughout the study, prednisolone therapy adherence was high. The doses used throughout the 6-week period were sufficient to achieve a substantial anti-inflammatory effect, as there was a significant reduction in pericardial constriction. The reduction in the incidence of constrictive pericarditis also translated to fewer hospitalizations in the prednisolone-treated group. This is important because pericardiectomy is associated with high perioperative morbidity and mortality, and cardiac surgery is not widely available in many parts of sub-Saharan Africa with limited health care resources. The study also revealed a positive association between prednisolone therapy and HIV-related cancer. These results are consistent with two previous studies of HIV-associated TB, in which cases of Kaposi's sarcoma occurred only in the prednisolone-treated groups [24,25]. However, the association of HIV-related cancer with *Mycobacterium indicus pranii* immunotherapy observed in this study has not been reported previously. It is possible that adjunctive glucocorticoids and *Mycobacterium indicus pranii* act synergistically to increase the risk of cancer in immunosuppressed patients. Unfortunately, the available data on the interaction between *Mycobacterium indicus pranii* immunotherapy and adjunctive glucocorticoid therapy are limited [26].

8.1.5 Study limitations

This study had a number of limitations that also require comment. First, a diagnosis of TB either in the pericardium or elsewhere in the body was made in only one-quarter of the patients. This is because the diagnosis of extrapulmonary TB is challenging, and only a small proportion of such cases are treated on the basis of a definite diagnosis. Thus, one interpretation of the results may be that the intervention was ineffective due to the limited number of patients with diagnosed tuberculous pericarditis. However, this is unlikely as the results for those with definite TB and those with probable TB were consistent. Second, although the estimation of the sample size needed for this study was based on the clinical case definition of tuberculous pericarditis, it was expected that a small proportion of cases would have an alternative cause of pericarditis. This was indeed the case, with a small proportion (less than 2%) of patients having a diagnosis other than TB. Third, the trial was powered for a rate of nonadherence of 10% in the active-treatment groups. Although this rate was almost achieved in the prednisolone group (11%), the nonadherence rate was 21% in the *Mycobacterium indicus pranii* group, owing mainly to injection-site side effects. Therefore, the power of the study may have been diminished by the high nonadherence rates with respect to the analysis of the primary outcome in the *Mycobacterium indicus pranii* group. Finally, an interaction may have occurred between adjunctive prednisolone and *Mycobacterium indicus pranii*, which could result in each one either increasing or reducing the effects of the other, because prednisolone is immunosuppressive and *Mycobacterium indicus pranii* is immunostimulatory [26].

8.1.6 Study conclusions

In conclusion, *Mycobacterium indicus pranii* administered for 3 months combined with adjunctive prednisolone therapy for 6 weeks did not have a positive effect on the combined outcome of death from any cause, constrictive pericarditis, or cardiac tamponade requiring pericardiocentesis. There was an increased risk of HIV-related cancer when both therapies were administered in HIV-positive patients. However, the incidence of hospitalization and pericardial constriction were reduced through the use of adjunctive glucocorticoids. In addition, the beneficial effects of prednisolone with respect to hospitalization and pericardial constriction were similar in HIV-negative and HIV-positive patients.

CHAPTER 9

Human immunodeficiency virus–related heart disease

Friedrich Thienemann[1], Melinda Jane Carrington[2], Karen Sliwa[3], Mpiko Ntsekhe[4], and Simon Stewart[2]

[1] University of Cape Town, South Africa
[2] Australian Catholic University, Melbourne, Victoria, Australia
[3] University of Cape Town, South Africa; University of the Witwatersrand, Johannesburg, South Africa
[4] University of Cape Town/Groote Schuur Hospital, Cape Town, South Africa

9.0 Introduction

The Heart of Soweto Study has contributed to an improved, if not definitive, understanding of both communicable and noncommunicable forms of heart disease in the sub-Sahara African context. In this chapter the nexus between the underlying scourge of HIV/AIDS in communities such as Soweto and the range of related heart disease presentations (noting the specific focus on HIV cases and ACS presentations to be described in Chapter 10) is described. These data provide an important perspective on (and even counterpoint) to this phenomenon relative to reports derived from other developing countries and indeed high-income countries where affected cases are closely monitored and optimally treated [27].

9.1 The nexus between HIV/AIDS and heart disease in an urban African community

Sliwa K, Carrington MJ, Becker A, Thienemann F, Ntsekhe M, Stewart S. Contribution of the HIV/AIDS syndrome epidemic to de novo presentations of heart disease in the Heart of Soweto Study cohort. *European Heart Journal* 2012; 33(7):866–74. [1]

9.1.1 Study background

The worldwide pandemic of HIV is reported to contribute to 35 million new cases and 1.6 million deaths (2012). Sub-Saharan Africa alone accounts for almost two-thirds of all people living with HIV [28], although population infection rates have diverged as different public health policies have been implemented. As HIV infects the entire human immune system and various different organs, it increases one's chances of becoming infected with a number of different diseases. Even though CAD is a major public health concern in developed countries in post-HAART, the cardiac manifestations that are most associated with HIV in sub-Saharan Africa are PH, pericardial disease, and CMO [29–32]. However, as this population is constantly in a phase of transition, previous reports provide limited insight into cardiac manifestations in South Africa [33].

9.1.2 Study aims

The Heart of Soweto Study provided an opportunity to investigate previous HIV-related heart disease observation, as well as the demographic and clinical characteristics of the case presentations [13,34,35]. Therefore, the aim of this study was to examine the Heart of Soweto registry (see Section 3) in order to gain knowledge of the impact of HIV/AIDS on heart disease presentations in a typical African urban community at high risk of exposure to the virus. The study also focused on the potential impact of concurrently prescribed HAART.

9.1.3 Study methods

During the period 2006 to 2008 a total of 5,238 de novo patients presented to the Cardiology Unit of the Chris Hani Baragwanath Hospital in Soweto. Along with detailed clinical profiling (see Section 3), HIV status was documented and subject to clinical follow-up depending on case presentation, without enforcing mandatory reporting and testing (noting the sensitivity of HIV status in this context).

9.1.4 Study findings

In total, 518 (9.7%) of the 5,328 patients presenting with newly diagnosed heart disease were determined to be HIV positive; of these 403 (77.8%) underwent HIV testing at the time of diagnosis. Overall, 170 (42.2%) patients who were tested were newly discovered as HIV positive and received HIV counseling. As shown in Table 9.1, 320 (61.8%) HIV-positive patients were women and 500 (96.5%) were of African ancestry. HIV-positive patients were more likely to present with more severe anemia (p<0.001), more preserved estimated glomerular filtration rate (p<0.001), a higher heart rate (p<0.001), more LV systolic dysfunction (p=0.036) associated with lower mean LVEF (p=0.002) and to present as NYHA Class II or higher than the rest of the study cohort. At the same time, they presented with lower BMI (p<0.001) and lower BP (p<0.001 for systolic and diastolic BP). Figure 9.1 shows the primary diagnoses among HIV-positive patients, with HIV-related CMOs being the most common (37.8%) and CHD being the least common (0.4%). Relative to the rest of the study cohort, HIV-positive patients were more likely to present with cerebrovascular disease (p=0.002), HIV-related CMO (p<0.001), and pericarditis (p<0.001).

Table 9.1 Patients' demographic and clinical characteristics and primary diagnosis.

	HIV-Positive Patients (n = 518)	Remaining de novo Patients (n = 4,810)
Demographic characteristics		
African ancestry	500 (96.5%)	4,126 (85.8%)
Age (years)	39 ± 13	53 ± 17
Born in Soweto	195 (37.6%)	1,730 (36.0%)
Education (<6-years)	203 (39.2%)	2,061 (42.9%)
Women	320 (61.8%)	2,850 (59.3%)
Clinical characteristics		
Anemia	157 (30.3%)	767 (16.0%)
BMI (kg/m²)	24.4 ± 4.3	28.6 ± 7.5
Systolic BP (mm Hg)	119 ± 22	134 ± 27
Diastolic BP (mm Hg)	72 ± 14	76 ± 15
Median eGFR	105 (84–137)	85 (63–108)
Heart rate (beats/min)	99 ± 22	84 ± 19
LV end-diameter diastole (mm)	49 ± 9	47 ± 11
LV end-diameter systole (mm)	35 ± 11	34 ± 12
LVEF (%)	52 ± 16	55 ± 16
LV systolic dysfunction	148 (28.6%)	1,041 (21.6%)
RV systolic pressure (≥35 mm Hg)	51 (9.8%)	393 (8.2%)
NYHA Class II, III, Or IV	400 (77.2%)	3,245 (67.5%)
Palpitations	289 (55.8%)	2,513 (52.3%)
Primary diagnosis		
Cerebrovascular disease	18 (3.5%)	69 (1.4%)
CAD	14 (2.7%)	567 (11.8%)
HIV-related CMO	196 (37.8%)	0 (0%)
Hypertension	42 (8.1%)	38 (0.8%)
Pericarditis	65 (12.6%)	58 (1.2%)
RHF	34 (6.6%)	311 (6.5%)
Valve disease	58 (11.2%)	668 (13.9%)

9.1.4.1 HIV-related dilated CMO

As shown in Table 9.2, those presenting with an HIV-related dilated CMO were predominantly women (59.7%) and of African ancestry (98.5%). Affected women were more likely to have a BMI >30 (OR 3.47, 95% CI 1.06–11.5; p = 0.024) and affected men to report cigarette smoking (OR 8.63, 95% CI 4.45–16.8; p < 0.0001). Pharmacological therapy most commonly comprised loop diuretics (prescribed in 50.5% of cases) in addition to spironolactone (35.2%), a beta blocker (29.1%), an ACE inhibitor (26%), aspirin (14.8%), and digoxin (12.2%).

HIV-related PAH was found in 42 patients, with more men than woman affected (73.8%). Men were significantly older (51 ± 18 versus 39 ± 14 years; p < 0.0001); however, there were no differences in clinical parameters according to the presence or absence of HAART. Out of 581 de novo patients who were

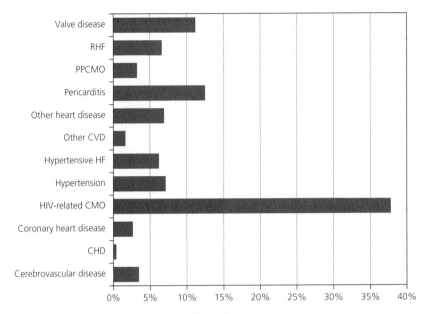

Figure 9.1 HIV-positive patient's primary diagnosis.

diagnosed with CAD, 14 (2.4%) patients were found to be HIV positive (mean age of 41 ± 13 years and the majority being of African ancestry).

9.1.5 Study interpretation

As originally reported, this was the largest study of HIV-related cardiac manifestations in sub-Saharan Africa. As in previous reports [31], concurrent HIV infection was most commonly associated with pericardial disease (2.4% of all case presentations) and HIV-related CMO (3.7%) and to a much lesser extent with CAD and PAH (0.8% and 0.3%) [13,34]. Encouragingly, the much-predicted "tsunami" of HIV-related cardiac cases had yet to appear at the time of this study. However, a number of aspects around the study findings require further consideration and research given the size of the underlying problem and the potential for future cardiac cases. The complex interplay between HAART and cardiac function is yet to be fully elucidated. However, CMO is known to be a late-stage manifestation of HIV infection, being a trigger for HAART independent of the CD4 count [36,37]. Its etiology and pathogenesis is poorly described, with multiple factors seemingly in play. These include (a) direct HIV infection of the myocardial cells, (b) opportunistic infection with other pathogens, (c) an autoimmune response, (d) concurrent drug abuse and/or cardiotoxicity, (e) malnutrition, and (f) endocrine disturbances [38–40]. It is of clinical significance that the incidence of HIV-related CMO has declined with the introduction of HAART in high-income countries [41]. In contrast to this phenomenon, it has been predicted that HAART will increase the number of cases of ACS in treated individuals. This is discussed in

Table 9.2 HIV-related CMO patients' demographic and clinical characteristics.

	Women (n = 117)	Men (n = 79)	All (n = 196)
Demographic characteristics			
African ancestry	115 (98.3%)	78 (98.7%)	193 (98.5%)
Age, years	39 ± 13	45 ± 13	41 ± 13
Born in Soweto	49 (41.9%)	31 (39.2%)	80 (40.8%)
Education (<6 years)	41 (35.0%)	37 (46.8%)	78 (39.8%)
Women	117 (100%)	0 (0%)	117 (59.7%)
Clinical characteristics			
Anemia	36 (30.8%)	21 (26.6%)	57 (29.1%)
BMI >30 (kg/m²)	15 (12.8%)	3 (3.8%)	18 (9.2%)
Cigarette smoking	33 (28.2%)	61 (77.2%)	94 (48.0%)
Median eGFR (IQR)	97 (76–128)	102 (76–140)	99 (76–133)
Heart rate (beats/min)	104 ± 23	100 ± 18	102 ± 21
LVEF (%)	47 ± 17	43 ± 17	46 ± 17
LV systolic dysfunction	66 (56.4%)	53 (67.1%)	119 (60.7%)
LV diastolic dysfunction	64 (54.7%)	52 (65.8%)	116 (59.2%)
LV end-diameter diastole (mm)	49 ± 8.7	54 ± 8.4	51 ± 9.2
LV end-diameter systole (mm)	37 ± 11	40 ± 11	39 ± 12
NYHA Class II, III or IV	102 (87.2%)	66 (83.5%)	168 (85.7%)
Palpitations	84 (71.8%)	36 (45.6%)	120 (61.2%)
RHF	24 (20.5%)	11 (13.9%)	35 (17.9%)
Other complications			
Cerebrovascular disease	3 (2.6%)	2 (2.5%)	5 (2.6%)
Hypertension	18 (15.4%)	16 (20.3%)	34 (17.4%)
Pericardial effusion	18 (15.4%)	13 (16.5%)	31 (15.8%)
RHF	24 (20.5%)	11 (13.9%)	35 (17.9%)
Type 2 diabetes	3 (2.6%)	3 (3.8%)	6 (3.1%)
Valve dysfunction	32 (27.4%)	30 (38.0%)	62 (31.6%)
Prescribed medication			
ACE inhibitor	30 (25.6%)	21 (26.6%)	51 (26.0%)
Aspirin	13 (11.1%)	16 (20.3%)	29 (14.8%)
Beta-blockers	35 (29.9%)	22 (27.9%)	57 (29.1%)
Digoxin	20 (17.1%)	4 (5.1%)	24 (12.2%)
Loop diuretic	59 (50.4%)	40 (50.6%)	99 (50.5%)
Spironolactone	39 (33.3%)	30 (38.0%)	69 (35.2%)

greater detail in Chapter 10. However, it is important to note that HIV infection may independently predispose toward coronary events via a combination of endothelial dysfunction, a proinflammatory state, dyslipidemia, and thrombosis [31,42–44]. Similarly, HAART has the potential to induce an adverse metabolic phenotype leading to an AMI (particularly with prolonged therapy); however, these data are particularly important in described cardiac manifestations relating to HIV/AIDS in a largely HAART-untreated population. They provide important insights into the direct cardiac consequences of HIV infection. While HIV/AIDS has already affected >5.5 million individuals in South Africa [31], it is expected to increase dramatically in the future.

9.1.6 Study limitations

Beyond the broader limitations of the overall study, there were a number of specific limitations relating to the study of HIV and heart disease. First, this study consisted of patients who were seeking specialist care at the hospital at the time of recruitment; therefore, these patients presented with more advanced forms of heart disease. Second, definitive HIV status for each patient was not validated; however, more definitive investigation of HIV status occurred when clinically indicated. More important, this was not a study of HIV-positive patients investigated for cardiac abnormalities and/or established heart disease.

9.1.7 Study conclusions

Despite these important limitations, these data provide an important historical context to the status of the HIV pandemic and related manifestations of cardiac disease in South Africa and wider sub-Saharan Africa. Immediately following the study period, the South African government initiated a national program of HAART application in those infected with HIV. As noted in the original report, this will hopefully have a mitigating effect on presentations of HIV-related CMO and pericardial effusion/pericarditis. Given the complexities of the underlying infection and its treatment, ongoing surveillance is required to document and respond to the impact of wider HAART implementation on lipid levels and atherosclerotic events in treated individuals. As described in Chapter 6, these findings have important clinical and public health implications for sub-Saharan Africa, the wider African continent, and other parts of the world in epidemiological transition where a confluence of noncommunicable and communicable forms of heart disease is starting to emerge.

S4.2 Infectious heart disease in Africa—not just a historical footnote

When considering study findings focused on acquired forms of heart disease in pediatric patients, presented in Section 2, and the additional data presented in this section of an equivalent substantive burden of infectious forms of heart disease (with typically poor outcomes) in the adult population, it is clear that there is a long way to go before communicable heart disease becomes a rare and historical footnote, as it has in many high-income countries. Tuberculous pericarditis is the most common and significant cause of pericardial disease in sub-Saharan Africa and other regions of the world where TB is endemic. Importantly, it is a major cause of cardiac morbidity and mortality. Coinfection with HIV occurs in close to two-thirds of patients with tuberculous pericarditis and is an important determinant of outcomes and response to adjunctive therapy. This was demonstrated in the large IMPI randomized controlled trial, which compared two independent immune modulators—*Mycobacterium indicus pranii* and prednisolone—to placebo. In this multicenter study conducted across the African continent, neither therapy reduced the composite outcome of death, constrictive pericarditis, or cardiac tamponade requiring pericardiocentesis. In those who were HIV infected, while both interventions increased the risk of developing HIV-associated malignancies, adjunctive prednisolone alone reduced the rate of constrictive pericarditis and hospitalizations. In those who were HIV uninfected, rates of constrictive pericarditis and hospitalization were significantly reduced by corticosteroids with little evidence of any significant adverse effects. Equivalent to the innovative research and trials around understanding and treating PPCMO in African women (see Section 1), these findings strengthen the need for greater investment in African-specific research for African-specific health issues. Much of the clinical evidence and treatments for heart disease from high-income countries focus on noncommunicable disease. Without a "healthy" commercial market, there is less incentive (beyond charitable organizations) to invest in treatments that will predominantly benefit Africans—and yet the health benefits would be substantial and profound.

References

1 Carapetis JR. *The Current Evidence of the Burden of Group A Streptococcal Disease*. Geneva: World Health Organization, 2004.

2 Carapetis JR, Steer AC, Mulholland EK, Weber M. The global burden of group A streptococcal diseases. *Lancet Infect Dis*. 2005;5:685–94.

3 Carapetis JR. Rheumatic heart disease in developing countries. *N Engl J Med*. 2007;357:439–41.

4 Otto CM. Valvular stenosis and valvular regurgitation. *Textbook of Clinical Echocardiography*, 3rd ed. Philadelphia: Elsevier Saunders, 2004. p. 281–328.

5 Tibazarwa KB, Volmink JA, Mayosi BM. Incidence of acute rheumatic fever in the world: a systematic review of population-based studies. *Heart*. 2008;94(12):1534–40.

6 Clur SA. Frequency and severity of rheumatic heart disease in the catchment area of Gauteng hospitals, 1993–1995. *S Afr Med J*. 2006;96(3 Pt 2):233–7.

7 Nkomo VT, Gardin JM, Skelton TN, Gottdiener JS, Scott CG, Enriquez-Sarano M. Burden of valvular heart diseases: a population-based study. *Lancet*. 2006;368(9540):1005–11.

8 Perez de Isla L, Zamorano J, Quezada M, Almeria C, Rodrigo JL, Serra V, et al. Functional mitral regurgitation after a first non-ST-segment elevation acute coronary syndrome: contribution to congestive heart failure. *Eur Heart J*. 2007;28(23):2866–72.

9 Ypenburg C, Lancellotti P, Tops LF, Boersma E, Bleeker GB, Holman ER, et al. Mechanism of improvement in mitral regurgitation after cardiac resynchronization therapy. *Eur Heart J*. 2008;29(6):757–65.

10 Troughton RW, Asher CR, Klein PA. Pericarditis. *Lancet*. 2004;363(9410):717–27.

11 Mayosi BM. Contemporary trends in the epidemiology and management of cardiomyopathy and pericarditis in sub-Saharan Africa. *Heart*. 2007;93(10):1176–83.

12 Damasceno A, Mayosi BM, Sani M, Ogah OS, Mondo C, Ojji D, et al. The causes, treatment, and outcome of acute heart failure in 1006 Africans from 9 countries. *Arch Intern Med*. 2012;172(18):1386–94.

13 Sliwa K, Wilkinson D, Hansen C, Ntyintyane L, Tibazarwa K, Becker A, et al. Spectrum of heart disease and risk factors in a black urban population in South Africa (the Heart of Soweto Study): a cohort study. *Lancet*. 2008;371(9616):915–22.

14 Ntsekhe M, Mayosi BM. Tuberculous pericarditis with and without HIV. *Heart Failure Reviews*. 2013;18(3):367–73.

15 Mayosi BM, Burgess LJ, Doubell AF. Tuberculous pericarditis. *Circulation*. 2005;112(23):3608–16.

16 Mayosi BM, Wiysonge CS, Ntsekhe M, Gumedze F, Volmink JA, Maartens G, et al. Mortality in patients treated for tuberculous pericarditis in sub-Saharan Africa. *S Afr Med J*. 2008;98(1):36–40.

17 Mutyaba AK, Balkaran S, Cloete R, du Plessis N, Badri M, Brink J, et al. Constrictive pericarditis requiring pericardiectomy at Groote Schuur Hospital, Cape Town, South Africa:

The Heart of Africa: Clinical Profile of an Evolving Burden of Heart Disease in Africa, First Edition.
Edited by Simon Stewart, Karen Sliwa, Ana Mocumbi, Albertino Damasceno, and Mpiko Ntsekhe.
© 2016 John Wiley & Sons, Ltd. Published 2016 by John Wiley & Sons, Ltd.

causes and perioperative outcomes in the HIV era (1990–2012). *J Thorac Cardiovasc Surg.* 2014;148(6):3058–65 e1.

18 Mayosi BM, Ntsekhe M, Volmink JA, Commerford PJ. Interventions for treating tuberculous pericarditis. *Cochrane Database Syst Rev.* 2002(4):CD000526.

19 Ntsekhe M, Wiysonge C, Volmink JA, Commerford PJ, Mayosi BM. Adjuvant corticosteroids for tuberculous pericarditis: promising, but not proven. *QJM.* 2003;96(8):593–9.

20 Critchley JA, Young F, Orton L, Garner P. Corticosteroids for prevention of mortality in people with tuberculosis: a systematic review and meta-analysis. *Lancet Infect Dis.* 2013;13(3):223–37.

21 Gupta A, Ahmad FJ, Ahmad F, Gupta UD, Natarajan M, Katoch V, et al. Efficacy of Mycobacterium indicus pranii immunotherapy as an adjunct to chemotherapy for tuberculosis and underlying immune responses in the lung. *PLoS One.* 2012;7(7):e39215.

22 Mathur A, Mallia MB, Subramanian S, Banerjee S, Sarma HD, Kothari K, et al. Preparation and in vivo evaluation of (99 m)TcN-tertiary butyl xanthate as a potential myocardial agent. *Appl Radiat Isot.* 2006;64(6):663–7.

23 Saini V, Raghuvanshi S, Talwar GP, Ahmed N, Khurana JP, Hasnain SE, et al. Polyphasic taxonomic analysis establishes Mycobacterium indicus pranii as a distinct species. *PLoS One.* 2009;4(7):e6263.

24 Elliott AM, Halwiindi B, Bagshawe A, Hayes RJ, Luo N, Pobee JO, et al. Use of prednisolone in the treatment of HIV-positive tuberculosis patients. *Q J Med.* 1992;85(307–308):855–60.

25 Elliott AM, Luzze H, Quigley MA, Nakiyingi JS, Kyaligonza S, Namujju PB, et al. A randomized, double-blind, placebo-controlled trial of the use of prednisolone as an adjunct to treatment in HIV-1-associated pleural tuberculosis. *J Infect Dis.* 2004;190(5):869–78.

26 Mayosi BM, Ntsekhe M, Bosch J, Pogue J, Gumedze F, Badri M, et al. Rationale and design of the Investigation of the Management of Pericarditis (IMPI) trial: a 2 x 2 factorial randomized double-blind multicenter trial of adjunctive prednisolone and Mycobacterium w immunotherapy in tuberculous pericarditis. *Am Heart J.* 2013;165(2):109–15 e3.

27 Thienemann F, Sliwa K, Rockstroh JK. HIV and the heart: the impact of antiretroviral therapy: a global perspective. *Eur Heart J.* 2013;34(46):3538–46.

28 Joint United Nations Programme on HIV/AIDS (UNAIDS). *Global Report: UNAIDS Report on the Global AIDS Epidemic 2013.* UNAIDS, 2013.

29 Becker AC, Sliwa K, Stewart S, Libhaber E, Essop AR, Zambakides CA, et al. Acute coronary syndromes in treatment-naïve black South Africans with human immunodeficiency virus infection. *J Interv Cardiol.* 2010;23(1):70–7.

30 Khunnawat C, Mukerji S, Havlichek D, Jr., Touma R, Abela GS. Cardiovascular manifestations in human immunodeficiency virus-infected patients. *Am J Cardiol.* 2008;102(5):635–42.

31 Ntsekhe M, Mayosi BM. Cardiac manifestations of HIV infection: an African perspective. *Nat Clin Pract Cardiovasc Med.* 2009;6(2):120–7.

32 Reinsch N, Neuhaus K, Esser S, Potthoff A, Hower M, Brockmeyer NH, et al. Prevalence of cardiac diastolic dysfunction in HIV-infected patients: results of the HIV-HEART study. *HIV Clin Trials.* 2010;11(3):156–62.

33 Vedanthan R, Fuster V. Cardiovascular disease in Sub-Saharan Africa: a complex picture demanding a multifaceted response. *Nat Clin Pract Cardiovasc Med.* 2008;5(9):516–7.

34 Stewart S, Carrington M, Pretorius S, Methusi P, Sliwa K. Standing at the crossroads between new and historically prevalent heart disease: effects of migration and socio-economic factors in the Heart of Soweto cohort study. *Eur Heart J.* 2011;32(4):492–9.

35 Stewart S, Libhaber E, Carrington M, Damasceno A, Abbasi H, Hansen C, et al. The clinical consequences and challenges of hypertension in urban-dwelling black Africans: insights from the Heart of Soweto Study. *Int J Cardiol.* 2011;146(1):22–7.

36 Bijl M, Dieleman JP, Simoons M, van der Ende ME. Low prevalence of cardiac abnormalities in an HIV-seropositive population on antiretroviral combination therapy. *J Acquir Immune Defic Syndr*. 2001;27(3):318–20.

37 World Health Organization. Antiretroviral therapy for HIV infection in adults and adolescents: recommendations for a public health approach. Revision. *World Health Organization*, 2006.

38 Monsuez JJ, Escaut L, Teicher E, Charniot JC, Vittecoq D. Cytokines in HIV-associated cardiomyopathy. *Int J Cardiol*. 2007;120(2):150–7.

39 Patel RC, Frishman WH. Cardiac involvement in HIV infection. *Med Clin North Am*. 1996;80(6):1493–512.

40 Wu TC, Pizzorno MC, Hayward GS, Willoughby S, Neumann DA, Rose NR, et al. In situ detection of human cytomegalovirus immediate-early gene transcripts within cardiac myocytes of patients with HIV-associated cardiomyopathy. *AIDS*. 1992;6(8):777–85.

41 Barbaro G. HIV-associated cardiomyopathy etiopathogenesis and clinical aspects. *Herz*. 2005;30(6):486–92.

42 D.A.D. Study Group, Friis-Moller N, Reiss P, Sabin CA, Weber R, Monforte A, et al. Class of antiretroviral drugs and the risk of myocardial infarction. *N Engl J Med*. 2007;356(17): 1723–35.

43 Mulligan K, Grunfeld C, Tai VW, Algren H, Pang M, Chernoff DN, et al. Hyperlipidemia and insulin resistance are induced by protease inhibitors independent of changes in body composition in patients with HIV infection. *J Acquir Immune Defic Syndr*. 2000;23(1):35–43.

44 Riddler SA, Smit E, Cole SR, Li R, Chmiel JS, Dobs A, et al. Impact of HIV infection and HAART on serum lipids in men. *JAMA*. 2003;289(22):2978–82.

SECTION 5

Noncommunicable disease

Albertino Damasceno

Universidade Eduardo Mondlane, Maputo, Mozambique

S5.1 A new health phenomenon in Africa—noncommunicable diseases

Noncommunicable diseases are new phenomena in the disease pattern of African countries. Their appearance in most African countries is recent, but their relative burden is different, undoubtedly due to the diverse economic profiles of those countries and their relative phases of epidemiologic transition [1–3]. Both stroke and ACS are increasing in frequency. Nevertheless, if we could synthesize the phenomena for the African continent we would say that the major cause of vascular end organ damage seen in sub-Saharan Africa is still precipitated by highly preventable strokes. In contrast, ACSs are an increasing but still infrequent clinical phenomenon in this setting. Specifically speaking about stroke, an important issue was highlighted in a recent paper analyzing the global burden of stroke worldwide [4]. Not only is stroke incidence increasing in LMIC (while decreasing in high-income countries), but this incidence rate has also exceeded by 20% the equivalent rates observed in high-income countries [4]. Another recently published paper reported on the first population survey of the incidence of stroke in Africa [5]. Undertaken in Tanzania, this seminal study revealed that the incidence of stroke in Dar es Salaam far exceeds the rate observed in the black African population of Manhattan, which in turn is double the incidence of the white population in the same place [5]. These two papers highlight the enormous burden of stroke in Africa and the need to build both research and clinical capacity to tackle the individual and societal consequences that burden engenders. Looking to the clinical characteristics of stroke in Africa, the two most important aspects are the younger age of incidence and the higher prevalence of the most devastating of stroke events—hemorrhagic episodes [6]. Most African studies show that stroke events occur 10 years before their onset

The Heart of Africa: Clinical Profile of an Evolving Burden of Heart Disease in Africa, First Edition.
Edited by Simon Stewart, Karen Sliwa, Ana Mocumbi, Albertino Damasceno, and Mpiko Ntsekhe.
© 2016 John Wiley & Sons, Ltd. Published 2016 by John Wiley & Sons, Ltd.

in high-income countries. Accordingly, a large percentage of de novo strokes occur before the age of 45 years in those of African ancestry – the equivalent, negative impact on individual and societal productivity and wealth potential being that much more profound than in high-income countries. In simple terms, this means that in Africa, stroke kills and disables people in the active phase of life, exacerbating the economic burden of already poor families. The other important factor is the high prevalence of hemorrhagic strokes. While in most high-income countries hemorrhagic stroke accounts for less than 10% of stroke cases, in several African studies this proportion was as high as 40% [7]. These two characteristics reflect the phenomenon of epidemiologic transition currently underway in most African countries.

As described in Section 3, hypertension is extremely prevalent and poorly controlled in most sub-Saharan African countries; the affected population is young, and diabetes and dyslipidemia, although increasing, remain less frequent than in high-income countries [8]. As will be described in Chapter 13, cases of hypertensive HF are likely to rise. However, stroke is already a major consequence of uncontrolled hypertension across the continent. Hemorrhagic stroke carries a higher mortality rate than its ischemic counterpart, and stroke patients in Africa are admitted to general wards where basic but specific treatments of the acute phase simply do not exist. These are probably the two most crucial contributors to the high mortality rate of stroke in Africa.

On this basis, this section presents two streams of research in this context. Chapter 10 presents a body of research focusing on the prevalence and characteristics of ACS in those captured by the Heart of Soweto Study and subjected to more intensive clinical and basic research profiling. In contrast, Chapter 11 summarizes the results of a population study of stroke in the city of Maputo, Mozambique. Both research programs, in addition to the key publications highlighted above, have been instrumental in highlighting the evolving issue of stroke and ACS from a uniquely African context.

S5.1.1 Geographical context

Section 5 of this book begins in Chapter 10 with the South African subset of an international multicenter registry before moving to two studies based in Soweto (for profiles of Soweto and South Africa, see Section 1). Chapter 11 shifts to the southeastern section of the continent, highlighting the Mozambican capital city of Maputo (for an introduction to Mozambique, refer to Section 2).

Maputo is the capital, largest city, and administrative hub of Mozambique. With a population of approximately 1.87 million individuals, Maputo is home to 56 ethnic groups and many associated native languages, while Portuguese is the official language [9]. Due to rapid expansion, the city is facing increased pressure on critical infrastructure, and around three-quarters of the population are housed in informal or unplanned settlements in suboptimal environmental conditions, with associated negative health implications [10]. Health systems and other basic public services are also overburdened, and high unemployment and food insecurity are continuing concerns [11,12]. However, levels of literacy and educational attainment are reported to be higher in Maputo than in neighbouring areas, although this is subject to notable gender inequality, which also affects health education and access to health care [13]. Average life expectancy in Maputo is 57 years [14,15], and close to 20% of residents aged 15 or above are infected with HIV/AIDS [16]. However, rates of infant and child mortality in the city are lower than reported in other parts of Mozambique [17].

CHAPTER 10

Acute coronary syndrome in the African context

Anthony Becker

University of the Witwatersrand, Johannesburg, South Africa

10.0 Introduction

In this chapter we summarize the findings of one of the first published registries examining the management and subsequent health outcomes of patients admitted to hospital for ACS in South Africa—a subset analysis of the wider, international ACCESS (Acute Coronary Events—a Multinational Survey of Current Management Strategies) registry. In contrast to the description of registry data, we also describe a sequential series of prospective studies from an area of high HIV prevalence, exploring the relationship between HIV infection and CAD from clinical and angiographic features through to the etiopathogenic link between HIV infection and atherothrombosis.

10.1 Management of ACS in South Africa: the ACCESS registry

Schamroth C & the ACCESS South Africa Investigators. Management of ACS in South Africa: Insights from the ACCESS (Acute Coronary Events—a multinational survey of current management strategies) registry. *Cardiovascular Journal of Africa* 2012; 23(7):365–70.

10.1.1 Study background

As described in Section 3, the pattern of CVD (including AMI) and its associated major risk factors (including hypertension, dyslipidemia, cigarette smoking, diabetes, and physical inactivity) varies according to the economic stage and development of a country due to epidemiological transition [1–3]. This means that sub-Saharan Africa is likely to experience an evolving but inherently heterogeneous burden of noncommunicable forms of heart disease in particular over the next decade or so.

The Heart of Africa: Clinical Profile of an Evolving Burden of Heart Disease in Africa, First Edition.
Edited by Simon Stewart, Karen Sliwa, Ana Mocumbi, Albertino Damasceno, and Mpiko Ntsekhe.

As also noted previously, notwithstanding the important evidence from the African INTERHEART study around common pathways to AMI [18], the majority of information pertaining to the prevention and management of heart disease is obtained from developed/Westernized countries. Such information is not readily applicable to resource-poor regions of the world [19–24]. Therefore, there is a need to establish registries in developing countries to increase awareness of the burden of heart disease and other common forms of CVD and to inform the application of preventive and management strategies applicable to the local health care environment.

10.1.2 Study aims

The overall aim of the ACCESS registry was to advance the understanding of the epidemiology, management/treatment, and 1-year outcomes of ACS across a range of LMIC, including South Africa.

10.1.3 Study methods

ACCESS was a prospective, observational, multinational registry in patients hospitalized for an acute coronary event. Overall, patients were enrolled from 134 sites in 19 countries in North and South Africa, Latin America, and the Middle East. As per convention, ACS encompassed the following diagnoses—unstable angina, non-ST segment elevation myocardial infarction (NSTEMI), and ST segment elevation myocardial infarction (STEMI). For the purpose of this chapter, the results primarily focus on the South African cohort. Patient eligibility criteria included age ≥21 years, presence of ischemic symptoms associated with ACS within 24 hours of hospitalization, presence of cardiac-associated changes on ECG, medical documentation of CAD, and an increase in a cardiac biochemical marker of myocardial necrosis. Patients were excluded if they presented with symptoms precipitated by a secondary condition, such as noncardiac trauma, HF, or anemia, or if they were participating in concomitant clinical trials.

10.1.4 Study findings

A total of 12,068 patients were enrolled in the ACCESS registry from January 2007 to January 2008. From this, 642 (5.3%) patients composed the South African cohort, 615 (95.8%) of whom were confirmed to have ACS. Complete follow-up data at 1 year was available for 548 (89.1%) patients due to the fact that 35 (5.7%) had died and 32 (5.2%) were lost to follow-up (see Figure 10.1). At hospital discharge, the most common diagnosis was non–ST-segment elevation ACS (59.9% of patients) including (32.4%) and unstable angina (26.4%). Within the South African cohort, 36 (5.9%) patients were of African ancestry, 66 (10.7%) were of mixed descent, 140 (22.8%) were Asian, and 373 (60.7%) were Caucasian. The population consisted of 467 (75.9%) men with a mean age of 58.0 ± 12.1 years. STEMI patients were younger than the rest (mean age 54.4 years versus 60.5 years).

As shown in Table 10.1, 345 (56.1%) of the South African patients had dyslipidemia, 320 (52.0%) had a family history of CVD, 287 (46.7%) had a history of angina,

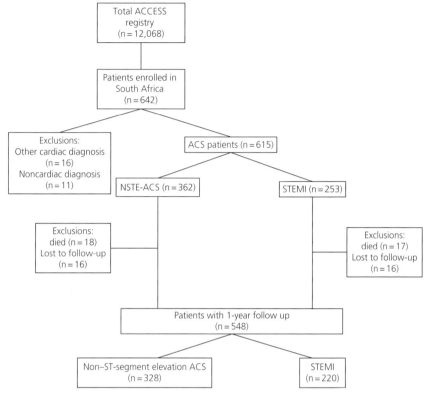

Figure 10.1 Study flow chart.

and 181 (29.4%) had myocardial infarction (MI). When compared to the entire ACCESS cohort, more patients in the South African cohort had prior coronary artery bypass graft (CABG) surgery (10.2% versus 4.9%), prior percutaneous coronary intervention (PCI) (19.0% versus 12.2%), and were current smokers (43.9% versus 39.1%). However, there were fewer patients with diabetes (23.9% versus 34.8%) but an almost equal amount of those with hypertension (55.6% versus 55.1%). Forty-nine percent of patients reported either moderate or heavy alcohol intake, and were all predominately overweight (BMI 28.4 ± 5.2kg/m², with only 25% of patients having a BMI below 25 kg/m². Women with STEMI had a larger waist circumference than the rest (98.6 ± 3.6 cm versus 95.1 ± 14.0 cm), while men with STEMI had a smaller waist circumference than the rest (99.9 ± 12.6 cm versus 103.1 ± 12.5 cm).

10.1.4.1 Acute management

Overall, South African patients were treated far more aggressively than the remainder of the registry cohort. Specifically, 18% of South African patients received thrombolytic therapy (most commonly streptokinase [55%]), which was consistent with the overall ACCESS cohort. Alternatively, a higher proportion underwent

Table 10.1 Patients' baseline characteristics according to the South African cohort and the entire ACCESS Registry.

	South Africa			Entire ACCESS Registry (n = 12,068)
	NSTE-ACS (n = 362)	STEMI (n = 253)	All (n = 615)	
Discharge diagnosis				
History of Angina	216 (59.7%)	71 (28.1%)	287 (46.7%)	5,293 (43.8%)
BMI (kg/m²)	28.7	28.1	28.4	27.0
Congestive HF	27 (7.5%)	9 (3.6%)	36 (5.9%)	640 (5.3%)
Current smoking	133 (36.7%)	135 (53.6%)	268 (43.9%)	4,730 (39.1%)
Diabetes	97 (26.8%)	50 (19.8%)	147 (23.9%)	4,208 (34.8%)
Dyslipidemia	228 (63.0%)	117 (46.2%)	345 (56.1%)	4,864 (40.3%)
Family history of CVD	194 (53.6%)	126 (49.8%)	320 (52.0%)	3,728 (30.8%)
Hypertension	238 (65.7%)	104 (41.1%)	342 (55.6%)	6,655 (55.1%)
MI	119 (32.9%)	62 (24.5%)	181 (29.4%)	2,588 (21.4%)
Peripheral arterial disease	18 (5.0%)	8 (3.2%)	26 (4.2%)	541 (4.4%)
Prior CABG	57 (15.7%)	6 (2.4%)	63 (10.2%)	602 (4.9%)
Prior PCI	85 (23.5%)	32 (12.6%)	117 (19.0%)	1,483 (12.2%)
Prior stent	75 (20.7%)	26 (10.3%)	101 (16.4%)	N/A
Stroke/TIA	6 (1.7%)	4 (1.6%)	10 (1.6%)	493 (4.0%)

coronary angiography (93% versus 58%), PCI (53.7% versus 35.3%) with a stent applied in 94.2% versus 33.2% of cases (drug-eluting in 58% versus 44% of these cases), and CABG (14.6% versus 5.7%). Although they subsequently received similar levels of aspirin (94% versus 93.1%) and unfractionated heparin (39.7% versus 39.5%), South African patients were more likely to receive low-molecular-weight heparin (73.5% versus 60.9%).

10.1.4.2 Posthospital management

At hospital discharge the vast majority of South African patients were prescribed statin and aspirin (93.3% and 92.6% respectively). Other commonly prescribed cardio-protective agents included a beta blocker (67.4%), an ACE inhibitor (61.4%), and/or calcium channel blockers (13.6%). Overall, 91 (16.6%) patients had at least one further cardiac-related hospitalization within 12 months. Unstable angina was the cause for rehospitalization in 49 (8.9%) patients and occurred in a median of 166 days after the index hospitalization. Six and four patients were readmitted to hospital for a STEMI and non–ST-segment elevation ACS, respectively. Six patients also reported a transient ischemic attack (TIA) or stroke following hospitalization, and 14 were readmitted for HF. At 12 months, the majority of patients in both groups were still taking their prescribed medications: aspirin (80.2%), statin (77.3%), beta-blockers (53.8%), ACE-inhibitors (46%), and calcium channel blockers (10.3%).

10.1.4.3 Case fatality

Thirty-day mortality was 2.4% in those presenting with STEMI, compared to 1.7% for the rest. Subsequently, 35 patients (5.7%) died within 12 months, comprising sudden cardiac death (n = 12), fatal MI (n = 8), non-CVD-related (n = 6), stroke (n = 2), and unknown (n = 7). As expected, 12-month case-fatality was higher for those diagnosed with STEMI (6.7% versus the rest 5.0%).

10.1.5 Study interpretation

This is the first South African-based ACS registry to document the demographics and management strategies used in patients admitted to hospital (although a minority were of African ancestry). Those admitted with STEMI were younger and were more likely to smoke cigarettes; the remainder were more likely to present with preexisting risk factors including hypertension, diabetes, and/or dyslipidemia. The use of appropriate ancillary drug therapy in hospital and on discharge was in line with registries from developed countries; however, the use of calcium channel blockers was low (13%). Antithrombotic therapy use was in accordance with clinical guidelines; however, the use of clopidogrel (or other adenosine diphosphate (ADP)-receptor blockers) at discharge was lower in the South African cohort compared to the entire ACCESS registry (62% versus 76%). The reasons for this are not entirely clear [25].

10.1.6 Study limitations

The limitations noted in this study were that patients seeking health care were only the minority who had access to private health care funding. Second, patients had to provide consent and be alive in order participate in the study; therefore, it represents more the demographics of survivors of acute ACS as it excludes any hospitalized patients who died shortly after arriving. Last, during the study period, guidelines changed; therefore, some data may be outdated.

10.1.7 Study conclusions

In conclusion, these data describing the management of ACS from a South African context demonstrated higher levels of angiography and revascularization relative to the wider ACCESS registry cohort. Readmission rates for recurrent ischemic events and bleeding were comparatively low, with a similar pattern for the 12-month mortality rate. As in other studies of longer-term secondary prevention, the reduction in appropriate treatment over time is of concern. These data highlight the need to develop more cost-effective primary and secondary prevention strategies to both prevent the expected rise in cases of AMI and other forms of ACS in South Africa and beyond and to maximize the application of proven treatments following appropriate hospital management.

10.2 ACS in treatment-naïve black South Africans with human immunodeficiency virus infection

Becker AC, Sliwa K, Stewart S, Libhaber E, Essop AR, Zambakides CA, Essop MR. Acute coronary syndromes in treatment-naïve black South Africans with human immunodeficiency virus infection. *Journal of Interventional Cardiology* 2010; 23(1):70–77.

10.2.1 Study background

As reported in previous studies, the prevalence of CAD among people of African ancestry is slowly increasing [26] and is particularly alarming when considering the status of HIV in South Africa [27]. Although cardiac complications of HIV infection are described thoroughly [28], opinions still conflict on whether HIV-positive patients have a higher ACS incidence. Autopsy studies have reported high atherosclerotic CAD rates in HIV-positive patients when compared to aged-matched HIV-negative patients [29]. Adverse metabolic phenotypes, including endothelial dysfunction and a prothrombotic state, as well as dyslipidemia and insulin resistance, are induced by protease inhibitors as part of HAART [28,30,31]. A strong association between premature CAD and HAART has been reported [32]; however, whether prolonged exposure to protease inhibitors increases the risk of ACS remains the subject of debate [33]. The lack of data for HAART cases presenting with CAD and HIV infection has limited the capacity to clarify the role of HIV in the development of premature CAD.

10.2.2 Study aims

The aim of the study was to determine the risk factors, clinical presentation, and coronary angiographic features within the HAART-naïve HIV-positive patient population presenting with ACS, and compare this to their HIV-negative counterparts in Soweto, South Africa. We hypothesized that the risk profile and clinical characteristics of HIV-positive patients would differ markedly from their HIV-negative counterparts, particularly with respect to the underlying morphology of coronary lesion(s) and thrombus formation.

10.2.3 Study methods
10.2.3.1 Study design and patient enrollment

Ethics approval was obtained to conduct a prospective single-center study at the Chris Hani Baragwanath Hospital, Soweto. A total of 60 patients were recruited to participate in the study, and all provided informed consent prior to baseline data collection. The study was conducted between March 2004 and February 2008, where all presenting patients with ACS were screened for HIV infection. Thirty consecutive HIV-positive patients presenting with ACS were enrolled. For each HIV-positive patient with ACS, an HIV-negative patient with ACS was selected as a case-control comparator. An angiographic follow-up was planned for all patients receiving a coronary stent at a minimum of 6 months postprocedure. Patients underwent testing to diagnose ACS based on current guidelines [34,35]. They also underwent blood tests to positively identify the HIV virus by examining plasma HIV RNA levels and determining CD4 counts by flow cytometry. Conventional risk factors for arterial thrombosis were documented along with history of opportunistic infections and/or HIV-related malignancies and CDC disease stage [36] in the HIV-positive group. Patients were designated as having comorbidities such as diabetes, hypertension, or dyslipidemia if they were being treated concurrently for these conditions or if they were diagnosed with the condition on hospital admission. Patients underwent anthropometric testing, were assessed for risk factors for ACS (i.e., smoking, family history of disease, hypertension), and also underwent a series of questions and/or measurements to determine their level of other coronary risk factors (i.e., postmenopausal state, family history of CAD, and abdominal obesity). All baseline and subsequent follow-up testing was conducted at the Chris Hani Baragwanath cardiac clinic.

Single-vessel disease was defined as a single major epicardial coronary artery with a stenosis of ≥50% and multivessel disease as ≥2 major epicardial arteries with stenosis ≥50%. The infarct-related artery was defined by reviewing each patient's angiogram, ECG, and/or echocardiogram. An artery was defined as infarct related if a thrombus or ruptured plaque was present, or if the two above-mentioned diagnostic tests implicated the same "coronary territory." The infarct-related artery was defined as "angiographically normal" if the contour was smooth with no angiographic features of atherosclerotic disease in any of the coronary arteries. Angiographic classification of the infarct-related artery thrombus burden was based on a previously published descriptive model [37]. Initial thrombolysis in MI flow grade in the infarct-related artery was defined based on previous findings [38]. PCI interventions were defined as the accomplishment of normal coronary flow with a residual stenosis of ≤50% and no complications.

10.2.3.2 Study definitions

Binary angiographic in-stent restenosis was defined as a >50% diameter stenosis at angiographic follow-up. In-stent restenosis was further defined as focal or diffuse according to a previously proposed classification [39]. Target lesion revascularization was defined as any repeat revascularization of the infarct-related artery involving the stent and/or its 5-mm proximal or distal edges. Major adverse cardiovascular events were defined as death, non-fatal MI, or target lesion revascularization.

10.2.4 Study findings

In total, 60 ACS patients were analyzed during this study: 30 HIV-positive patients and 30 HIV-negative patients. Overall, these 60 patients represented 8.9% of the total patients presenting with ACS during the study period (n = 673).

10.2.4.1 Clinical and demographic characteristics according to HIV status

As shown in Table 10.2, the HIV-negative patients were significantly more likely to have type 2 diabetes (p = 0.05), hypertension (p = 0.0001), multiple risk factors (p = 0.0182), and other coronary risk factors (p = 0.0001), with a higher BMI

Table 10.2 ACS patients' clinical features according to HIV status.

	HIV positive (n = 30)	HIV negative (n = 30)
Demographic profile		
African ancestry	30 (100%)	30 (100%)
Age (years)	43 ± 7	54 ± 13
Men	20 (66.7%)	18 (60.0%)
Coronary risk factors		
Cigarette smoking	22 (73.3%)	10 (33.3%)
Type 2 diabetes	1 (3.3%)	7 (23.3%)
Hypertension	7 (23.3%)	23 (76.7%)
Total cholesterol (mmol/L)	3.6 ± 1.0	4.6 ± 1.4
LDL cholesterol (mmol/L)	2.2 ± 0.9	3.0 ± 1.2
HDL cholesterol (mmol/L)	0.8 ± 0.3	1.1 ± 0.4
Triglycerides (mmol/L)	1.4 ± 0.8	1.1 ± 0.4
Multiple risk factors	8 (26.7%)	18 (60.0%)
Other coronary risk factors	2 (6.7%)	16 (53.3%)
Clinical features		
BP (mm Hg)	132 ± 31/86±22	145 ± 37/89 ± 18
Pulse rate (beats/min)	91 ± 22	91 ± 29
BMI (kg/m²)	25 ± 5	28 ± 5
Waist to hip ratio	0.91 ± 0.06	0.95 ± 0.05
Abdominal circumference (cm)	85 ± 10	100 ± 15

(p = 0.01) and abdominal circumference (representing abdominal obesity, p = 0.0003) when compared to the HIV-positive patients. However, HIV-positive patients were significantly more likely than HIV-negative patients to report cigarette smoking (p=0.002). No study patients reported drug abuse with the exception of one HIV-negative patient who reported the use of cocaine.

Although not reaching significance, more HIV-positive patients received clopidogrel (66.7% versus 43.3%, p=0.10) and thrombolytic therapy as an initial strategy (30% versus 16.7%). All patients were administered 300 mg of aspirin on admission followed by 150 mg daily thereafter. They were also administered weight-adjusted antithrombotic therapy, and 25 patients in each group received beta blockers and statins.

10.2.4.2 Initial angiographic features

HIV-positive patients were more likely to have single vessel disease (80% versus 60%, p=0.08), an angiographically normal infarct-related artery (46.7% versus 13.3%, p=0.005), a thrombus in multiple arteries (10% versus 0%, p=0.24), and a large thrombus burden (43.3% versus 16.7%, p=0.02). Figures 10.2 and 10.3 provide angiographic images of a thrombus in an otherwise angiographically normal infarct-related artery.

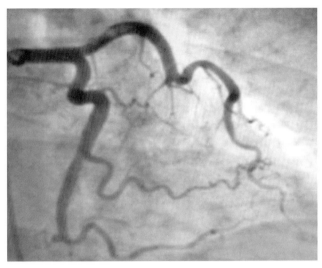

Figure 10.2 Angiographic image of thrombus in an otherwise angiographically normal left anterior descending coronary artery in a 43-year-old HIV-positive man presenting with a STEMI. Source: Becker et al., 2010 [29] (S4.3 References). Reproduced with permission of Wiley.

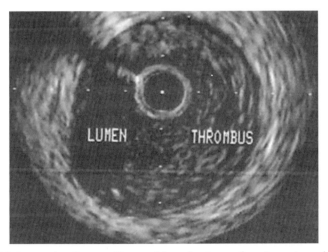

Figure 10.3 Intravascular ultrasound image of thrombus in an otherwise angiographically normal left anterior descending coronary artery depicted in Figure 10.2. Source: Becker et al., 2010 [29] (S4.3 References). Reproduced with permission of Wiley.

10.2.4.3 Coronary intervention

PCI was the most commonly used treatment strategy in both groups, with similar usage of bare metal stents and excellent procedural success rates in both HIV-positive and -negative groups (100% versus 72.7%, p=0.36). HIV-negative patients were, however, more likely to have pre-PCI thrombolysis in MI 0 flow (83.3% versus 22.2%, p=0.0007). Surgical revascularization was undertaken in 2 of the 30 (6.7%) HIV-negative patients compared to none in the HIV-positive cohort.

10.2.4.4 Clinical outcomes

As shown in Table 10.3, the HIV-positive patients were found to have significantly higher rates of major adverse cardiovascular events (46.7% versus 16.7%, p=0.026) and target lesion revascularization (16.7% versus 0%, p=0.05). HIV-positive patients also tended to have higher rates of mortality (30.0% versus 16.7%) and nonfatal MI (3.3% versus 0%). Mortality in the HIV-positive group was attributed to cardio-embolic stroke (one patient), massive pulmonary embolus (one patient), cardiogenic shock (two patients), and unknown causes (five patients). In the HIV-negative group, mortality was attributed to cardiogenic shock (one patient), fatal stroke (one patient), recurrent MI (one patient), suicide (one patient), and unknown causes (one patient).

10.2.4.5 Angiographic follow-up

In total, angiographic follow-up was performed in 55% of the patients who received bare metal stents in both the HIV-positive group (5 of 9 [55.6%]) and the HIV-negative group (6 of 11 [54.6%]). Binary angiographic restenosis in those who received bare metal stents occurred in 100% of the HIV-positive group

Table 10.3 ACS patients' long-term outcomes according to HIV status.

	HIV positive (n=30)	HIV negative (n=30)
Clinical outcomes at 48 months		
Major adverse cardiovascular events	14 (46.7%)	5 (16.7%)
Mortality	9 (30.0%)	5 (16.7%)
Nonfatal MI	1 (3.3%)	0 (0%)
Target lesion revascularization	5 (16.7)	0 (0%)
Angiographic follow-up		
Patients originally receiving bare metal stents	9 (30.0%)	11 (36.7%)
Patients eligible for follow-up angiography	5/9 (55.6%)	6/11 (54.6%)
Duration of follow-up angiogram, months	7 ± 5	11 ± 3
Binary in-stent restenosis	5/5 (100%)	3/6 (50.0%)
Focal	0/5 (0%)	1/3 (33.3%)
Diffuse	5/5 (100%)	2/3 (66.7%)
Composite target lesion revascularisation	5/9 (55.6%)	0/11 (0%)

compared to 50% of the HIV-negative group (see Table 10.3). Among the HIV-positive group with binary angiographic restenosis, all had a type 3 diffuse proliferative with evidence of ischemia and received target lesion revascularization, one patient with an angioplasty alone and four others with a drug eluting stent. Among the HIV-negative group, one patient (17%) had type 1C focal body restenosis, and two patients (33%) presented with a type 4 diffuse proliferative pattern. Due to the lack of objective evidence of reversible ischemia on nuclear perfusion imaging, no target lesion revascularization was performed among HIV-negative patients.

10.2.5 Study interpretation

As this study was conducted during a period in South Africa when HAART was not routinely available, we were able to document the clinical presentations of HIV-positive patients of African ancestry with ACS in the Soweto community without the confounding effects of HAART. These results showed that HIV-negative patients presented with more prevalent classical risk factors for ACS [40]. However, consistent with other studies [41], HIV-positive patients demonstrated higher rates of cigarette smoking. They were also found to be predominantly male, younger in age, and have lower high-density lipoprotein (HDL) levels, which is also consistent with previous studies [41]. However, no HIV-positive patients reported IV drug abuse, nor did they have opportunistic infections or HIV-related malignancies. We reported a higher burden of large thrombus in the infarct-related artery of HIV-positive patients, suggesting a prothrombotic state [31,42,43].

10.2.6 Study limitations

Beyond the limitations noted in Chapter 9, this was a relatively small cohort that permitted detection of only major differences between the groups. Moreover, not all patients with bare metal stents inserted as part of percutaneous coronary angioplasty underwent repeat angiography, affecting the reliability of the data regarding in-stent restenosis.

10.2.7 Study conclusions

Despite the limitations, it could be concluded that HAART-naïve HIV-positive South African patients of African ancestry presenting with ACS exhibit different clinical and angiographic features than do HIV-negative patients. Factors including younger age, a predominance of men, high rates of cigarette smoking, and lower HDL levels suggest a prothrombotic state that requires further investigation. As modifiable cardiovascular risk factors in the HIV-positive group were identified in this study, it shows that cigarette smoking may contribute to the pathogenesis of ACS and is a vital target to reduce cardiovascular risk. The management of HIV-positive patients (both pre- and post-treatment) should be an important focus when completing cardiovascular risk assessment and primary prevention strategies.

10.3 The thrombotic profile of treatment-naïve HIV-positive South Africans of African ancestry with ACS

Becker AC, Jacobson B, Singh S, Sliwa K, Stewart S, Libhaber E, Essop MR. **The thrombotic profile of treatment-naïve HIV-positive black South Africans with acute coronary syndromes.** *Clinical and Applied Thrombosis/Hemostasis* 2011; 17(3):264–72.

10.3.1 Study background

Previous studies provide evidence that venous thromboembolic complications are induced by HIV infection, malignancies, or can be increased from HAART (incidence ranging from 0.3% and 8%) [31,44]. HIV infection is known to cause endothelial cell and platelet activation, which has been shown to increase cardiovascular events [45,46]. Although lupus anticoagulants and antiphospholipid antibodies are prevalent in HIV-infected patients, their association with thrombosis is unknown [47]. It is also unclear whether thrombosis risk is higher among treatment-naïve HIV-infected patients. What is known is that treatment-naïve HIV-positive patients of African ancestry presenting with ACS are younger with less traditional risk factors but more thrombotic burden than their HIV-negative counterparts, suggesting the possibility of a prothrombotic state [48].

10.3.2 Study aims

The aim of the study was to compare the thrombotic profile of treatment-naïve HIV-positive patients of African ancestry presenting with ACS with that of HIV-negative patients. It was hypothesized that thrombophilia would be present among HIV-positive patients on laboratory screening.

10.3.3 Study methods
10.3.3.1 Patient enrollment and thrombophilic screening

During the period of March 2004 to February 2008, 30 consecutive HIV-positive patients of African ancestry presenting with ACS were enrolled from the Cardiology Department at Chris Hani Baragwanath Hospital, Soweto. For each HIV-positive patient presenting with an ACS, we selected a non-HIV patient of African ancestry with an ACS as a case control comparator. In addition, any HIV-positive patient without an ACS matched for sex, age, and ethnicity were recruited from the HIV clinic for non-ACS but HIV-positive comparisons. Blood was obtained from each patient and was then stored, transported, and analyzed by the National Health Services Laboratory. Patients were classified as having other coronary risk factors if they reported a premature CAD family history, chronic kidney disease, abdominal obesity, and/or were postmenopausal. All patients provided informed consent before enrollment and ethics approval was obtained through the University of Witwatersrand.

10.3.4 Study findings

10.3.4.1 Clinical profile and thrombotic profile of ACS patients

As shown in Table 10.4, the HIV-negative patients presenting with ACS were significantly more likely to present with type 2 diabetes (23.3% versus 3.3%, p=0.03), hypertension (76.7% versus 23.3%, p=0.0001), elevated LDL-cholesterol (p=0.0032), elevated HDL-cholesterol (p=0.0006), elevated BMI (p=0.008), and other coronary risk factors (53.3% versus 6.7%, p=0.0001). Alternatively, HIV-positive patients were significantly more likely to smoke cigarettes (33.3% versus 73.3%, p=0.004). Among the entire cohort, 15 patients were not tested due to 10 deaths and 5 patients lost to follow-up. Therefore, 21 out of 30 (70%) HIV-positive patients with ACS and 24 out of 30 (80%) HIV-negative patients with ACS completed thrombotic screens. Overall, HIV-positive patients with ACS had higher frequencies of antiphospholipid antibodies (anticardiolipin immunoglobulin-G [46.7% versus 10%, p=0.003]) compared to the HIV-negative patients with ACS, as well as lower levels of protein-C (82 versus 108 IU/dL, p=0.0003) and higher levels of Factor VIII (201 versus 136 IU/dL, p=0.0011).

10.3.4.2 Platelet studies

Overall, 21 of 30 (70%) and 24 of 30 (80%) HIV-positive and negative ACS patients respectively completed platelet reactivity studies using light transmission aggregometry. Among HIV-positive patients, 16 of 21 (76.2%) were using 150 mg of aspirin per day and 2 of 21 (9.5%) were using 75 mg of clopidogrel per day. Among the HIV-negative patients, 22 of 24 (91.7%) were using 150 mg of aspirin per day and 4 of 24 (16.7%) were using 75 mg of clopidogrel per day. HIV-positive patients who were using aspirin were more likely to show evidence of aspirin resistance with >20% aggregation to arachidonic acid compared to the HIV-negative patients (3 of 16 [18.8%] versus 2 of 22 [9.1%], not significant). However, of the patients using clopidogrel in both groups, approximately half exhibited evidence of clopidogrel resistance with normal aggregation to ADP (not significant). In the patients not taking aspirin or clopidogrel, the response to agonists was normal with no platelet hyper-reactivity in either group.

10.3.4.3 HIV-positive clinical and thrombotic profile

As shown in Table 10.5, the HIV-positive patients presenting with ACS had a significantly higher CD4 count (230 [30–1356] versus 125 cells/ml³ [6–1041], p=0.0126) and were more likely to report cigarette smoking (73.3% versus 36.7%%, p=0.0026) when compared with the HIV-positive controls. However, HIV-positive patients with ACS tended to have higher viral loads (54,000 [25–11×105] versus 29,000 [25–7×105]) and AIDS-defining criteria (70% versus 36.7%, p=0.01) when compared with the HIV-positive controls. Overall, 21 (70%) HIV-positive patients presenting with ACS and 29 (96.7%) HIV-positive controls completed thrombotic screens at 6 weeks follow-up. Overall, both groups had similar frequencies of antiphospholipid antibodies. Mean protein-C levels were lower in the HIV-positive control group (82±22 versus 92±19 IU/dL, p=0.0163).

Table 10.4 ACS patients' clinical and thrombotic characteristics according to HIV status.

	HIV Positive Patients with ACS (n = 30)	HIV Negative Patients with ACS (n = 30)
Demographic profile		
African ancestry	30 (100%)	30 (100%)
Age (years)	43 ± 7	54 ± 13
Men	20 (66.7%)	18 (60.0%)
Coronary risk factors		
Cigarette smoking	22 (73.3%)	10 (33.3%)
Type 2 diabetes	1 (3.3%)	7 (23.3%)
Hypertension	7 (23.3%)	23 (76.7%)
Total cholesterol (mmol/L)	3.6 ± 1.0	4.6 ± 1.4
LDL cholesterol (mmol/L)	2.2 ± 0.9	3.0 ± 1.2
HDL cholesterol (mmol/L)	0.8 ± 0.3	1.1 ± 0.4
Triglycerides (mmol/L)	1.4 ± 0.8	1.1 ± 0.4
BMI (kg/m^2)	25 ± 5	28 ± 5
Other coronary risk factors	2 (6.7%)	16 (53.3%)
Thrombotic screen at baseline	30 (100%)	30 (100%)
Hemoglobin (g/dL)	13.6 ± 2.8	14.5 ± 1.8
Platelet count (× 10^9/L)	301 ± 113	302 ± 72
Antiphospholipid antibody frequencies		
Anticardiolipin (immunoglobulin-G)	14 (46.7%)	3 (10.0%)
Anticardiolipin (immunoglobulin-M)	3 (10.0%)	1 (3.3%)
Anticardiolipin (immunoglobulin-A)	0 (0%)	3 (10.0%)
Anti-ß-2 glycoprotein (immunoglobulin-G)	11 (36.7%)	6 (20.0%)
Anti-ß-2 glycoprotein (immunoglobulin-M)	3 (10.0%)	0 (0%)
Anti-ß-2 glycoprotein (immunoglobulin-A)	7 (23.3%)	12 (40.0%)
Antiprothrombin (immunoglobulin-G)	26 (86.7%)	6 (20.0%)
Antiprothrombin (immunoglobulin-M)	2 (6.7%)	0 (0%)
Antiprothrombin (immunoglobulin-A)	2 (6.7%)	1 (3.3%)
Thrombotic screen 6 weeks post event	21 (70.0%)	24 (80.0%)
Fibrinogen (g/L)	3.5 ± 1.0	3.9 ± 2.2
D-Dimer quantitative (mg/L)	0.42 (0.2-2.49)	0.28 (0.2-3.08)
Antithrombin (IU/dL)	101 ± 19	103 ± 15
Protein-C (IU/dL)	82 ± 22	108 ± 20
Protein-S (IU/dL)	91 ± 29	107 ± 25
Activated protein-C	2.6 ± 0.5	2.8 ± 0.5
Factor VIII (IU/dL)	201 ± 87	136 ± 45
Von Willebrand factor antigen	225 ± 64	197 ± 84
Von Willebrand factor activity	108 ± 7	105 ± 12
Lupus anticoagulant	0 (0%)	0 (0%)

Table 10.5 HIV-positive patients' clinical and thrombotic characteristics according to ACS status.

	HIV-Positive Patients with ACS (n = 30)	HIV-Positive Controls (n = 30)
Demographic profile		
African ancestry	30 (100%)	30 (100%)
Age (years)	43 ± 7	41 ± 8
Men	20 (66.7%)	19 (63.3%)
HIV-related factors		
CD4 (cells/mL^3)	230 (30–1356)	125 (6–1041)
Viral load (RNA, copies/mL)	29,000 (25–7×10^5)	54,000 (25–11×10^5)
AIDS-defining criteria	11 (36.7%)	21 (70.0%)
Coronary risk factors		
Cigarette smoking	22 (73.3%)	11 (36.7%)
Type 2 diabetes	1 (3.3%)	0 (0%)
Hypertension	7 (23.3%)	2 (6.7%)
Total cholesterol (mmol/L)	3.6 ± 1.0	3.7 ± 0.8
LDL cholesterol (mmol/L)	2.2 ± 0.9	2.0 ± 0.5
HDL cholesterol (mmol/L)	0.8 ± 0.3	1.0 ± 0.5
Triglycerides (mmol/L)	1.4 ± 0.8	1.4 ± 0.8
BMI (kg/m^2)	25 ± 5	21 ± 4
Other coronary risk factors	2 (6.7%)	0 (0%)
Thrombotic screen at baseline	30 (100%)	30 (100%)
Hemoglobin (g/dL)	13.6 ± 2.8	12.6 ± 2.3
Platelet count (× 10^9/L)	301 ± 113	252 ± 83
Antiphospholipid antibody frequencies		
Anticardiolipin (immunoglobulin-G)	14 (4.67%)	17 (56.7%)
Anticardiolipin (immunoglobulin-M)	3 (10.0%)	4 (13.3%)
Anticardiolipin (immunoglobulin-A)	0 (0%)	0 (0%)
Anti-ß-2 glycoprotein (immunoglobulin-G)	11 (36.7%)	10 (33.3%)
Anti-ß-2 glycoprotein (immunoglobulin-M)	3 (10.0%)	2 (6.7%)
Anti-ß-2 glycoprotein (immunoglobulin-A)	7 (23.3%)	8 (26.7%)
Antiprothrombin (immunoglobulin-G)	26 (86.7%)	29 (96.7%)
Antiprothrombin (immunoglobulin-M)	2 (6.7%)	0 (0%)
Antiprothrombin (immunoglobulin-A)	2 (6.7%)	3 (10.0%)
Thrombotic screen 6 weeks follow-up	21 (70.0%)	29 (96.7%)
Fibrinogen (g/L)	3.5 ± 1.0	3.6 ± 0.9
D-Dimer quantitative (mg/L)	0.42 (0.2–2.49)	0.34 (0.2–5.47)
Antithrombin (IU/dL)	101 ± 19	113 ± 19
Protein-C (IU/dL)	82 ± 22	92 ± 19
Protein-S (IU/dL)	91 ± 29	85 ± 23
Activated protein-C	2.6 ± 0.5	2.6 ± 0.4
Factor VIII (IU/dL)	201 ± 87	228 ± 130
Von Willebrand factor antigen	225 ± 64	252 ± 119
Von Willebrand factor activity	108 ± 7	104 ± 9
Lupus anticoagulant	0 (0%)	1 (3.3%)

10.3.4.4 Platelet studies

Overall, 21 (70%) and 28 (93.3%) HIV-positive patients presenting with and without ACS, respectively, completed light transmission aggregometry. Most notably (beyond that described above) among HIV-positive controls, 27 of 28 (96.4%) were not using aspirin, and of these, 8 of 27 (29.6%) showed a "flat" response to arachidonic acid in the absence of antiplatelet drugs, while 19 (70.4%) showed a normal aggregation response to agonists.

10.3.5 Study interpretation

HIV-negative patients presenting with ACS were more likely to exhibit traditional risk factors for AMI and higher protein-C levels when compared with HIV-positive patients presenting with ACS. HIV-positive patients presenting with ACS were more likely to report cigarette smoking and have elevated factor VIII levels, antiphospholipid antibody frequencies, and greater evidence of thrombophilia. The low HDL levels found in the HIV-positive patients presenting with ACS may also contribute to thrombotic risk and have commonly been noted in treatment-naïve HIV-infected patients [49,50]. Decreased protein-C levels and elevated factor VIII levels as seen in the HIV positive patients with ACS are consistent with a thrombophilic state. This is consistent with previous studies, which have reported that protein-C deficiency and increased clotting factor VIII are well-known venous thromboembolic risk factors [51,52]. The relationship between decreased protein-C levels and elevated factor VIII in arterial thrombosis is less clear but has been described in the pathogenesis of myocardial infarction in young patients with otherwise normal coronary arteries [53,54]. The significance of the raised antiphospholipid antibodies in the HIV-positive group with ACS remains unclear and requires further investigation. To potentially heighten thrombotic risk, it is known that HIV-positive patients have high degrees of endothelial activation when compared with HIV-negative patients [55–57]. In this study, we found that although von Willebrand factor antigen levels were higher in the HIV-positive group, statistical significance was not reached.

10.3.6 Study limitations

A few limitations are worth noting: (a) the sample size was relatively small, making it challenging to detect minor differences between the groups; (b) not all patients underwent thrombotic screening, which weakens the study's accuracy; and (c) direct comparison of the thrombotic profiles of the two HIV groups was difficult due to the imperfect matching of the groups with respect to degree of immunosuppression.

10.3.7 Study conclusions

In conclusion, treatment-naïve HIV-positive patients presenting with ACS display risk factors and thrombotic profiles that are distinct from HIV-negative patients. Consistent with other studies, HIV-positive patients are younger, more commonly cigarette smokers, and exhibit fewer traditional risk factors than do HIV-negative patients. They do, however, show evidence of a prothrombotic state, given the findings of lower protein-C levels, higher factor VIII levels, and elevated antiphospholipid antibodies, which need further investigation to determine their potential causal nature. It is possible that the pathogenesis of thrombosis is multifactorial in these patients with the interaction of conventional risk factors and HIV-specific coagulation abnormalities. To this extent, smoking is the most modifiable risk factor and thus an important target for cardiovascular risk reduction in this population. As an additional note to this study and its conclusions, a further study was undertaken to investigate the role of antiphospholipid antibodies as a risk factor for ACS in patients of African ancestry presenting with minimal traditional risk factors. It was hypothesized that HIV-positive patients with ACS would have a higher prevalence of antiphospholipid antibodies and the antiphospholipid syndrome when compared to HIV negative patients, and that antiphospholipid antibodies would be causally related to thrombosis and ACS. However, it was demonstrated (in this same group of patients) that antiphospholipid antibodies are unlikely to be linked to ACS; they are more likely an epiphenomenon of the HIV infection itself. Based on these findings, Figure 10.4 summarizes the pathogenesis of atherothrombosis in the context of HIV infection.

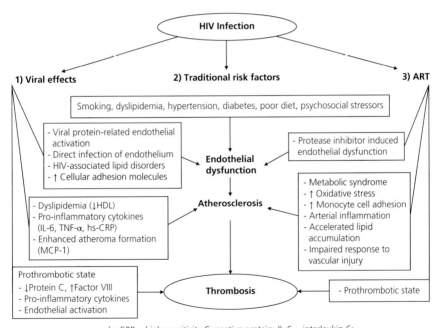

hs-CRP = high sensitivity C reactive protein; IL-6 = interleukin-6;
MCP-1 = macrophage chemoattractant protein-1;
TNF-α = tumour necrosis factor-α

Figure 10.4 The pathogenesis of atherothrombosis and HIV infection.

CHAPTER 11
Stroke in the African context

Albertino Damasceno

Universidade Eduardo Mondlane, Maputo, Mozambique

11.0 Introduction

In this chapter we describe the results of an epidemiologic study to evaluate the hospital incidence rate of stroke, its main clinical characteristics, and the in-hospital and 28-day mortality. A standard methodology was used to allow comparisons with similar studies from other parts of the world, as well as with future studies in Maputo. Based in the capital of Mozambique, this prospective study involved hospitalized or ambulatory patients, all of whom were followed for 28 days; the vast majority of stroke diagnoses (including stroke type) were based on CT scan or necropsy. These new data highlighted a number of novel (to Africa) aspects around the epidemiology and impact of stroke.

11.1 An epidemiological study of stroke hospitalizations in Mozambique

Damasceno A, Gomes J, Azevedo A, Carrilho C, Lobo V, Lopes H, Madede T, Pravinrai P, Silva-Matos C, Jalla S, Stewart S, Lunet N. An epidemiological study of stroke hospitalisations in Maputo, Mozambique. *Stroke* 2010; 41:2463–69.

11.1.1 Study background

There are approximately 15 million new acute stroke cases every 12 months worldwide, with the majority of cases residing in low- and middle-income countries [58]. This is due to extended life expectancy and rising exposure to major risk factors of stroke, such as smoking, obesity, diabetes, and hypertension [59]. Stroke, which frequently reduces patients' quality of life through cognitive and motor impairment and is ranked globally as the second leading cause of mortality,

The Heart of Africa: Clinical Profile of an Evolving Burden of Heart Disease in Africa, First Edition.
Edited by Simon Stewart, Karen Sliwa, Ana Mocumbi, Albertino Damasceno, and Mpiko Ntsekhe.
© 2016 John Wiley & Sons, Ltd. Published 2016 by John Wiley & Sons, Ltd.

has recently become a concern in sub-Saharan Africa [59,60]. The impact of stroke in African countries is increasing due to a rising prevalence of hypertension associated with a very poor level of awareness and control. At the same time, there is limited access to health services and pharmacological treatment, poor standards of care, and delay in seeking acute hospital treatment [61].

Approximately one-third of the Mozambican adult population is hypertensive; of these, less than 10% receive pharmacological treatment [62]. With stroke risk factors adding a concern, 4.8% of the Mozambique population is obese [63] and approximately 30% smoke cigarettes [64]. In 1994, cerebrovascular disease was reported to be the sixth cause of mortality among individuals aged 15 to 59 years and was ranked first among individuals aged ≥60 years in Maputo [60]. In order to meet the increasing health service needs of the Maputo population, stroke surveillance is vital to plan future resource necessity [61].

11.1.2 Study aims
By utilizing the WHO's STEPwise approach to Stroke Surveillance methodology [64], the study aimed to evaluate and estimate the new cases of stroke hospitalization, the epidemiological stroke event features, and the 28-day case-fatality rate and disability status in Maputo, Mozambique.

11.1.3 Study methods
11.1.3.1 Patient enrollment
During a full year, in the period of August 2005 to July 2006, all private or governmental hospital patients who had encountered a first-ever or recurrent stroke event and who had been residing in Maputo for ≥12 months were registered for the study. When new symptoms occurred in the same arterial distribution ≥29 days previously, or in a different arterial distribution caused by a former event <28 days previously, these were recorded as a recurrent stroke event [65]. Alternatively, events that occurred before the study period were referred to as old stroke events and were not included in the study analysis. When stroke-related events likely to be associated with HIV infection were suspected, the patients' status of HIV infection was evaluated. However, all stroke events were recorded regardless of their HIV status.

11.1.3.2 Data collection
When stroke patients approached a private or governmental hospital, they were administered the STEPS Stroke survey, which included demographic and clinical questions. Trained interviewers were responsible for data collection and were positioned at the Maputo Central Hospital's emergency department, as well as trained nurses in other emergency departments and trained physicians with cerebrovascular disease experience in medical wards.

First-ever and recurrent stroke events were self-reported by the patients as well as by the analysis of medical records, necropsy reports, and CT-scan images by physicians. Pharmacological treatment and assessment, biomedical tests, and in-hospital complications were recorded. Diabetes, hypertension, dyslipidemia, and AF were either self-reported or assessed through different analysis methods, including the prescription of pharmacological treatment, evaluation of questionnaires, and performing 12-lead ECG. Ethics approval was obtained, along with informed consent from all study patients.

11.1.4 Study findings

Figure 11.1 shows the schema of study participation. A total of 825 patients with reported stroke-related events were analyzed. Of these, 174 (21.1%) patients were excluded from the study; this was due to 40 (23%) patients reported old strokes, 39 (22.4%) had TIA, 27 (15.5%) had HIV-related cerebral infection, 5 (2.9%) had trauma, 8 (4.6%) had hypoglycemia, 5 (2.9%) had cerebral tumors, 14 (8%) were nonresidential Maputo patients, and 36 (20.7%) were excluded for other reasons. Overall, therefore, 651 (78.9%) of 825 patients had a clinically confirmed stroke-related event and were formally included in the study. Of these, 531 (81.6%) were classified as first-ever/de novo stroke events. Only 50 (17.7%) patients were clinically diagnosed without a CT scan or necropsy, 543 (83.4%) were confirmed by CT scan, and 58 (8.9%) were confirmed by necropsy examination. From these, 8 (1.3%) subarachnoid hemorrhages, 242 (40.3%) hemorrhagic events, and 351 (58.4%) ischemic events were identified. Of clinical and epidemiologic significance, more ischemic (42% versus 13.4%) and hemorrhagic events occurred as first-ever stroke presentations (36.1% versus 4.2%).

As shown in Table 11.1, there were similar numbers of men and women, and the majority were of African ancestry (94.5%). Significantly, 12.9% of the stroke-related events occurred in patients aged ≤45 years. Those who arrived at the hospital on the same day as their onset of stroke symptoms represented just

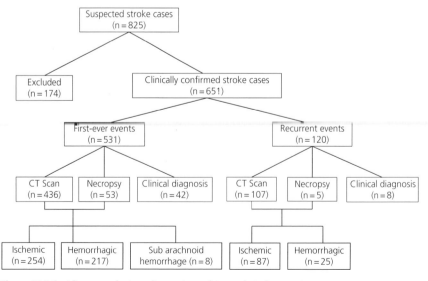

Figure 11.1 Incidence, exclusion, diagnosis, and type of stroke events.

Table 11.1 Patients' prehospital characteristics according to type of case presentation.

	First-Ever Events		Recurrent Events		All Events (n=651)
	Ischemic (n=264)	Hemorrhagic (n=217)	Ischemic (n=87)	Hemorrhagic (n=25)	
Women	124 (47.0%)	96 (44.2%)	47 (54.0%)	15 (60.0%)	309 (47.5%)
Age (years)	60.5±13.8	54.7±11.5	63.9±11.8	57.2±11.8	59.1±13.2
African ancestry	249 (94.3%)	212 (97.7%)	77 (88.5%)	23 (92.0%)	615 (94.5%)
Education					
None	77 (29.2%)	55 (25.4%)	27 (31.1%)	7 (28.0%)	182 (28.0%)
1–4 years	90 (34.1%)	68 (31.3%)	31 (35.6%)	9 (36.0%)	218 (33.5%)
5 years	49 (18.6%)	35 (16.1%)	9 (10.3%)	5 (20.0%)	104 (16.0%)
Time to stroke presentation					
Same day	131 (49.6%)	155 (71.4%)	46 (52.9%)	16 (64.0%)	380 (58.4%)
1 day poststroke	55 (20.8%)	45 (20.7%)	21 (24.1%)	6 (24.0%)	140 (21.5%)
2–7 days poststroke	63 (23.9%)	13 (6.0%)	17 (19.5%)	3 (12.0%)	108 (16.6%)
Prestroke disability					
0–2 (minimal)	253 (97.4%)	215 (99.5%)	68 (78.2%)	21 (84.0%)	618 (94.9%)
Risk factors					
Hypertension	213 (86.6%)	196 (95.6%)	80 (93%)	24 (96.0%)	561 (91.2%)
Cigarette smoking	27 (10.5%)	18 (8.5%)	4 (4.8%)	3 (12.0%)	62 (9.8%)
Dyslipidemia	37 (15.4%)	23 (12.3%)	11 (13.9%)	4 (17.4%)	82 (14.3%)
Diabetes	40 (15.8%)	20 (9.8%)	16 (19.3%)	3 (12.0%)	87 (14.1%)
AF	16 (6.2%)	3 (1.4%)	13 (15.7%)	1 (4.4%)	38 (6.1%)

over half of the patients (58.4%). At the other end of the spectrum, 3.5% arrived >7 days after symptom onset. Overall, 177 (27.2%) and 171 (26.3%) of those with ischemic and hemorrhagic events, respectively, presented at the hospital on the same day as symptom onset. Far more de novo stroke patients arrived at the hospital on the day of symptom onset compared to those with a recurrent event (43.9% versus 9.5%). With regard to risk factors, hypertension was noted in 91.2% of the patients while AF was present in 6.1%.

As shown in Table 11.2, case-fatality rates were high with a differential pattern according to ischemic versus hemorrhagic strokes and de novo versus recurrent events. Overall, 254 (39%) patients died during the 28-day follow-up, hemorrhagic strokes were related to 2- to 3-fold higher case-fatality rate, and median in-hospital stay was 6 days for the entire cohort.

11.1.5 Study interpretation

Overall, 148.7/100,000 residents in Maputo per year required medical care for stroke and for hemorrhagic events; this resulted in in-hospital mortality of 50%, with case fatality rising to 70% by 28 days. These data confirm the serious impact

Table 11.2 Patients' short-term stroke-related case-fatality.

	First-Ever Events % (95% CI)		Recurrent Events % (95% CI)		All Events (n=651)
	Ischemic (n=264)	Hemorrhagic (n=217)	Ischemic (n=87)	Hemorrhagic (n=25)	
In-hospital mortality (%)	17.4 (13.0–22.5)	47.9 (41.1–54.8)	24.1 (15.6–34.5)	52.0 (31.3–72.2)	33.3 (29.7–37.1)
7-day case fatality (%)	16.2 (11.9–22.2)	52.9 (43.0–65.1)	17.3 (10.2–29.2)	31.9 (15.2–67.2)	32.9 (28.4–38.0)
14-day case fatality (%)	26.0 (20.2–33.4)	69.0 (57.0–83.5)	36.5 (25.1–53.3)	63.1 (35.5–100)	47.7 (42.1–54.1)
28-day case fatality (%)	27.4 (21.4–35.1)	72.3 (59.8–87.5)	40.7 (28.2–58.7)	70.8 (40.6–100)	49.6 (43.8–56.2)

of stroke on a population with high levels of often undetected and untreated hypertension, and complement more recent population incidence data derived from Tanzania [5]. However, as discussed in more detail below, it is clear that the hospital event-rates for stroke arising from this population may be conservative given a number of influential clinical, socioeconomic, and cultural factors that require consideration.

Despite the above factors, this study revealed much higher rates of stroke than the previous STEPS Stroke Multicenter survey [61]. However, both the high stroke incidence rate and the high proportion of hemorrhagic stroke events in Maputo are largely supported by the high prevalence of hypertension in Mozambique [62]. In agreement with these data, a contemporary, single-center study of hospital stroke presentations in South Africa reported that just over one quarter of presentations were hemorrhagic (27%), with a mean age of 51 years among those of African ancestry [59]. Previous studies report similarly high stroke-related case-fatality rates [59,66,67]. Poor survival rates reflect the limited pharmacological, technical, and human resources available to administer optimal treatment options. In Maputo, stroke patients are cared for in a general medical ward instead of in stroke units, where only one CT scan device is available for 1 million inhabitants. Furthermore, these data highlight gaps in secondary prevention due to insufficient access to treatment and monitoring of health conditions postdiagnosis. These data also emphasize the limited number of institutions available to rehabilitate individuals if they survive a primary stroke event. Physical rehabilitation therapy was offered to the patients free of charge; however, patients were required to fund their own transportation, restricting access to the minority with sufficient means to bear that cost. Overall, these findings are in agreement with previously reported results that the population of Mozambique is at a higher risk of adult mortality compared to other countries [68].

11.1.6 Study limitations

Importantly, these figures do not take into account additional stroke cases among those not residing in Maputo for more than 12 months. A small in-hospital stay fee was charged (as per the health system in Mozambique), but individuals with limited means and/or resources did not pay. Accessing hospital care with limited transport options is always challenging, and so these data remain conservative in terms of estimating the number and impact of stroke cases in this setting. The possibility of patients seeking health care in hospitals outside Maputo is highly unlikely as there are limited hospitals with no emergency medicine available to serve a population 10% larger and spreading over an area 87-fold larger than Maputo City [69,70]. Alternatively, owing to African culture (regarding stroke as a supernatural force and therefore requiring attention by a traditional healer [71]), local customs may have limited the number of stroke presentations to participating hospitals. From a clinical perspective, small hemorrhagic events may also have been missed in patients scanned long after the stroke event; however, the proportion of CT scans performed >7 days after stroke was relatively low and thus is unlikely to meaningfully influence the research estimates.

11.1.7 Study conclusions

In conclusion, the study's surveillance approach strategy revealed a high incidence of stroke and related morbidity and mortality in Maputo, Mozambique. Given the rigorous methods used to derive such data, there is an opportunity to compare and contrast stroke-related events both within (on a historical basis) and without (in comparison to similarly derived data from other populations) the target population. Overall, these data reveal the deadly impact of stroke in Mozambique and wider sub-Saharan Africa, highlighting important issues around future stroke prevention (hypertension being a major target), life-saving treatments, and health services, as well as longer-term rehabilitation programs to mitigate the burden in vulnerable populations.

S5.2 Beyond counting cases: The next steps to improve health outcomes in stroke and beyond

After describing a troubling epidemiologic and clinical picture of stroke and indeed ACS, it is appropriate to outline some measures that could improve the situation. Stroke mortality reflects the control rate of hypertension in the community. Collectively, we need first to increase the awareness levels of hypertension in Africa to further increase its control rate. In countries such as Seychelles where this was achieved, researchers have already observed a decrease in the mortality rate of stroke [72]. The second measure is the creation of small and simple stroke units in the main hospitals where stroke patients can be admitted and undergo simple but efficacious procedures that are life saving. A small and simple unit with standard protocols and with personnel prepared for and dedicated to this type of patient has proved to be economically effective [73]. The same considerations around primary prevention and the need to develop a regional/national network of clinics to deal with an increasing and deadly caseload of ACS in younger African men and women may well emerge in the next decade or so. As discussed in Chapter 6, when combined with stroke events, there is a real potential for AMI and other forms of ACS to become the predominant forms of noncommunicable heart disease in sub-Saharan Africa, with more women and younger individuals affected relative to high-income countries.

References

1 van Rooyen JM, Kruger HS, Huisman HW, Wissing MP, Margetts BM, Venter CS, et al. An epidemiological study of hypertension and its determinants in a population in transition: the THUSA study. *J Hum Hypertens*. 2000;14(12):779–87.

2 Yusuf S, Reddy S, Ounpuu S, Anand S. Global burden of cardiovascular diseases: Part II. Variations in cardiovascular disease by specific ethnic groups and geographic regions and prevention strategies. *Circulation*. 2001;104(23):2855–64.

3 Yusuf S, Reddy S, Ounpuu S, Anand S. Global burden of cardiovascular diseases: Part I. General considerations, the epidemiologic transition, risk factors, and impact of urbanization. *Circulation*. 2001;104(22):2746–53.

4 Feigin VL, Forouzanfar MH, Krishnamurthi R, Mensah GA, Connor M, Bennett DA, et al. Global and regional burden of stroke during 1990–2010: findings from the Global Burden of Disease Study 2010. *Lancet*. 2014;383(9913):245–54.

5 Walker R, Whiting D, Unwin N, Mugusi F, Swai M, Aris E, et al. Stroke incidence in rural and urban Tanzania: a prospective, community-based study. *Lancet Neurol*. 2010;9(8):786–92.

6 O'Donnell MJ, Xavier D, Liu L, Zhang H, Chin SL, Rao-Melacini P, et al. Risk factors for ischaemic and intracerebral haemorrhagic stroke in 22 countries (the INTERSTROKE study): a case-control study. *Lancet*. 2010;376(9735):112–23.

7 Adoukonou TA, Vallat JM, Joubert J, Macian F, Kabore R, Magy L, et al. Management of stroke in sub-Saharan Africa: current issues. *Rev Neurol (Paris)*. 2010;166(11):882–93.

8 Ntsekhe M, Damasceno A. Recent advances in the epidemiology, outcome, and prevention of myocardial infarction and stroke in sub-Saharan Africa. *Heart*. 2013;99(17):1230–5.

9 Barros CP, Chivangue A, Samagaio A. Urban dynamics in Maputo, Mozambique. *Cities*. 2014;36:74–82.

10 Andersen JE, Jenkins P. *Urban Development in Maputo: Strategic Action Planning on a Tight Budget*. Cities, Health and Wellbeing. 2011.

11 Jones L, Roux J-P, Scott C, Tanner T. *Climate and Development Outlook: Stories of Change from CDKN*. Climate and Development Knowledge Network, 2014.

12 Raimundo I, Crush J, Pendleton W. The State of Food Insecurity in Maputo, Mozambique. African Food Security Urban Network (AFSUN), 2014 Contract No.: 20.

13 United Nations Human Settlements Programme: Regional and Technical Cooperation Division. *Mozambique Cities Profile*. United Nations Human Settlements Programme (UN-HABITAT), 2010.

14 Instituto Nacional de Estatística (INE). *Estatísticas Distritais (Estatísticas do Distrito de Cidade De Maputo) 2011*. Maputo, Mozambique: INE, 2012.

15 Instituto Nacional de Estatística de Moçambique (INE). Indicadores 2014. Available from: http://www.ine.gov.mz/pt/DataAnalysis.

16 Health Mo. *National Survey of Prevalence, Behavioral Risks, and Information about HIV and AIDS in Mozambique*. Maputo: Ministry of Health, 2010.

17 Macassa G, Ghilagaber G, Charsmar H, Walander A, Sundin O, Soares J. Geographic differentials in mortality of children in Mozambique: their implications for achievement of Millennium Development Goal 4. *J Health Popul Nutr.* 2012;30(3):331–45.

18 Steyn K, Sliwa K, Hawken S, Commerford P, Onen C, Damasceno A, et al. Risk factors associated with myocardial infarction in Africa: the INTERHEART Africa study. *Circulation.* 2005;112(23):3554–61.

19 Eagle KA, Goodman SG, Avezum A, Budaj A, Sullivan CM, Lopez-Sendon J, et al. Practice variation and missed opportunities for reperfusion in ST-segment-elevation myocardial infarction: findings from the Global Registry of Acute Coronary Events (GRACE). *Lancet.* 2002;359(9304):373–7.

20 Fox KA, Goodman SG, Anderson FA, Jr., Granger CB, Moscucci M, Flather MD, et al. From guidelines to clinical practice: the impact of hospital and geographical characteristics on temporal trends in the management of acute coronary syndromes. The Global Registry of Acute Coronary Events (GRACE). *Eur Heart J.* 2003;24(15): 1414–24.

21 Hasdai D, Behar S, Wallentin L, Danchin N, Gitt AK, Boersma E, et al. A prospective survey of the characteristics, treatments and outcomes of patients with acute coronary syndromes in Europe and the Mediterranean basin: the Euro Heart Survey of Acute Coronary Syndromes (Euro Heart Survey ACS). *Eur Heart J.* 2002;23(15):1190–201.

22 Kotseva K, Wood D, De Backer G, De Bacquer D, Pyorala K, Keil U, et al. EUROASPIRE III: a survey on the lifestyle, risk factors and use of cardioprotective drug therapies in coronary patients from 22 European countries. *Eur J Cardiovasc Prev Rehabil.* 2009; 16(2):121–37.

23 Kumar A, Fonarow GC, Eagle KA, Hirsch AT, Califf RM, Alberts MJ, et al. Regional and practice variation in adherence to guideline recommendations for secondary and primary prevention among outpatients with atherothrombosis or risk factors in the United States: a report from the REACH Registry. *Crit Pathw Cardiol.* 2009;8(3):104–11.

24 Patel MR, Chen AY, Roe MT, Ohman EM, Newby LK, Harrington RA, et al. A comparison of acute coronary syndrome care at academic and nonacademic hospitals. *Am J Med.* 2007;120(1):40–6.

25 Yusuf S, Zhao F, Mehta SR, Chrolavicius S, Tognoni G, Fox KK, et al. Effects of clopidogrel in addition to aspirin in patients with acute coronary syndromes without ST-segment elevation. *N Engl J Med.* 2001;345(7):494–502.

26 Stewart S, Wilkinson D, Hansen C, Vaghela V, Mvungi R, McMurray J, et al. Predominance of heart failure in the Heart of Soweto Study cohort: emerging challenges for urban African communities. *Circulation.* 2008;118(23):2360–7.

27 UNAIDS. AIDS by the Numbers 2015. Available from: http://www.unaids.org/sites/default/files/media_asset/AIDS_by_the_numbers_2015_en.pdf (Accessed February 2016).

28 Hsue PY, Waters DD. What a cardiologist needs to know about patients with human immunodeficiency virus infection. *Circulation.* 2005;112(25):3947–57.

29 Morgello S, Mahboob R, Yakoushina T, Khan S, Hague K. Autopsy findings in a human immunodeficiency virus-infected population over 2 decades: influences of gender, ethnicity, risk factors, and time. *Arch Pathol Lab Med.* 2002;126(2):182–90.

30 Hsue PY, Hunt PW, Sinclair E, Bredt B, Franklin A, Killian M, et al. Increased carotid intima-media thickness in HIV patients is associated with increased cytomegalovirus-specific T-cell responses. *AIDS.* 2006;20(18):2275–83.

31 Saif MW, Greenberg B. HIV and thrombosis: a review. *AIDS Patient Care STDS.* 2001;15(1): 15–24.

32 Henry K, Melroe H, Huebsch J, Hermundson J, Levine C, Swensen L, et al. Severe premature coronary artery disease with protease inhibitors. *Lancet.* 1998;351(9112):1328.

33 Friis-Moller N, Sabin CA, Weber R, d'Arminio Monforte A, El-Sadr WM, Reiss P, et al. Combination antiretroviral therapy and the risk of myocardial infarction. *N Engl J Med.* 2003;349(21):1993–2003.

34 Bertrand ME, Simoons ML, Fox KA, Wallentin LC, Hamm CW, McFadden E, et al. Management of acute coronary syndromes in patients presenting without persistent ST-segment elevation. *Eur Heart J.* 2002;23(23):1809–40.

35 Van de Werf F, Ardissino D, Betriu A, Cokkinos DV, Falk E, Fox KA, et al. Management of acute myocardial infarction in patients presenting with ST-segment elevation: The Task Force on the Management of Acute Myocardial Infarction of the European Society of Cardiology. *Eur Heart J.* 2003;24(1):28–66.

36 Matsuda J, Gotoh M. Classification system for HIV infection by CDC. *Nihon Rinsho.* 1993;51(Suppl):243–8.

37 Gibson CM, de Lemos JA, Murphy SA, Marble SJ, McCabe CH, Cannon CP, et al. Combination therapy with abciximab reduces angiographically evident thrombus in acute myocardial infarction: a TIMI 14 substudy. *Circulation.* 2001;103(21):2550–4.

38 TIMI Study Group. The Thrombolysis in Myocardial Infarction (TIMI) trial. Phase I findings. *N Engl J Med.* 1985;312(14):932–6.

39 Mehran R, Dangas G, Abizaid AS, Mintz GS, Lansky AJ, Satler LF, et al. Angiographic patterns of in-stent restenosis: classification and implications for long-term outcome. *Circulation.* 1999;100(18):1872–8.

40 Mineo C, Deguchi H, Griffin JH, Shaul PW. Endothelial and antithrombotic actions of HDL. *Circ Res.* 2006;98(11):1352–64.

41 Hsue PY, Giri K, Erickson S, MacGregor JS, Younes N, Shergill A, et al. Clinical features of acute coronary syndromes in patients with human immunodeficiency virus infection. *Circulation.* 2004;109(3):316–9.

42 Aboulafia DM, Mitsuyasu RT. Hematologic abnormalities in AIDS. *Hematol Oncol Clin North Am.* 1991;5(2):195–214.

43 Zon LI, Arkin C, Groopman JE. Haematologic manifestations of the human immune deficiency virus (HIV). *Br J Haematol.* 1987;66(2):251–6.

44 Shen YM, Frenkel EP. Thrombosis and a hypercoagulable state in HIV-infected patients. *Clin Appl Thromb Hemost.* 2004;10(3):277–80.

45 Hwang SJ, Ballantyne CM, Sharrett AR, Smith LC, Davis CE, Gotto AM, Jr., et al. Circulating adhesion molecules VCAM-1, ICAM-1, and E-selectin in carotid atherosclerosis and incident coronary heart disease cases: the Atherosclerosis Risk In Communities (ARIC) study. *Circulation.* 1997;96(12):4219–25.

46 Sudano I, Spieker LE, Noll G, Corti R, Weber R, Luscher TF. Cardiovascular disease in HIV infection. *Am Heart J.* 2006;151(6):1147–55.

47 Abuaf N, Laperche S, Rajoely B, Carsique R, Deschamps A, Rouquette AM, et al. Autoantibodies to phospholipids and to the coagulation proteins in AIDS. *Thromb Haemost.* 1997;77(5):856–61.

48 Becker AC, Sliwa K, Stewart S, Libhaber E, Essop AR, Essop MR. Acute coronary syndromes in black South African patients with human immunodeficiency virus infection: the clinical and angiographic features. *Circulation.* 2008;118(12).

49 Bukrinsky M, Sviridov D. Human immunodeficiency virus infection and macrophage cholesterol metabolism. *J Leukoc Biol.* 2006;80(5):1044–51.

50 Mujawar Z, Rose H, Morrow MP, Pushkarsky T, Dubrovsky L, Mukhamedova N, et al. Human immunodeficiency virus impairs reverse cholesterol transport from macrophages. *PLoS Biol.* 2006;4(11):e365.

51 Boekholdt SM, Kramer MH. Arterial thrombosis and the role of thrombophilia. *Semin Thromb Hemost.* 2007;33(6):588–96.

52 Koster T, Blann AD, Briet E, Vandenbroucke JP, Rosendaal FR. Role of clotting factor VIII in effect of von Willebrand factor on occurrence of deep-vein thrombosis. *Lancet.* 1995; 345(8943):152–5.

53 Peterman MA, Roberts WC. Syndrome of protein C deficiency and anterior wall acute myocardial infarction at a young age from a single coronary occlusion with otherwise normal coronary arteries. *Am J Cardiol.* 2003;92(6):768–70.

54 Tiong IY, Alkotob ML, Ghaffari S. Protein C deficiency manifesting as an acute myocardial infarction and ischaemic stroke. *Heart.* 2003;89(2):E7.

55 Feffer SE, Fox RL, Orsen MM, Harjai KJ, Glatt AE. Thrombotic tendencies and correlation with clinical status in patients infected with HIV. *South Med J.* 1995;88(11):1126–30.

56 Klein SK, Slim EJ, de Kruif MD, Keller TT, ten Cate H, van Gorp EC, et al. Is chronic HIV infection associated with venous thrombotic disease? A systematic review. *Neth J Med.* 2005;63(4):129–36.

57 Lafon ME, Steffan AM, Royer C, Jaeck D, Beretz A, Kirn A, et al. HIV-1 infection induces functional alterations in human liver endothelial cells in primary culture. *AIDS.* 1994;8(6): 747–52.

58 Murray CJ, Lopez AD. Alternative projections of mortality and disability by cause 1990–2020: Global Burden of Disease Study. *Lancet.* 1997;349(9064):1498–504.

59 Connor MD, Walker R, Modi G, Warlow CP. Burden of stroke in black populations in sub-Saharan Africa. *Lancet Neurol.* 2007;6(3):269–78.

60 Dgedge M, Novoa A, Macassa G, Sacarlal J, Black J, Michaud C, et al. The burden of disease in Maputo City, Mozambique: registered and autopsied deaths in 1994. *Bull World Health Organ.* 2001;79(6):546–52.

61 Truelsen T, Heuschmann PU, Bonita R, Arjundas G, Dalal P, Damasceno A, et al. Standard method for developing stroke registers in low-income and middle-income countries: experiences from a feasibility study of a stepwise approach to stroke surveillance (STEPS Stroke). *Lancet Neurol.* 2007;6(2):134–9.

62 Damasceno A, Azevedo A, Silva-Matos C, Prista A, Diogo D, Lunet N. Hypertension prevalence, awareness, treatment, and control in Mozambique: urban/rural gap during epidemiological transition. *Hypertension.* 2009;54(1):77–83.

63 Gomes A, Damasceno A, Azevedo A, Prista A, Silva-Matos C, Saranga S, et al. Body mass index and waist circumference in Mozambique: urban/rural gap during epidemiological transition. *Obes Rev.* 2010;11(9):627–34.

64 Padrao P, Silva-Matos C, Damasceno A, Lunet N. Association between tobacco consumption and alcohol, vegetable and fruit intake across urban and rural areas in Mozambique. *J Epidemiol Community Health.* 2011;65(5):445–53.

65 Farooq MU, Chaudhry AH, Amin K, Majid A. The WHO STEPwise approach to stroke surveillance. *J Coll Physicians Surg Pak.* 2008;18(10):665.

66 Garbusinski JM, van der Sande MA, Bartholome EJ, Dramaix M, Gaye A, Coleman R, et al. Stroke presentation and outcome in developing countries: a prospective study in the Gambia. *Stroke.* 2005;36(7):1388–93.

67 Rosman KD. The epidemiology of stroke in an urban black population. *Stroke.* 1986; 17(4):667–9.

68 Rajaratnam JK, Marcus JR, Levin-Rector A, Chalupka AN, Wang H, Dwyer L, et al. Worldwide mortality in men and women aged 15–59 years from 1970 to 2010: a systematic analysis. *Lancet.* 2010;375(9727):1704–20.

69 Instituto Nacional de Estatística. III Recenseamento Geral de População e Habitação, 2007. 2007. Available from: http://www.ine.gov.mz/censo2007.

70 Infraestruturas das unidades sanitárias do serviço nacional de saúde, 2004–2008. 2008. Available from: www.Ine.Gov.Mz/sectorias_dir/saude_dir/iussns04_08.

71 Mshana G, Hampshire K, Panter-Brick C, Walker R. Urban-rural contrasts in explanatory models and treatment-seeking behaviours for stroke in Tanzania. *J Biosoc Sci.* 2008; 40(1):35–52.

72 Stringhini S, Sinon F, Didon J, Gedeon J, Paccaud F, Bovet P. Declining stroke and myocardial infarction mortality between 1989 and 2010 in a country of the african region. *Stroke.* 2012;43(9):2283–8.

73 de Villiers L, Kalula SZ, Burch VC. Does multidisciplinary stroke care improve outcome in a secondary-level hospital in South Africa? *Int J Stroke.* 2009;4(2):89–93.

SECTION 6
Heart failure

Simon Stewart

Australian Catholic University, Melbourne, Victoria, Australia

S6.1 The many faces of HF in Africa

In this section of the book, the various manifestations of HF in the sub-Saharan African context are presented, providing an important counterpoint to that presented from a Western, high-income perspective. Despite some controversy over the true spectrum of HF in high-income regions of the world including Europe and North America, due to the influence of clinical trials and registries reporting from specialist cardiology centers (perhaps with a natural focus on middle-aged men presenting with an ischemic CMO), it is clear from whole population data that HF predominantly affects men and women alike beyond the age of 65 years and is a major cause of morbidity and mortality [1–5]. In recent years, the rate of incident HF admissions has declined and the overall rate (per head of population) has plateaued and even declined in some age groups; with notable shifts in the pattern of HF-related morbidity due to CAD associated with heart failure with reduced ejection fraction (HFrEF). These trends are counterpointed by an increasing number of heart failure with preserved ejection fraction (HFpEF) cases associated with uncontrolled hypertension in older individuals (particularly women). We know this because of an early recognition that HF posed a significant threat to aging populations in whom antecedent risk factors remained high, but the risk of dying prematurely from an AMI was declining [3,6]. In simple terms, the "Cinderella" of heart disease was no longer being ignored and has been closely monitored for more than two decades.

The temptation, of course, is to assume that epidemiology and subsequent treatment of HF derived from large-scale clinical trials will apply uniformly across the globe. However, in the sub-Saharan Africa context, this would be a mistake. As described by Falase and Ogah [7], the predominance of CAD and its chronic manifestation ischemic CMO in the Western world was contrasted by historical lows in Africa. For more than 50 years the pattern of HF in Africa was

The Heart of Africa: Clinical Profile of an Evolving Burden of Heart Disease in Africa, First Edition.
Edited by Simon Stewart, Karen Sliwa, Ana Mocumbi, Albertino Damasceno, and Mpiko Ntsekhe.
© 2016 John Wiley & Sons, Ltd. Published 2016 by John Wiley & Sons, Ltd.

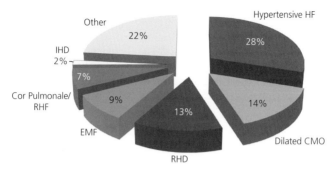

S6.1 Major causes of heart failure presentations in Nigeria in the late 1960s.

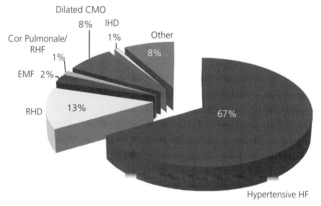

S6.2 Major causes of heart failure presentations in Nigeria in 2010.

remarkably stable with hypertensive HF an important but nondominant contributor to HF cases, given the contribution of the dilated CMOs, RHD, EMF and cor pulmonale/RHF. These conditions reflected a combination of infectious and genetic pathways to the syndrome. As described in Section 1, cases of PPCMO among young African women remains an ongoing and significant contributor to HF cases in Africa. At the same time, the typical Ischemic CMOs seen in the Western world and the subject of clinical trials feeding the evidence base to improve typically poor survival rates and prevent progressive cardiac dysfunction/recurrent episodes of acute heart failure (AHF) remained scarce in those of African ancestry. Overall, however, HF cases were relatively rare in sub-Saharan Africa, at least from a reported and research perspective. The following chapters quickly dispel the myth that HF is rare in Africa. Indeed, there are now many pathways (both communicable and noncommunicable) to the syndrome, and these pose an increasing challenge to resource-poor health care systems throughout the continent.

S6.1.1 Geographical context

The final section of this book spans several regions of the continent, commencing with the twelve-country THESUS-HF registry and concluding with the four-country Pan African Pulmonary Hypertension Cohort (PAPUCO) registry. Chapter 12 introduces us to Abeokuta, a Nigerian city that also features in Chapters 13 and 14, while the Nigerian capital, Abuja, is highlighted in Chapter 13 (for a country-level profile of Nigeria, refer to Section 2). Cameroon (see Section 2) is revisited in Chapter 14, and Chapter 13 includes a final return to South African Soweto (see Section 1).

Abuja, the capital city of Nigeria, is reported to be the fastest-growing city in Africa, with an urbanization rate of 8.32% per annum [8,9]. With over 3 million permanent residents, Abuja's daytime population often reaches 7 million [9,10]. The consequence of this rapid growth and urbanization is that the city's administration is struggling to manage the increasing difficulties of providing basic housing and public services [9]. Despite a national health care system, the level of overall government contribution to health services is low, and private out-of-pocket payments compose almost 70% of costs [11]. A lack of human and technical resources, particularly in maternal health [12] and specialty areas such as cardiology [11,13] contributes to health outcomes that do not match the region's economic growth [13].

Abeokuta is the capital city of Ogun State, located in southwest Nigeria. Currently estimated at approximately 1 million individuals, the population of Abeokuta is rising rapidly [14,15]. The majority of residents do not have access to social health insurance, and health care costs are typically borne out of pocket [16]. However, strong family ties ensure that poorer patients are generally assisted by wealthier relatives [16]. The Federal Medical Centre in which the Abeokuta-based studies featured in this book were undertaken is the only tertiary hospital in the city, receiving referrals from across the city and state as well as from neighboring states [16].

CHAPTER 12

Acute heart failure

Mahmoud Sani[1], Dike Bevis Ojji[2], Anastase Dzudie[3],
and Okechukwu Samuel Ogah[4]

[1] Bayero University Kano/Aminu Kano Teaching Hospital, Kano, Nigeria
[2] University of Abuja Teaching Hospital, Abuja, Nigeria
[3] Hospital General de Douala, Douala, Littoral, Cameroon
[4] University College Hospital, Ibadan, Oyo, Nigeria

12.0 Introduction

AHF is a major cause of morbidity and mortality in high-income countries. The most common reason for hospital admission in patients over the age of 65 years, it is also associated with staggering management costs [17,18]. Moreover, the prognosis of patients admitted with AHF remains dismal, with over 20% experiencing recurrent HF admissions and over 20% dying during the first year after initial admission [17]. Patients with recent hospitalizations for AHF are at high risk for future cardiovascular events and death [19]. In contrast to the state of treatment for CHF, advances in the management of AHF have been limited even while its incidence in developed countries increases. Although AHF is common, the data on its clinical presentation, characteristics, and outcomes in low- to middle-income regions such as sub-Saharan Africa remains limited [20]. Historically, HF cases in sub-Saharan Africa are largely attributable to the major nonischemic causes, with hypertensive heart disease, RHD, and CMO accounting for over 75% of cases in most series. CAD remains an uncommon cause of HF, with no apparent increase in its contribution to African cases. Of concern, many causes of HF including RHD, idiopathic dilated CMO, EMF, and PPCMO present in young and middle-aged individuals, in contrast to the pattern in developed countries where HF is a disease of the elderly [21,22]. Finally, the contribution of cor pulmonale and pericarditis to around 20% of cases of HF reflects the continuing impact of TB on heart disease across the continent [23–27]. However, as outlined in previous chapters of this book, epidemiological transition has changed the landscape of risk and heart disease and presentations of AHF in sub-Saharan Africa. Countries in this region are currently experiencing one of the most rapid epidemiological transitions characterized by increasing urbanization and changing lifestyle factors [28], which in turn have increased the incidence of noncommunicable diseases, especially CVD. As a result, HF due to underlying myocardial ischemia/LV dysfunction secondary to

The Heart of Africa: Clinical Profile of an Evolving Burden of Heart Disease in Africa, First Edition.
Edited by Simon Stewart, Karen Sliwa, Ana Mocumbi, Albertino Damasceno, and Mpiko Ntsekhe.
© 2016 John Wiley & Sons, Ltd. Published 2016 by John Wiley & Sons, Ltd.

IHD and/or AF in obese individuals may well become more common in sub-Saharan Africa. In this chapter we describe the causes and treatment of AHF as well as the morbidity and mortality of its sufferers on the African continent.

12.1 A landmark registry of AHF in sub-Saharan Africa: THESUS-HF

Damasceno A, Mayosi BM, Sani M, Ogah O, Mondo C, Ojji D, Dzudie A, Yonga G, Abou Ba S, Maru F, Alemayehu B, Edwards C, Davison B, Cotter G, Sliwa K. The causes, treatment, and outcomes of acute heart failure in 1006 Africans from 9 countries: results of the sub-Saharan Africa Survey of Heart Failure. *Archives of Internal Medicine* 2012; 172(18):1386–94. [29]

12.1.1 Study background
Previous HF studies in sub-Saharan Africa were largely clinical and necropsy studies [21]. The Heart of Soweto Study (see Chapter 6) is the largest clinical and echocardiographic study from the region in recent times [30]. Other smaller clinical and echocardiographic studies on the continent have been conducted [31–34], but the majority provided cross-sectional views of HF presentations from single communities. Furthermore, no study had focused on acute presentations of HF in sub-Saharan Africa. THESUS-HF was the first prospective multicenter and multi-country registry to document the characteristics and outcomes of acute presentations of HF from nine sub-Saharan African countries.

12.1.2 Study aims
The aim of the study was to determine the pattern (including morbidity and mortality) of AHF in sub-Saharan Africa as well as to investigate the causes and available treatments of this condition.

12.1.3 Study methods
12.1.3.1 Patient enrollment
THESUS-HF was conducted during the period July 2007 to June 2010. Patients aged >12 years presenting to 12 cardiology centers in sub-Saharan Africa with dyspnea and subsequently diagnosed with AHF were entered into the registry. Excluded patients were those also presenting with severe renal failure, STEMI, hepatic failure, nephrotic syndrome, or hypoalbuminemia. The 12 centers were located in Senegal, Sudan, Ethiopia, Nigeria, Kenya, Uganda, Cameroon, South Africa, and Mozambique. However, Senegal, Ethiopia, and Kenya were late in joining the study and thus had a shorter enrollment period. All participating centers included a physician trained in clinical cardiology and echocardiography, and demographic and clinical data were collected on standardized case report forms. Ethics approval and informed consent were obtained prior to implementation.

Information collected included demographic data, detailed medical history, vital signs (i.e., BP, heart rate, respiratory rate, and temperature), and signs and symptoms of HF (oxygen saturation, intensity of edema and rales, body weight, and levels of orthopnea). Assessments were performed at admission and days 1, 2, and 7 (or discharge if earlier). ECGs were conducted and read using standard reference ranges. A detailed echocardiographic assessment was performed if not completed in the month prior to admission. The probable primary cause of HF was provided by the investigators, based on the ESC guidelines [35] as applied in the chronic HF cohort of the Heart of Soweto Study [30]. Information on readmissions and death, with respective reasons and cause, was collected through the 6-month follow-up. Outcomes of interest were readmission or death through 60 days, and death through 180 days. HIV status was recorded for patients who were suspected of infection and consented to testing.

12.1.4 Study findings

As shown in Figure 12.1, a total of 1,011 patients were enrolled in the study, for which 1,006 case reports were received and included in published analyses. The majority of patients were enrolled from Kano, Nigeria (n = 205), followed by Abeokuta, Nigeria (n = 200); Kampala, Uganda (n = 154); Douala, Cameroon (n = 90); Johannesburg, South Africa (n = 82); Maputo, Mozambique (n = 76); Khartoum, Sudan (n = 72); Cape Town, South Africa (n = 50); Nairobi, Kenya (n = 32); Abuja, Nigeria (n = 25); Dakar, Senegal (n = 15); and Addis Ababa, Ethiopia (n = 10).

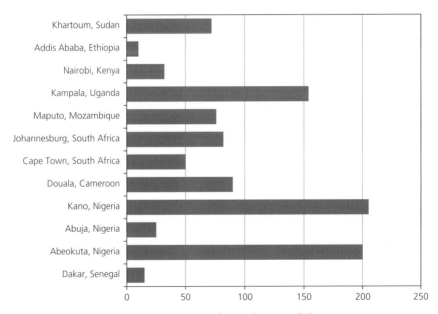

Figure 12.1 Distribution of AHF patients according to the 12 cardiology centres.

As shown in Table 12.1, the majority of patients were of African ancestry (97.8%, p=0.47) with a mean age of 52.3±18.3 years. Women were more likely to be HIV positive (p=0.75), to present with AF (p=0.03) and anemia (p=0.43), and to exhibit higher BMI (p=0.08), heart rate (p=0.003), and LVEF (p=0.002) when compared with men. Men were more likely to present with hyperlipidemia (p=0.09), hypertension (p=0.004), and a history of smoking (p<0.001), and to exhibit higher creatinine (p<0.001), serum urea nitrogen (p<0.001), and hemoglobin levels (p<0.001), as well as marginally higher systolic (p=0.06) and diastolic BP (p=0.08) levels.

12.1.4.1 Causes and therapies for HF

The predominant cause of HF in this study cohort was hypertension in 453/998 (45.4%). This was followed by idiopathic dilated CMO in 118/998 (18.8%) and RHD in 143/997 (14.3%). A range of other causes contributing to fewer than 1 in 10 cases included IHD in 77/999 (7.7%), PPCMO in 77/1,002 (7.7%), pericardial effusion tamponade 68/999 (6.8%), HIV-related CMO in 26/1,000 (2.6%), and EMF in 13/1,000 (1.3%). Critically, the causes of AHF varied from country to country. Hypertension was the most common cause in Nigeria, Mozambique,

Table 12.1 Patients' demographic and clinical characteristics.

	Women (n=512)	Men (n=494)	All (n=1,006)
Demographic characteristics			
Age (years)	50.7±19.5	54.0±16.9	52.3±18.3
African ancestry	497 (97.7%)	486 (98.4%)	984 (97.8%)
Clinical characteristics			
AHF admissions <12 months	0.34±0.78	0.41±0.77	0.37±0.78
LVEF (%)	41.1±16.6	37.8±16.2	39.5±16.5
Anemia	79 (15.5%)	68 (13.8%)	147 (14.6%)
AF	107 (20.9%)	77 (15.6%)	184 (18.3%)
BMI (kg/m^2)	25.7±11.6	24.7±4.9	25.2±9.0
Type 2 diabetes history	56 (11.0%)	58 (11.7%)	114 (11.3%)
History of hypertension	259 (50.7%)	296 (59.9%)	556 (55.3%)
History of cigarette smoking	13 (2.5%)	85 (17.2%)	98 (9.7%)
Heart rate, beats/min	105.7±21.6	101.6±21.4	103.7±21.6
Systolic BP (mm Hg)	128.4±33.3	132.4±33.7	130.4±33.5
Diastolic BP (mm Hg)	83.2±20.7	85.5±21.2	84.3±20.9
Cholesterol level (mg/dL)	155.2±49.1	160.0±59.0	157.6±54.2
Hyperlipidemia	38 (7.4%)	52 (10.5%)	90 (9.0%)
Creatine kinase level (U/L)	210.8±473.9	259.4±412.6	232.2±447.7
Sodium level (mEq/L)	135.3±6.8	134.9±6.5	135.1±6.6
eGFR (mL/min/1.73 m^2)	81.4±44.4	85.3±51.4	83.3±48.0
Serum urea nitrogen level (mg/dL)	30.2±27.7	41.1±38.9	35.6±34.1
Renal dysfunction	38 (7.4%)	35 (7.1%)	73 (7.3%)
Blood glucose level (mg/dL)	109.5±54.9	109.7±44.0	109.7±49.7
Hemoglobin level (g/dL)	11.8±2.5	12.6±2.6	12.2±2.6
Seropositive for HIV	35/260 (13.5%)	30/240 (12.5%)	65/500 (13.0%)
White blood cell count (No./μL)	7014±4581	7484±3505	7,699±4,092

Uganda, Cameroon, and Senegal; idiopathic dilated CMO in Ethiopia and Sudan; IHD in Kenya; and RHD in South Africa. Consistent with the management of AHF elsewhere in the world, initial IV management included furosemide in 92.9% at baseline and the decreasing to 22.9% at the 7-day follow-up, followed by digoxin (13.7%), nitrate therapy (7.9%), dobutamine (5.1%), and dopamine (5%). Mechanical ventilation was required in only a small proportion (0.6%) of cases. Similarly, oral therapy typically comprised an ACE inhibitor/angiotensin II receptor blockers, followed by an aldosterone inhibitor, digoxin, aspirin, loop diuretics, beta blockers, statins, anticoagulants, nitrates, and hydralazine.

12.1.4.2 Patient follow-up and outcomes
Overall, 578 of 1,006 (57.5%) patients completed the assessment at 1-month follow-up. Subsequently, 461 (45.8%) were followed as planned at 6 months. A total of 159 (15.8%) patients died prior to the 6-month follow-up assessment, 316 (31.4%) had a last date known alive, and 70 (7%) were lost to follow-up. The main clinical outcomes observed in the study are shown in Table 12.2.

12.1.5 Study interpretation
This study was the first and largest international registry to report on AHF in sub-Saharan Africa. A major finding from this study was the relative youth of AHF patients in Africa (median age of 55 years) compared with a typical median age of in 66 to 70 years reported in high-income countries [36]. Although AHF appeared to affect men and women equally, the causes and characteristics differed between the sexes. Importantly, hypertension was revealed as the predominant cause of AHF, accounting for three-quarters of cases when combined with other common causes, such as idiopathic dilated CMO and RHD. The remainder of AHF cases were attributable to a variety of conditions (including PPCMO, EMF, and CAD). As outlined in Section 3 and to be discussed in the next chapter (Chapter 13), hypertension and hypertensive heart disease represent an enormous health burden within urban African communities in particular. The current data reinforce the urgent need to tackle hypertension in a sustained and systematic manner to

Table 12.2 Clinical outcomes reported from the THESUS-HF registry.

Outcome	Women (n=511)	Men (n=494)	All (n=1,006)
Initial hospital stay (days)	9.1±8.1	9.4±10.4	9.2±9.3
Inpatient mortality	18 (3.5%)	24 (4.9%)	42 (4.2%)
Readmission <60 days	8.5% (95% CI 6.2, 11.6)	9.7% (95% CI 7.2, 13.1)	9.1% (95% CI 7.3, 11.3)
Death <60 days	10.2% (95% CI 7.7,13.4)	11.0% (95% CI 8.4, 14.3)	10.6% (95% CI 8.7, 12.8)
Death or readmission <60 days	14.5% (95% CI 11.6,18.2)	16.6% (95% CI 13.5, 20.5)	15.6% (95% CI 13.3, 18.1)
Death <180 days	17.4% (95% CI 14.1, 21.4)	18.3% (95% CI 14.9, 22.4)	17.8% (95% CI 15.4, 20.6)

prevent more advanced cases of heart disease with their associated high levels of morbidity and mortality.

As the transition of socioeconomic changes slowly spreads across Africa, the non-communicable forms of heart disease may continue to increase (see Chapter 6). In contrast to the data reported in the Heart of Soweto Study (see Chapter 9), just under 3% of cases in this registry were found to be HIV positive; these results require careful interpretation given selective screening practices for HIV. The major outcomes revealed in this study, including the high rates of in-hospital and 6-month mortality, were strikingly similar to those of previous studies conducted in the United States and Europe. However, overall, morbidity and mortality rates were lower than those reported elsewhere in the world [36–38], undoubtedly reflecting a different spectrum of causality and acuity of presentations. Turning to treatment for AHF, nonischemic HF patients reported a high use of aspirin; however, the use of beta blockers was relatively low for the proportion of patients who presented with systolic dysfunction. These observations will assist future studies to improve the implementation of evidence-based treatments for AHF in the setting of sub-Saharan Africa, as well as represent a useful platform to continuously monitor the evolution of AHF in the region by supporting regional/national surveillance strategies. In addition, the combination of hydralazine hydrochloride and nitrates, which has been shown to be effective in patients of African ancestry but is rarely used in the sub-Saharan region [39,40] is being investigated in AHF patients in THESUS-HF Registry centers.

12.1.6 Study limitations

It was found that studies conducted in other regions had a higher follow-up rate compared to THESUS-HF. This was due most patients not having telephones, making them difficult to track when follow-up data were being collected.

12.1.7 Study conclusion

In conclusion, presentations of AHF in the THESUS-HF cohort (a representative sample of case presentations across the African continent) predominantly involved relatively young patients with underlying hypertension as the most likely AHF antecedent. AHF results in a high incidence of rehospitalization and mortality. Future studies should focus on addressing the causes and creation of awareness programs in order to reduce the incidence of AHF in sub-Saharan Africa.

12.2 Gender differences in AHF presentations in THESUS-HF

Ogah O, Davison B, Sliwa K, Mayosi BM, Damasceno A, Sani M, Mondo C, Dzudie A, Ojji D, Kouam C, Suliman A, Schrueder N, Yonga G, Abdou Ba S, Maru F, Alemayehu B. Gender differences in clinical characteristics and outcome of acute heart failure in sub-Saharan Africa: results of the THESUS-HF study. *Clinical Research in Cardiology* 2015; 104(6):481–90. [41]

12.2.1 Study background

The groundbreaking THESUS-HF (outlined above) provided an important overview of AHF presentations across the African continent. A high representation of women (relative to reports from other regions predominantly focusing on AHF secondary to myocardial ischemia/LV systolic dysfunction) with potentially different etiologies to men prompted a formal analysis of these data according to gender.

12.2.2 Study aims

The aim of the study, therefore, was to investigate potential sex differences through the examination of clinical characteristics, prognosis, and treatment of HF patients using primary data from the THESUS-HF Registry [29].

12.2.3 Study methods

The primary methods for the THESUS-HF Registry are outlined earlier in this chapter. For this report, data were analyzed on a sex-specific basis and compared accordingly.

12.2.4 Study findings

Figure 12.1 shows the recruitment of AHF patients from the 12 cardiology centers in sub-Saharan Africa, and the overall demographic profile of study patients has been presented earlier. Additional demographic characteristics are shown in Table 12.3, demonstrating potentially important differences in case presentation according to sex. Men were significantly older, had more previous admissions for HF, and were more likely to report a functional status of NYHA Class III/IV one month prior to admission (p=0.022). They also presented with more peripheral edema (p=0.0394) compared with women. However, women were more likely to report a history of valvular heart disease (VHD) (p<0.0001), to have AF, and to present with a higher respiratory rate (p=0.0484).

12.2.4.1 Cardiac function

On echocardiography, men had significantly larger volumes/values in respect to left atrial area (p=0.039), interventricular septal thickness in diastole (p=0.025), posterior wall thickness at end diastole (p=0.0106), LV internal diameter in diastole (p<0.0001) and in systole (p<0.0001) and E/A ratios (p=0.0039), and more impaired systolic function (based on significantly lower LVEF: p<0.0001) when compared with women. Alternatively, women were more likely to present with a higher E-wave deceleration time (p=0.0466), A-wave duration (p=0.0423), and mitral stenosis (p<0.0001).

12.2.4.2 Health outcomes

Overall, despite differing etiologies, there were no significant sex-based differences with respect to index hospital stay, inpatient case-fatality, recurrent hospital stay, and mortality during 6-month follow-up, although all of these parameters tended to be higher in men than women.

12.2.5 Study interpretation

Overall, the specific characteristics of AHF patients in sub-Saharan Africa differed according to sex. More men were aged >50 years, with AHF more common among women aged <50 years. This finding was at odds with data from Japan and Europe, although the women patients in those studies were older [42–45], perhaps attributable to the youth of Africa's population as a whole relative to high-income countries [21,23]. A history of the commonly identified risk factors and precursors for HF in high-income countries (including smoking, hypertension, and CAD) was more frequently observed in men. This, in turn, was reflected in higher underlying cardiac dysfunction in men, although not reaching statistical significance. These findings reinforce the different pathways to HF in sub-Saharan Africa and the need for prevention (and management) strategies that may well be optimally determined by sex. Certainly, there is more evidence for the effective

Table 12.3 Patients' demographic characteristics of the THESUS-HF registry.

Characteristic	Women (n = 511)	Men (n = 494)	All (n = 1,006)
Mean age (years)	50.7	54.0	52.4
>65 years	135 (26.4%)	134 (27.1%)	269 (26.7%)
Clinical profile			
CMO	216 (42.3%)	200 (40.5%)	416 (41.4%)
Cor pulmonale	36 (7.1%)	36 (7.3%)	72 (7.2%)
Dementia	13 (2.5%)	9 (1.8%)	22 (2.2%)
Depression	18 (3.5%)	15 (3.0%)	33 (3.3%)
CAD	36 (7.1%)	46 (9.3%)	82 (8.2%)
Malignancy	8 (1.6%)	5 (1.0%)	13 (1.3%)
Pacemaker	0 (0%)	4 (0.8%)	4 (0.4%)
Pericardial disease	24 (4.7%)	29 (5.9%)	53 (5.3%)
Peripheral vascular disease	3 (0.6%)	9 (1.8%)	12 (1.2%)
Stroke	15 (2.9%)	10 (2.0%)	25 (2.5%)
VHD	159 (31.1%)	113 (22.9%)	272 (27.1%)
NYHA functional class <1 month prior admission			
II	170 (33.3%)	133 (26.9%)	303 (30.1%)
III	98 (19.2%)	118 (23.9%)	217 (21.6%)
IV	10 (2.0%)	18 (3.6%)	28 (2.8%)
Signs and symptoms on admission			
Systolic BP (mm Hg)	128.5±33.4	132.4±33.7	130.4±33.5
Diastolic BP (mm Hg)	83.2±20.7	85.5±21.2	84.3±20.9
Pulse pressure (mm Hg)	45.4±20.0	47.0±19.4	46.2±19.7
Heart rate (beats/min)	105.7±21.6	101.6±21.4	103.7±21.6
Orthopnea	2.29±0.75	2.33±0.76	2.31±0.76
Peripheral edema	1.78±1.03	1.87±1.05	1.83±1.04
Rales	1.70±0.94	1.66±0.90	1.68±0.92
Respiratory rate, beats/min	31.3±8.3	30.0±7.5	30.7±7.9
Temperature (°C)	36.6±0.6	36.7±0.7	36.7±0.6

management of (so-called) HFrEF (derived from mainly North American and European trials involving relatively young men) than HFpEF, the latter being more prevalent in older women in those countries [46,47]. These data suggest a real problem in applying evidence-based management of HF in the African context, particularly given the paucity of evidence to support acute manifestations of the syndrome [47]. The higher burden of valvular disease in women (who are generally young) highlights the need to strengthen strategies for the control of RHD in this group in order to prevent AHF across sub-Saharan Africa.

12.2.6 Study limitations

As this study was conducted in a tertiary hospital, the study findings may not reflect what happens in the secondary or primary health care services in these African countries. Therefore, this study only indicates what happens in these tertiary institutions. Invasive cardiac procedures were not available in many of the centers; therefore, many IHD patients may have been missed.

12.2.7 Study conclusions

In conclusion, this study revealed differences between men and women in the profile of AHF presentations in sub-Saharan Africa. Men presenting with HF were predominantly older than women and more likely to present with greater systolic dysfunction. These data are vital to understanding and responding to different patterns of heart disease and to their successful treatment on a sex-specific basis.

12.3 Prognostic significance of ECG abnormalities in THESUS-HF Registry

Dzudie A, Milo O, Edwards C, Cotter G, Davison BA, Damasceno A, Mayosi BM, Mondo C, Ogah O, Ojji D, Sani MU, Sliwa K. Prognostic significance of ECG abnormalities for mortality risk in acute heart failure: insight from the Sub-Saharan Africa Survey of Heart Failure (THESUS-HF). *Journal of Cardiac Failure* 2014; 20(1):45–52. [48]

12.3.1 Study background

The 12-lead ECG is a widely available, reasonably inexpensive, simple test that provides results instantly. The American Heart Association and European Society of Cardiology recommend an ECG as the initial test in HF patients [35,49] where most patients with HF due to systolic dysfunction have a significant abnormality on ECG [50]. Importantly, the current ECG criteria derived from North American and European studies may not be applicable to the African population. In the Heart of Soweto Study for example, up to 13% of the studied population presented with significant Q-waves in the absence of myocardial ischemia. The prognostic and diagnostic utility of the ECG in Africans with AHF has not been reported; consequently, THESUS-HF [29] collected clinical data in an African cohort of AHF patients during admission and after follow-up (as discussed above).

12.3.2 Study aims

The aim of the study was to assess the analytical utility of 12-lead ECG abnormalities among African patients with AHF in the THESUS-HF Registry.

12.3.3 Study methods

12.3.3.1 Study design and clinical setting

In addition to the methods described in Section 12.1.3, a 12-lead ECG was completed within approximately 2 weeks of admission and all ECGs were analyzed for rhythm or conduction abnormalities, using the Minnesota code classification system [51]. The following parameters were entered into the database registry together with other clinical data: heart rate; type of rhythm (junctional rhythm, AF, sinus rhythm, ventricular tachycardia, ventricular pacing, other supraventricular tachycardia, and 1st-, 2nd-, or 3rd-degree atrioventricular block); length of QRS, QT, and QTc intervals; Q-wave compatible with myocardial infarction as well as all other forms of Q-waves; and ST-T segment changes. All ECG abnormalities were then characterized as "major" or "minor."

12.3.4 Study findings

As outlined earlier, 1,006 patients were enrolled in THESUS-HF. 12-lead ECGs were recorded for 813 patients (of these, 523 [64.3%] were obtained within approximately 2 weeks of admission and were analyzed). Consistent with the overall cohort findings, hypertension (55.8%) was the most common concurrent diagnosis among study patients, followed by type 2 diabetes (10.5%), HIV infection (8.8%), cor pulmonale (7.3%), and malignancy (4.5%).

12.3.4.1 12-lead ECG findings

Sinus rhythm and AF were found in 329 (75.1%) and 121 (23.6%) patients, respectively. Other ECG abnormalities common to those with HF included LVH in 158 (30.6%), left bundle branch block in 42 (8.1%), and right bundle branch block in 26 (5.0%) patients. Overall, 511 (out of 523 patients, 97.7%) had one or more ECG abnormality. Corrected QT intervals were measured for all patients, and after separating patients into two groups according to sex, only 7 out of 254 (2.8%) men had a borderline to abnormal QTc (>430 ms), while only 6 out of 267 (2.3%) women had a borderline to abnormal QTc (>450 ms).

12.3.4.2 Health outcomes according to ECG findings

Overall, 80 (15.3%) patients died prior to completion of the 6-month assessment and 261 (49.9%) completed the 6-month assessment. Of those subject to active follow-up at 6 months, 63 patients had a readmission and 77 died (17.5% case-fatality at 6 months). An increasingly higher ventricular rate was associated with increasing risk of readmission and case-fatality, whereas sinus rhythm was associated with lower risk. Figure 12.2 displays the results of survival analyses according to underlying rhythm and heart rate, with differential survival rates evident on this basis.

Overall, QT duration and QRS width were not linked with either readmission through 2 months or mortality through 6 months, nor with composite outcome

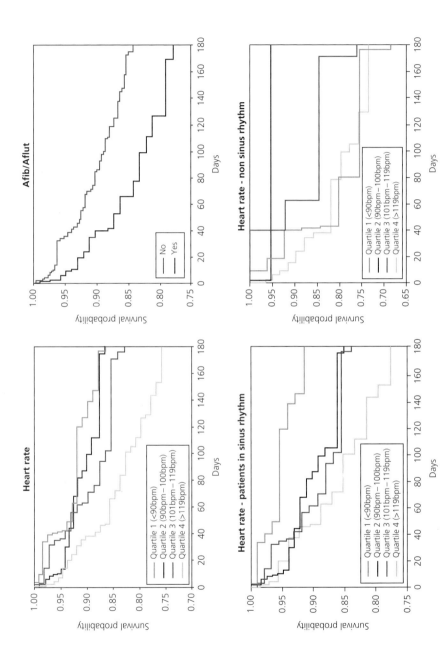

Figure 12.2 Kaplan-Meier estimates of 6-month survival according to ECG findings. Adapted from Dzudie et al., 2014 [48]. Reproduced with permission of Elseiver.

of mortality. Ischemic and bundle branch block fluctuations were not significantly connected with either outcome. After multivariable adjustment, lack of Q-waves and sinus rhythm associated with MI were the only ECG variables associated with mortality or readmission within 2 months or 6 months (see Table 12.4).

12.3.5 Study interpretation

Overall, a prevalence of 97.7% of ECG abnormalities (associated with a high risk for adverse outcomes) was found among the study cohort of AHF patients in the nine African countries participating in THESUS-HF. The main ECG abnormalities

Table 12.4 Predictors of mortality within 6 months.

Baseline Characteristic	Univariate Model	Multivariate Model
	Hazard Ratio (95% CI)	Hazard Ratio (95% CI)
Men	1.05 (0.67–1.64)	1.04 (0.63–1.72)
Edema	2.34 (1.34–4.08)	2.20 (1.17–4.14)
Heart rate	1.84 (1.22–2.78)	1.43 (0.93–2.19)
History of cor pulmonale	2.71 (1.45–5.05)	2.09 (1.04–4.23)
History of malignancy	6.05 (2.21–16.59)	5.43 (1.83–16.08)
History of cigarette smoking	1.12 (0.51–2.44)	1.31 (0.56–3.08)
HIV infection	1.30 (0.62–2.72)	0.99 (0.43–2.27)
Orthopnea	2.36 (0.83–6.71)	2.22 (0.72–6.89)
Oxygen saturation	0.92 (0.80–1.07)	0.86 (0.72–1.04)
Rales	2.03 (1.15–3.59)	1.37 (0.71–2.65)
Systolic BP	0.85 (0.79–0.92)	0.88 (0.81–0.95)
Laboratory tests		
Creatinine	1.62 (1.11–2.35)	1.33 (0.93–1.91)
Hemoglobin	0.92 (0.84–1.01)	0.94 (0.84–1.04)
ECG parameters		
AF	1.53 (0.94–2.51)	—
Left Bundle Branch Block	1.00 (0.43–2.32)	—
LVH	0.52 (0.29–0.93)	—
QRS duration	0.94 (0.86–1.03)	—
QT	0.95 (0.88–1.04)	—
QTc	0.98 (0.95–1.01)	
Right Bundle Branch Block	0.77 (0.24–2.45)	—
Sinus rhythm	0.56 (0.35–0.90)	0.61 (0.36–1.02)
Ventricular rate (beats/min)	1.04 (1.00–1.09)	—
Other ECG abnormalities		
Isolated pathologic Q-waves	1.90 (0.47–7.73)	—
Nonspecific ST-T changes	1.45 (0.89–2.37)	1.57 (0.91–2.72)
Q-waves compatible with AMI	2.19 (1.34–3.57)	2.45 (1.39–4.32)
ST-segment depression ≥1 mm	0.48 (0.07–3.45)	—
ST-segment elevation ≥1 mm	1.90 (0.77–4.71)	—
T-wave inversion in ≥2 contiguous leads	0.55 (0.31–0.97)	—

found in this study included lack of sinus rhythm and Q-waves, as well as elevated heart rate. As concluded in previous studies, the presence of ECG abnormalities is associated with poor health outcomes [50,52]. Patients suffering from structural cardiac abnormalities such as VHD and reduced LVEF, as well as comorbidities such as type 2 diabetes (11%) and hypertension (56%) resulted in a high prevalence of abnormal ECGs. A normal ECG is thus uncommon in suspected HF patients and is also beneficial in confirming underlying CVD (noting the caveats around interpreting the "normal" African ECG arising from the Heart of Soweto Study [53]).

Only 90 (17.2%) patients were found to have Q-waves compatible with AMI, indicating that IHD is a rare cause of AHF in patients in African countries [20,22,29]. Patients with HF who are left untreated usually display an increased heart rate; however, the association with increased heart rate and mortality is due to highly severe neurohormonal activation and cannot go unnoticed [54]. The prevalence of left bundle branch block rate was relatively low (8%) compared with reports from European countries (16%–22%). Furthermore, left bundle branch block was not linked with increased mortality as has been found in Europe. This might be due to the variance in age groups and HF etiologies of the study populations [55–57]. Although an ECG is a widely available, reasonably inexpensive, simple test that provides instant results and is recommended by the American Heart Association and European Society of Cardiology, its value lies in excluding specific causes of AHF, such as life-threatening arrhythmias or AMI; it does not significantly aid the risk stratification of HF patients. Although an association between adverse outcomes and preserved systolic dysfunction has been described [58], other data involving AHF patients with an LVEF ≤40% QRS duration did not support this [59]. Turning to QTc abnormalities, although a previous study of almost 100 CHF patients reported prolonged QTc in more than half the cohort [60], the current African study revealed QTc prolongation in a minority of patients. Noting that a significant proportion of the cohort was hypertensive, it was predicted that this study would reveal a high prevalence of ECG signs of LVH. However, just under a third of patients met such criteria. Despite ECG-specified LVH being previously reported as an independent predictor of worse outcomes [61], this study found that African patients with LVH were at decreased risk of readmission and all-cause mortality through 2 months as well as mortality through 6 months. This result was unexpected and requires further analysis but raises the possibility that hypertensive HF has a comparatively benign prognosis in African cohorts.

12.3.6 Study limitations

There were a number of limitations noted in the study. First, only 523 ECGs were available from 1,006 patients; however, the patients with available ECGs had similar characteristics to the rest of the cohort. Second, there was a lack of standardization of the manner in which the ECGs were acquired. Third, there were data missing for other variables, which may have diluted the associations that were sought in this study. Fourth, cases of HF may have been missed due to no access to cardiac catheterization in a number of centers. Finally, ECG recordings were completed at 615 days and not absolutely on admission; therefore, this study undoubtedly missed transient ECG abnormalities.

12.3.7 Study conclusions

In conclusion, 98% of the African patients admitted for AHF presented with an abnormal ECG, and some of these abnormalities, such as nonsinus rhythm, higher heart rate, and presence of Q-waves, are associated with a high risk for adverse outcomes. Although ECGs should be regularly evaluated in AHF patients to confirm the presence of heart disease, ECG abnormalities among African AHF patients are nonspecific and do not significantly enhance the risk stratification among these patients.

12.4 Contemporary profile of AHF in Southern Nigeria

Ogah O, Stewart S, Falase A, Akinyemi J, Adegbite G, Alabi A, Ajani A, Adesina J, Durodola A, Sliwa K. Contemporary profile of acute heart failure in Southern Nigeria. Journal of the American College of Cardiology: Heart Failure 2014; 2(3):250–9. [16]

12.4.1 Study background

Although HF is known to be an important health issue in developed countries, it is now a major public health concern globally [62,63]. Due to the increasing burden of cardiovascular risk factors and the aging population, HF is increasing yearly, with a global estimate of 15 million diagnosed patients [64]. Although there are generous data available for the incidence and prevalence of HF in North America and Europe, there are limited equivalent data for sub-Saharan African countries such as Nigeria [20,21,36,65–68]. Previous studies conducted in Nigeria were implemented in the 1960s, 1970s, and 1980s when a diagnosis of HF was not confirmed by echocardiography [69–71]. Furthermore, there are limited data on acute clinical presentations of HF in Nigeria to be effectively compared with larger American and European populations [72].

12.4.2 Study aims

The aim of this study was to determine the causes and characteristics of AHF presentations in Abeokuta, Nigeria, as well as to assess the effects of demographic characteristics and epidemiological transition, through utilizing the Abeokuta HF Clinical Registry.

12.4.3 Study methods

During the period January 2009 to December 2010, all AHF patients with pre-established HF presenting to the Federal Medical Centre were enrolled for the study after providing informed consent. Patient data including demographic and clinical characteristics were collected for each patient through the use of case report forms, 12-lead ECG analysis, and echocardiography. All cases of AHF, both de novo presentations and recurrent decompensation with pre-established diagnoses of HF, were consecutively recruited into the registry. HF was diagnosed using the Framingham criteria as well as the European Society of Cardiology guidelines on diagnosis and treatment of AHF.

12.4.4 Study findings
12.4.4.1 Cohort profile
Of the total number of AHF patients admitted to the Federal Medical Centre, 9.4% (452) were enrolled in the study. As shown in Table 12.5, there was a similar distribution between men and women with regard to the number of patients residing in urban areas and a range of demographic and clinical parameters. Men, however, were more likely to have higher levels of education (p = 0.006) and unemployment (p = 0.002), as well as to report heavier alcohol intake (p < 0.001) and cigarette smoking (p = 0.006) and to exhibit underlying hypertension (p = 0.010).

Table 12.5 Patients' demographic and clinical characteristics.

Characteristic	Women (n = 204)	Men (n = 248)	All (n = 452)
Age (years)	55.7 ± 17.1	57.3 ± 13.4	56.6 ± 15.3
Unemployed	38 (18.6%)	25 (10.1%)	13 (2.9%)
Urban residence	153 (75.0%)	185 (74.6%)	388 (85.8%)
Alcohol intake (previous/current)	18 (8.8%)	148 (59.7%)	166 (36.7%)
Cigarette smoking	1 (0.5%)	14 (5.6%)	15 (3.3%)
Total cholesterol (mg/dL)	188.6 ± 64.8	164.1 ± 72.2	171.0 ± 70.5
BMI (kg/m^2)	23.7 ± 6.4	24.0 ± 5.1	23.9 ± 5.7
Obesity	20 (9.8%)	21 (8.5%)	41 (9.1%)
Family history of CVD	6 (2.9%)	8 (3.2%)	14 (3.1%)
Known type 2 diabetes	25 (12.3%)	20 (8.1%)	45 (10.0%)
Known hypertension	119 (58.3%)	174 (70.2%)	293 (64.8%)
Anemia (n = 382)	22 (12.4%)	18 (8.8%)	40 (10.5%)
Arthritis	35 (17.2%)	10 (4.0%)	64 (14.2%)
Asthma	6 (2.9%)	3 (1.2%)	9 (2.0%)
COPD	4 (2.0%)	12 (4.8%)	16 (3.5%)
Renal dysfunction (n = 366)	77 (47.0%)	97 (48.0%)	174 (47.5%)
HIV infection (n = 222)	1.9%	3.5%	2.7%
Pulse rate (beats/min) (n = 418)	96.3 ± 18.7	96.9 ± 17.9	96.6 ± 18.3
Systolic BP (n = 424; mm Hg)	136.2 ± 31.4	138.7 ± 32.2	137.5 ± 31.8
Diastolic BP (n = 424; mm Hg)	85.9 ± 19.4	88.5 ± 21.0	87.3 ± 20.3
NYHA functional class (n = 308)			
II	32 (15.7%)	47 (19.0%)	79 (25.7%)
III	134 (65.8%)	150 (60.5%)	284 (92.2%)
IV	38 (18.6%)	51 (20.4%)	89 (28.9%)
Days in hospital	6.48 ± 0.52	10.8 ± 0.78	11.4 ± 9.1

12.4.4.2 Signs of AHF

The most common signs of AHF were basal crepitation, followed by displaced apex beat, elevated jugular venous pressure, 3rd heart sound, peripheral edema, tender hepatomegaly, systolic murmur, gallop rhythm, ascites, pallor, fever, central cyanosis, diastolic murmur, splenomegaly, finger clubbing, and jaundice. The most common symptoms of AHF were cough, followed by dyspnea, orthopnea, paroxysmal nocturnal dyspnea, pedal edema, easy fatigability, palpitation, abdominal swelling, chest pain, headache, nausea, vomiting, and hemoptysis.

12.4.4.3 Precipitating factors for AHF and 12-lead ECG

Overall, 284 (62.8%) patients presented with chest pain, 200 (44.2%) with uncontrolled hypertension, 123 (27.3%) with AF, 33 (7.3%) with anemia, 25 (5.5%) with excessive physical activity, 10 (2.2%) with electrolyte imbalance, and 1 (0.2%) with AMI. With regard to the 12-lead ECG results, the majority of the patients displayed abnormal readings. Overall, 374 (82.7%) patients presented with LVH, 344 (76.1%) with axis deviations (most commonly left axis deviation), 315 (69.7%) with atrial enlargement, and 52 (11.5%) with AF.

12.4.4.4 Etiology of HF

The predominant etiology for HF among study patients was hypertensive HF, found in 335 (78.5%) patients. The remaining cases were attributable to dilated CMO in 34 (7.5%), cor pulmonale in 20 (4.4%), pericardial disease in 15 (3.3%), and RHD in 11 (2.4%) patients. As shown in Figure 12.3, men were more likely to present with hypertensive HF, dilated CMO, and IHD, while women were more likely to display pericardial disease and thyroid heart disease. However, there was a similar sex distribution for cor pulmonale, RHD, EMF, and adult CHD.

12.4.4.5 Echocardiography

On echocardiography, men were more likely to present with higher aortic root diameter, posterior wall thickness, LV septal wall thickness in diastole, LV mass, and indexes of LV systolic function when compared with women. As shown in Table 12.6, E/A ratios, LV internal diameter in diastole, and LV internal diameter in systole were more common among patients diagnosed with CMO, while fractional shortening and relative wall thickness was more frequent among patients diagnosed with cor pulmonale. Aortic root diameter, isovolumic relaxation time, and LV mass were more common in patients diagnosed with hypertensive HF, whereas deceleration time of E-velocity was more frequent among patients diagnosed with pericardial disease. Finally, interventricular septal wall thickness in diastole, LV mass index, and LV posterior wall thickness in diastole were more often observed in patients diagnosed with RHD.

12.4.4.6 Pharmacotherapy

Upon admission to the Federal Medical Centre, 431 (95.4%) patients were prescribed a diuretic agent, 419 (92.7%) an ACE inhibitor, 338 (74.7%) digoxin, 292 (64.7%) an anticoagulant agent, 78 (17.3%) a calcium-channel blocker, 54 (12%)

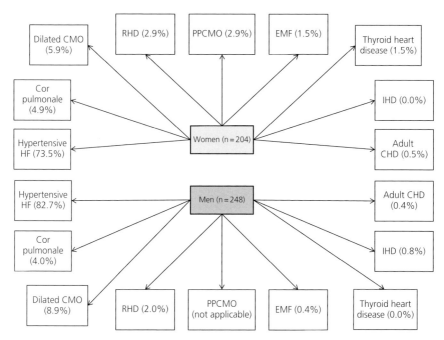

Figure 12.3 Etiology of AHF patients.

a centrally acting antihypertensive agent, and 42 (9.4%) a beta blocker. On hospital discharge, 448 (99.1%) patients were prescribed an ACE inhibitor, 398 (88.1%) a loop diuretic, 327 (72.3%) digoxin, 121 (26.8%) a long-acting calcium-channel blocker, 65 (14.4%) combined hydralazine and isosorbide dinitrate, and 41 (9.1%) a beta blocker.

12.4.4.7 Outcomes

In total, 17 (3.8%) patients died during the course of admission; of these, 7 (41.2%) patients died from cardiogenic shock, 5 (29.4%) from a fatal arrhythmia, 3 (17.7%) from pulmonary embolism, and 2 (11.8%) from stroke. Those patients who died were younger, predominantly women, and were most likely to have existing hypertension (52.9%) or dilated CMO (29.4%).

12.4.5 Study interpretation

This study revealed that AHF patients compose 10% of all medical admissions in Abeokuta, Nigeria, while 1 in 5 patients presenting with heart conditions are admitted into emergency medical centers [73]. The prevalence of hypertension in the region has risen from 8.6% in 1979 to 22.5% in 2011, with hypertension awareness, treatment, and management being relatively low and hypertension-specific complications being consequently high [74]. More than half of the study patients exhibited systolic HF, with hypertensive HF the most common etiology for AHF, consistent with studies in Cameroon [29], and IHD the least common.

Table 12.6 ECG characteristics according to etiological risk factors for HF.

	CMO (n=38)	Cor Pulmonale (n=26)	Hypertensive HF (n=355)	Pericardial Disease (n=15)	RH (n=11)
Aortic root diameter	2.89±0.48	2.93±0.11	3.10±0.50	2.76±0.39	2.90±0.42
Deceleration time of E velocity	114.6±41.4	113.9±64.6	144.3±57.6	184.9±91.0	154.0±36.2
E/A ratio	2.50±1.10	1.54±1.10	2.04±1.45	1.58±0.89	2.49±1.49
LVEF	35.4±16.2	52.6±14.6	42.9±16.5	50.3±16.5	58.6±10.5
Fractional shortening	14.3±8.20	25.5±9.0	17.9±8.70	21.8±9.2	25.9±6.0
Interventricular septal wall thickness (diastole)	1.13±0.28	1.18±0.43	1.35±0.37	1.18±0.23	1.46±0.37
Isovolumic relaxation time	109.9±38.4	107.2±29.1	116.4±34.8	89.0±8.7	92.0±7.0
Left atrial area (cm²)	26.7±6.1	24.8±4.3	26.6±8.1	21.5±4.2	33.5±12.0
Left atrial diameter	4.80±1.18	4.26±1.15	4.90±2.99	3.87±0.96	4.71±1.06
LV internal diameter (diastole)	6.19±0.75	4.59±1.28	5.52±1.49	4.14±0.70	5.72±0.94
LV internal diameter (systole)	5.33±0.87	3.42±1.23	4.57±1.43	3.05±0.48	4.50±1.01
LV mass index	79.9±31.1	77.1±34.5	90.4±37.7	38.4±11.0	93.4±24.2
LV posterior wall thickness (diastole)	1.05±0.35	1.04±0.16	1.19±0.36	0.96±0.18	1.21±0.30
Relative wall thickness	0.35±0.14	0.49±0.15	0.45±0.15	0.48±0.13	0.43±0.15

While studies in Japan, North America, and Europe reported AHF in older patients, the current data suggest that AHF primarily affects young and middle-aged individuals in this setting. This may be related to the predominance of hypertension in the AHF etiology of this population. The lower rate of HF in women relative to men was consistent with many previous reports (although differing from studies conducted in South Africa and Kenya [30,75,76]) and may reflect sex differences in health-seeking behaviors, as the "breadwinner" may be more likely to be sent to hospital when resources are limited. Similar to the findings of the Heart of Soweto Study, valvular dysfunction was common among the patients; however, the intrahospital mortality rates in the current cohort were lower than previous reports from sub-Saharan Africa [29,33,75,77]. The average length of hospital stay in this study was 11 days, which is longer than previous reports from sub-Saharan Africa and developed countries (4 to 7 days) [29,36], although shorter than the 13 days reported by a study in Cameroon [77]. The prescribed medications, such as ACE inhibitors and spironolactone, are consistent with patterns in developed countries. However, use of beta blockers or combined hydralazine and isosorbide was lower than in developed countries; this may be due to the reluctance of Nigerian physicians to commence such medications in severely ill patients with HF. This finding presents an opportunity for improved management of AHF patients in Abeokuta and wider Nigeria.

12.4.6 Study limitations

As the study was conducted in a tertiary institution, patients with milder forms of HF were likely to have been underrepresented. This study therefore contacted the clinic requesting referral of all HF patients. IHD patients may have also been underrepresented due to the lack of coronary angiography and the likelihood of sudden out-of-hospital deaths. Finally, nutritional deficiencies and malnutrition were not assessed as possible factors for the earlier development of HF in this population.

12.4.7 Study conclusions

In conclusion, AHF affects younger individuals of working age in Abeokuta, Nigeria, is more common in males, and is associated with severe signs and symptoms due to late presentation. Inpatient mortality in Nigeria is similar to that observed in studies conducted in other parts of the world. Hypertension has been projected to increase in African countries by 89% [78], particularly in Nigeria, which is the most populous country in the region. There is a need for future studies to investigate and implement primary prevention and health promotion strategies to combat hypertension among the population of Nigeria.

CHAPTER 13

Hypertensive heart failure

Dike Bevis Ojji[1], Mahmoud Sani[2], Anastase Dzudie[3],
and Okechukwu Samuel Ogah[4]

[1] University of Abuja Teaching Hospital, Abuja, Nigeria
[2] Bayero University Kano/Aminu Kano Teaching Hospital, Kano, Nigeria
[3] Hospital General de Douala, Douala, Littoral, Cameroon
[4] University College Hospital, Ibadan, Oyo, Nigeria

13.0 Introduction

In this chapter we describe three different studies (one from Soweto, South Africa, and the other two from Nigeria) examining the clinical spectrum and consequences of hypertension and hypertensive HF in the African context. As already outlined in Chapter 4, given elevated BP levels observed across the continent, hypertension may well pose the largest threat to the future health of the African population as it effectively combats infectious disease and increases its overall economic wealth. These studies (with comparison across two study findings) provide an important insight into the contemporary and likely future burden of hypertensive HF in sub-Saharan Africa.

13.1 Clinical consequences and challenges of hypertension in urban-dwelling black Africans

Stewart S, Libhaber E, Carrington MJ, Damasceno A, Abbasi H, Hansen C, Wilkinson D, Silwa K. The clinical consequences and challenges of hypertension in urban-dwelling black Africans: Insights from the Heart of Soweto Study. *International Journal of Cardiology* 2011; 146(1):22–27. [79]

13.1.1 Study background

At the time of this study (derived from the Heart of Soweto Study described in more detail in Chapter 6) it was noted that although data describing the broad pattern of hypertension in LMIC and sub-Saharan Africa are readily available [80], there are few studies examining the clinical consequences of undiagnosed/untreated and/or controlled hypertension in this context. In order to minimize the emergence of noncommunicable forms of CVD, it is critical to understand the consequences of undetected and untreated hypertension in vulnerable communities in urban

---

The Heart of Africa: Clinical Profile of an Evolving Burden of Heart Disease in Africa, First Edition.
Edited by Simon Stewart, Karen Sliwa, Ana Mocumbi, Albertino Damasceno, and Mpiko Ntsekhe.
© 2016 John Wiley & Sons, Ltd. Published 2016 by John Wiley & Sons, Ltd.

sub-Saharan Africa. During 2006, the clinical spectrum of CVD and its risk factors were reported in prevalent and incident cases of heart disease as part of the Heart of Soweto Study [22,81] (see Chapter 6 for full details). In patients of African ancestry, hypertension was diagnosed in more than half of the patients and was frequently associated with advanced forms of heart disease. Overall, hypertension was revealed as the most common diagnosis in the cohort [30].

13.1.2 Study aims

The primary aim of this study was to examine the clinical consequences of hypertension as manifested in advanced presentations of hypertensive heart disease in the setting of an urban African population in whom both epidemiological transition and a poor awareness and response to noncommunicable forms of heart disease might play an important role in generating a substantial health burden.

13.1.3 Study methods
13.1.3.1 Patient enrollment

The Heart of Soweto Study methods have been described in greater detail in Chapter 6. For these analyses, all de novo presentations to the Cardiology Unit of the Chris Hani Baragwanath Hospital in Soweto in the year 2006 that were of African ancestry and clinically diagnosed with hypertension were included. Of the total of 897 de novo patients with hypertension, 761 (84.8%) were of African ancestry and were included in the study [22]. Included patients comprised emergency patients who were referred directly to the Cardiology Unit with recognized CVD, those referred externally from local primary care clinics for more definitive examination and treatment, and those referred internally to the Cardiology Unit on an inpatient and outpatient basis. The clinical spectrum of study patients, therefore, ranged from those with uncomplicated hypertension being treated with combination antihypertensive therapy to first-ever diagnosed patients with advanced hypertensive heart disease yet to receive definitive treatment.

13.1.4 Study findings
13.1.4.1 Demographic and clinical characteristics

The study cohort included 482 (63.3%) women who were of a similar age profile (typically middle aged) to their male counterparts (mean age of 58.5 ± 14.9 years versus 58.0 ± 15.6 years). Overall, 168 (22.1%) patients reported a family history of CVD, with more women reporting the risk factor than men (OR 1.63, 95% CI 1.20–2.23: p=0.001). Men were more likely to have a cardiovascular risk factor other than hypertension (OR 1.86, 95% CI 1.29–2.69: p=0.001) and to smoke cigarettes (OR 4.72, 95% CI 3.44–6.45: p<0.0001). However, women were more likely to be obese (OR 2.66, 95% CI 1.83–3.86: p<0.001). As shown in Figure 13.1, HF was found to be more common among men (n=166 [59.5%] versus n=244 [50.1%]; p=0.018), as well as renal disease (n=30 [10.8%] versus n=39 [8.1%]; p=0.001). Overall there were minor sex differences with regard to structural valve disease, CAD, stroke, diabetes, and HIV infection.

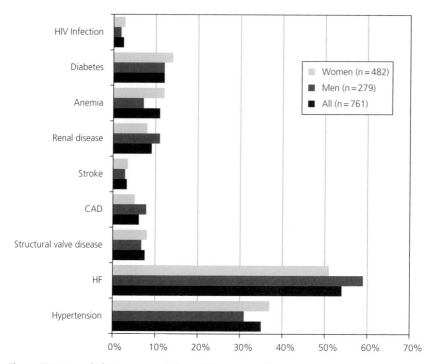

Figure 13.1 Comorbidities among study participants according to sex.

13.1.4.2 BP profile and management

BP profiles varied according to stage of treatment and presentation status. In total, 350 (46%) patients had a BP of ≥140/90 mm Hg and were considered to be hypertensive, while there was a weak association between systolic BP and age which was slightly stronger in men (p < 0.001) than in women (p = 0.042). Patients without progressive CVD presented with a significantly lower systolic (135 ± 27 versus 144 ± 28 mm Hg; p < 0.0001) but not diastolic BP. When presenting to the Cardiology Unit, it was found that 473 (62%) patients were currently on active antihypertensive therapy; the most commonly prescribed antihypertensive agents were calcium channel antagonists (20%), aldosterone inhibitor (20%), beta blockers (25%), ACE inhibitors (39%), and loop diuretics (49%). Overall, 384 (81.2%) patients were prescribed combination therapy, and 211 (44.6%) prescribed triple therapy. Combination therapy was associated with lower systolic BP (133 ± 29 versus 140 ± 28 mm Hg: p = 0.034) and diastolic BP (74 ± 17 versus 78 ± 16 mm Hg; p = 0.052). Those prescribed an aldosterone inhibitor (systolic BP 133 ± 24 versus 142 ± 30 mm Hg) or an ACE inhibitor (134 ± 27 versus 141 ± 29/74 ± 16 versus 79 ± 16 mm Hg: p < 0.001) had significantly lower BP profiles.

13.1.4.3 Hypertensive HF and other advanced forms of heart disease

Overall, 494 (65%) patients presented with progressive cardiovascular forms comprising a combination of stroke (3.3%), CAD (6.2%), renal disease (9.1%), anemia (11%), and most strikingly, hypertensive HF (54%). Echocardiography demonstrated that an additional 98 (13%) patients had abnormal valvular function. Overall, more than half (59%) of these were attributable to underlying structural valve disease. In addition, 258 (41%) patients displayed evidence of mildly impaired renal dysfunction and 150 (24%) had moderate to severe renal dysfunction indicative of progressive end organ damage. Although women were more likely than men to present with clinical symptoms, they were less likely to be diagnosed with renal disease (OR 0.47, 95% CI 0.30–0.73: p=0.001), and/or to present with HF (OR 0.85, 95% CI 0.75–0.97: p=0.018). Men were more likely to present with abnormal valvular function (OR 1.42, 95% CI 1.00–2.03: p=0.046).

13.1.4.4 Cardiac function

In total, 103 (24%) patients presented with evidence of RHF on ECG, 163 (24%) with diastolic dysfunction, 158 (24%) with moderate to severe systolic dysfunction, and 264 (39%) with LVH. Men displayed a significantly lower LVEF and larger LV dimensions, which increased their chance of presenting with impaired systolic function (OR 2.13, 95% CI 1.50–3.00; p<0.0001). Although there were minimal sex differences in LVH, women were less likely to present with any form of 12-lead ECG change (OR 0.57, 95% CI 0.36–0.88). The likelihood of presenting with concurrent systolic dysfunction and hypertension increased as patients grew older, in men, in those who smoked cigarettes, and in those with an elevated diastolic BP and heart rate. However, the likelihood of presenting with concurrent systolic dysfunction decreased with increasing systolic BP.

13.1.5 Study interpretation

This study prospectively analyzed the characteristics and consequences of hypertension in 761 urban-dwelling individuals of African ancestry presenting to a tertiary care center during 2006 [22]. In total, approximately 40% of patients presented with LVH and approximately 60% had previously undiagnosed heart and vascular disease [80]. These striking results were unfortunately consistent with the disturbingly low detection, treatment, and control levels of hypertension in Soweto and other parts of sub-Saharan Africa [80]. The findings confirm the importance of focusing on hypertension as a major contributor to avoidable noncommunicable heart disease—particularly in the form of hypertensive HF. Despite not providing a complete understanding of the history of hypertension leading to progressive heart disease in this African community, these data offer important insights for prevention strategies. The early signs of a hypertensive heart disease epidemic have been uncovered and will result in an escalating burden if primary and secondary prevention is not applied on a systematic basis. Fortunately, hypertension is readily detectable and can be controlled with inexpensive treatments [82,83]. Regardless of the population studied, hypertension is crucial to the subsequent vulnerability to and development of HF (particularly in the clinical context of LVH), although the pathways to HF are many and varied; further, the progression from concentric LVH to HF has not yet been recorded in Africa. Overall, 54% of the total study population presented with low to normal BP and advanced forms of heart disease. Consistent with previous reports [84], reasonably low levels of diagnosed anemia and renal disease were revealed. However, more than half of the patients had a combination of mild (41%) or moderate-to-severe (24%) renal dysfunction, and this was undoubtedly linked to their hypertension status as a marker of progressive end-organ damage.

13.1.6 Study limitations

There were a number of limitations noted in the study. First, not all hypertension patients in Soweto are managed by the Cardiology Unit at the Chris Hani Baragwanath Hospital, as patients of African ancestry rarely use private health care facilities, and it is possible that many patients were missed. Finally, clinical data were not captured for all patients in this study and therefore relied on clinical diagnosis.

13.1.7 Study conclusions

Previous findings from urban-dwelling areas in sub-Saharan Africa have demonstrated an increase in the prevalence of hypertension due to epidemiologic transition [80,85]. Overall, this study revealed that progressive forms of heart disease were a factor of undetected and untreated hypertension, most notably hypertensive HF. This observation was strengthened in later analyses of de novo presentations captured by the Heart of Soweto Study over a more prolonged period [86]. As an initial warning, these data reinforced the need to develop and implement cost effective prevention, screening and management programs in African communities to decrease the risk of developing hypertension in the first instance and to reduce the incidence of more advanced forms of heart disease (most notably hypertensive HF) in those already affected.

13.2 A predominance of hypertensive HF in the Abuja Heart Society cohort of urban Nigerians: A prospective clinical registry of 1,515 de novo cases

Ojji D, Stewart S, Ajayi S, Manmak M, Silwa K. A predominance of hypertensive heart failure in the Abuja Heart Society cohort of urban Nigerians: a prospective clinical registry of 1515 de novo cases. *European Journal of Heart Failure* 2013; 15(8):835–42. [87]

13.2.1 Study background

There have been substantive changes in global disease patterns, with non-communicable diseases emerging as a major cause of morbidity and mortality, due to the shift in epidemiological and demographical health determinants in LMIC [88,89].

Significantly, CVD is now more likely to occur in adults in sub-Saharan Africa than in residents of high-income countries [90]. Unfortunately, data on patterns of heart disease in sub-Saharan Africa remain limited, due to the continued underestimation of the future threat posed by the emergence of CVD and the concurrent emphasis on communicable diseases such as malaria and HIV/AIDS [90]. To our knowledge, the last available research on forms of heart disease in Nigeria was published in the 1970s.

13.2.2 Study aims

The aim of this study was to examine the pattern of heart disease in Abuja, Nigeria, one of the fastest growing and populous cities in Nigeria, as well as to compare the results with similar data obtained from the Heart of Soweto Study in South Africa.

13.2.3 Study methods
13.2.3.1 Patient enrollment

During the period April 2006 to April 2010, every consecutive patient referred for the first time to the Cardiology Unit of the University of Abuja Teaching Hospital was examined. Overall, 1,586 patients were enrolled; of these, 71 patients were excluded from the study as they did not present any signs or symptoms of CVD, leaving a total of 1,515 study patients. All patients provided informed consent before enrollment in the study.

13.2.4 Study findings

As shown in Table 13.1, women patients were more likely than men to present as obese (OR 1.78, 95% CI 1.20–2.34), with hypertension (OR 1.96, 95% CI 1.26–2.65), and with palpitations (OR 1.68, 95% CI 1.41–2.42). Alternatively, men were older (2 years); were more likely to present with diabetes (OR 1.77, CI 1.25–2.37), HF (OR 1.61, 95% CI 1.19–2.32), or stroke (OR 1.62, 95% CI 1.18–2.20); and were more likely to report cigarette smoking (OR 1.95, 95% CI 1.83–2.65).

As also shown in Figure 13.2, HF was found in 475 (31.1%) patients, with the most common cause of HF being hypertension (60.6%), followed by idiopathic dilated CMO (12%), rheumatic valvular disease (8.6%), and PPCMO (5.3%). Overall, there were no sex differences with regard to ECG presentation; however, echocardiographic findings showed that men were more likely than women to have larger ventricles and a lower mean LVEF.

13.2.4.1 Comparisons to the Heart of Soweto Study

When comparing results from the Heart of Soweto Study to the findings of this study (Table 13.2), it was found that Soweto patients mainly comprised women (62%), were 2 to 3 years older, and reported a greater number of multiple risk factors (58.6% versus 12%) than the Abuja patients. They also displayed higher rates of cigarette smoking (41.5% versus 7.6%), HFpEF (23.4% versus 5.7%), LV systolic dysfunction (26.1% versus 17.6%), angina/chest pain (28.3% versus 19.8%), anemia (9.8% versus 5.3%), renal dysfunction (7.2% versus 5.9%),

Table 13.1 Patients' demographic and clinical characteristics.

	Women (n = 768)	Men (n = 747)	Total (n = 1,515)
Demographic characteristic			
Age (years)	48.1±14.2	49.9±13.0	49.0±13.7
Family history of CVD	33 (4.3%)	43 (5.8%)	76 (5.0%)
History of cigarette smoking	96 (1.1%)	106 (14.2%)	115 (7.6%)
Clinical characteristic			
Hypertension	586 (76.3%)	397 (53.1%)	983 (64.9%)
Dyslipidemia	108/445 (24.3%)	96/476 (20.2%)	205/913 (22.5%)
BMI > 30 (kg/m²)	263 (34.2%)	136 (18.2%)	409 (27.0%)
Fasting blood sugar	5.5±2.6	5.7±2.7	5.6±2.6
Multiple risk factors	72 (9.4%)	110 (14.7%)	182 (12.0%)
Heart rate (beats/min)	85.5±18.3	80.2±17.2	82.9±18.3
Systolic BP (mm Hg)	136.1±27.2	138.1±28.5	137.1±27.9
Diastolic BP (mm Hg)	86.5±16.3	89.3±17.6	87.9±17.0
Structural valvular disease	22 (2.9%)	33 (4.4%)	55 (3.6%)
HF	261 (34.0%)	214 (28.6%)	475 (31.4%)
CAD	0 (0%)	3 (0.4%)	3 (0.2%)
Type 2 diabetes	40 (5.2%)	73 (9.8%)	113 (7.5%)
Stroke	22 (2.9%)	50 (6.7%)	72 (4.8%)
HIV infection	7 (0.91%)	10 (1.3%)	17 (1.1%)
Anemia	51 (6.6%)	30 (4.0%)	81 (5.3%)
Renal disease	329 (42.8%)	328 (43.9%)	657 (43.4%)
eGFR (mL/min/1.73 m²)	86.9±53.8	84.9±46.3	85.5±50.1
Chest pain/angina	153 (19.9%)	147 (19.7%)	300 (19.8%)
NHYA Class II/III-IV	30/92	27/76	57/168
Edema	389 (50.7%)	377 (50.5%)	766 (50.6%)
Palpitations	314 (40.9%)	219 (29.3%)	533 (35.2%)

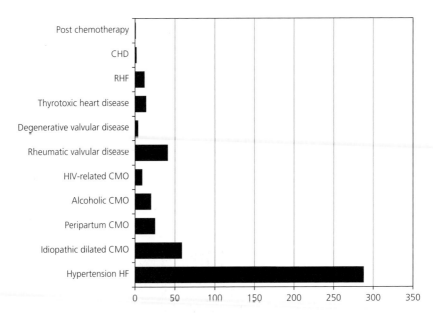

Figure 13.2 Pattern of HF in study patients.

Table 13.2 Patients' demographic and clinical characteristics according to the Abuja cohort and the Soweto cohort.

	Abuja Cohort (n = 1,515)	Soweto Cohort (n = 1,593)
Demographic characteristic		
Age (years)	49.0 ± 13.7	52.8 ± 17.1
Clinical characteristics		
History of CVD	76 (5.0%)	405 (25.4%)
Cigarette smoking	115 (7.6%)	661 (41.5%)
Hypercholesterolemia	205 (22.5%)	159 (10.0%)
Multiple risk factors	182 (12.0%)	933 (58.6%)
Type 2 diabetes	113 (7.5%)	165 (10.4%)
Bundle branch block on ECG	68 (5.1%)	124 (7.9%)
Heart rate (beats/min)	82.9 ± 18.3	86.0 ± 21.8
Systolic BP (mm Hg)	137.1 ± 27.9	130.0 ± 27.1
Diastolic BP (mm Hg)	87.9 ± 17.0	73.0 ± 16.6
HFpEF	87 (5.7%)	373 (23.4%)
LVEF	64.8 ± 20.6	53.0 ± 17.4
LV systolic dysfunction	266 (17.6%)	415 (26.1%)
AF	52 (3.9%)	102 (6.4%)
Anemia	81 (5.3%)	156 (9.8%)
Renal dysfunction	90 (5.9%)	115 (7.2%)
HIV infection	17 (1.1%)	74 (4.7%)
Angina/chest pain	300 (19.8%)	451 (28.3%)
NYHA Class III or IV	168 (11.1%)	486 (30.5%)
Edema	766 (50.6%)	494 (31.0%)

bundle branch block on 12-lead ECG (7.9% versus 5.1%), HIV infection (4.7% versus 1.1%), AF (6.4% versus 3.9%), and type 2 diabetes (10.4% versus 7.5%) when compared with the Abuja patients. However, the Abuja patients exhibited higher levels of hypercholesterolemia (22.5% versus 10%) and edema (50.6% versus 31%) relative to the Soweto patients.

13.2.5 Study interpretation

Overall, this Nigerian study revealed hypertension as the primary diagnosis in more than half of the study patients (more women than men) presenting at the Cardiology Unit of the University of Abuja Teaching Hospital. This finding was consistent with the results of the Heart of Soweto Study, where 64% of women and 36% of men presented newly diagnosed forms of CVD. As hypothesized, hypertension and hypertensive HF (with associated LVH) were the most common primary diagnoses, confirming previous observations that hypertension and its clinical consequences are common among those of African ancestry relative to other races. Abuja women were more likely than men to present with a primary diagnosis of hypertension, hypertensive LVH, obesity, palpitations, and anemia.

However, men were more likely to report cigarette smoking and to present with type 2 diabetes, HF, and history of stroke. Consistent with these observations, men had larger LV parameters and worse LV systolic function. The study sites selected in the Abuja study as well as the Heart of Soweto Study offer true representations of the community's spectrum of heart disease and provide indicators of more progressive heart disease cases. Higher levels of edema (indicative of congestion) and systolic and diastolic BP levels were found in Abuja; this can be explained by the sample's comprising only patients of African ancestry, while the Soweto cohort included different racial groups. Previous studies have reported a higher rate of fluid retention in cardiovascular patients of African ancestry compared to Asians and Caucasians, due to differences in salt-sensitive activation of the renin-angiotensin system [91]. Soweto patients displayed a higher prevalence of CAD when compared with the Abuja patients, attributable to a higher rate of risk factors such as cigarette smoking (41% versus 7.5%), type 2 diabetes (10.0% versus 7.5%), and perhaps HIV infection (5.0% versus 1.1%)—see Chapter 10. Hypertensive HF, RHF, and HF due to idiopathic dilated CMO were the three most common forms of HF in this study cohort. These results resembled those of the Heart of Soweto Study, with the exception of the finding of right-sided HF secondary to cor pulmonale as the third most common form of HF. In the Abuja study, right-sided HF occurred in 2.5% of the patients, contrasting with 27% in the Heart of Soweto patients. The higher prevalence of cor pulmonale and RHF in Soweto patients can likely be explained by a higher rate of smoking (41% versus 7.5%), more exposure to industrial pollutants, and a higher altitude of residence (see Chapter 15). The hypertension prevalence among the Abuja patients was 61%, consistent with previous reports [33,91], although slightly higher than the 53% prevalence reported in the Heart of Soweto Study (see Chapter 6). The prevalence of cigarette smoking (7.6%), hypercholesterolemia (22.5%), and type 2 diabetes (7.5%) in the Abuja study were lower than in Western communities, indicating a disease pattern in true transition. Overall, a significant proportion of Abuja patients were symptomatic on presentation, and the late presentation of HF patients explains the increasing rates of morbidity and mortality observed in this population.

13.2.6 Study limitations

As this study was conducted in a tertiary care facility, patients with milder forms of CVD may have been missed; therefore, the study data may underrepresent the Abuja population. In addition, Abuja patients may have approached other tertiary care facilities and have therefore not been captured.

13.2.7 Study conclusions

In conclusion, the most common cause of de novo HF presentations in Abuja, Nigeria, was hypertension, a finding that supports those of the earlier Heart of Soweto Study. These findings indicate the need for wider-ranging strategies to prevent, treat, and control the number of adults affected by hypertension and its clinical consequences, most notably hypertensive HF.

13.3 Hypertensive HF in Nigerian Africans

Ogah O, Sliwa K, Akinyemi J, Falase A, Stewart S. **Hypertensive heart failure in Nigerian Africans: insights from the Abeokuta Heart Failure Registry.** *Journal of Clinical Hypertension* 2015; 17(4):263–72. [92]

13.3.1 Study background

Hypertension is strongly associated with cardiovascular-related morbidity and mortality and is accountable for 7.5 million deaths worldwide [78,93,94]. Previous studies have demonstrated that the majority of these deaths occur in young to middle-aged individuals in developing countries and that hypertension is expected to rise by 89% in sub-Saharan Africa, compared to 24% in other countries [78,95]. Despite decreasing in many developed countries, mean systolic BP levels are on the rise in developing countries [93]. Given these findings and hypertension's status as the most common risk factor for heart disease in Nigeria, the scarcity of education, treatment, and management for hypertension and the associated increasing burden of hypertension-related complications are a serious concern [16,29,74,87,96,97].

13.3.2 Study aims

The aim of the study was to investigate the demographic and clinical characteristics and clinical outcomes among patients with hypertensive HF in Abeokuta, Nigeria.

13.3.3 Study methods

As described in greater detail in Chapter 12, as part of the Abeokuta HF Registry, a total of 452 HF patients were admitted to the Federal Medical Centre Abeokuta. Of these, 355 (78.5%) were known hypertensive heart disease cases (35 patients being excluded due to insufficient BP data). Patients were followed up at 1, 3, and 6 months to determine their well-being, medication prescription, rehospitalization history, and/or survival status.

13.3.4 Study findings

As shown in Table 13.3, women were more likely to be older, uneducated, and unemployed, while men were more likely to reside in a rural area. The majority of the cardiovascular risk factors and comorbidities were more prevalent in men, with the exception of asthma and arthritis, which were more frequent in women. Women were more likely to be overweight and obese, with a slightly longer length of admission and a higher pulse rate.

As shown in Table 13.4, women were more likely to present with impaired systolic function and evidence of LV dysfunction (including fractional shortening and abnormal LV filling patterns/geometry). In contrast, men were more likely to present with abnormalities in aortic root diameter, AF, longer QTc, LVH on 12-lead ECG (with strain patterns), and evidence of LV remodeling, including greater LV mass, interventricular septal wall thickness in diastole, and interventricular septal wall thickness in systole.

Table 13.3 Patients' demographic and clinical characteristics.

	Women (n = 136)	Men (n = 184)	All (n = 320)
Demographic characteristics			
Age (years)	60.6 ± 14.5	58.4 ± 12.4	59.3 ± 13.4
Rural resident	37 (27.2%)	48 (26.1%)	85 (26.6%)
Uneducated	49 (51.6%)	36 (27.1%)	85 (37.3%)
Cardiovascular risk factors and comorbidities			
Family history of CVD	7 (5.1%)	13 (7.1%)	20 (6.3%)
Cigarette smoker	7 (5.1%)	53 (28.8%)	60 (18.7%)
Type 2 diabetes	17 (12.5%)	22 (12.0%)	39 (12.2%)
BMI (kg/m^2)	24.5 ± 5.7	24.0 ± 5.0	24.2 ± 5.3
Asthma	4 (2.9%)	3 (1.6%)	7 (2.2%)
COPD	2 (1.5%)	6 (3.3%)	8 (2.5%)
HIV infection	1 (1.5%)	3 (3.4%)	4 (2.7%)
Clinical and laboratory characteristics			
NYHA class			
II	21 (15.4%)	36 (19.6%)	57 (17.8%)
III	92 (67.6%)	109 (59.2%)	201 (62.8%)
IV	23 (16.95)	39 (21.2%)	62 (19.4%)
Signs and symptoms			
Heart rate (beats/min)	94.7 ± 18.7	97.4 ± 19.1	96.2 ± 18.9
Systolic BP (mm Hg)	143.0 ± 19.4	143.8 ± 32.9	143.5 ± 32.1
Diastolic BP (mm Hg)	89.6 ± 19.4	91.1 ± 21.5	90.5 ± 20.6
Basal crepitation	110 (80.9%)	160 (87.0%)	270 (84.4%)
Hepatomegaly	85 (62.5%)	116 (63.0%)	210 (62.8%)
Leg edema	102 (75.0%)	140 (76.1%)	242 (75.6%)
Nocturnal cough	126 (92.6%)	166 (90.2%)	292 (91.3%)
Paroxysmal nocturnal dyspnea	111 (81.6%)	157 (82.1%)	262 (81.9%)
Raised Jugular Venous Pressure	82 (60.3%)	128 (69.6%)	210 (65.6%)
Third heart sound	92 (67.6%)	115 (62.5%)	207 (64.7%)
Laboratory findings			
Fasting glucose (mg/dL)	113.3 ± 56.2	113.4 ± 47.6	113.3 ± 51.2
Total cholesterol (mg/dL)	174.7 ± 68.6	162.9 ± 76.7	166.2 ± 74.1
eGFR	93.8 ± 50.7	95.2 ± 52.6	94.6 ± 51.7

13.3.4.1 Treatment patterns

Overall, 319 (99.1%) patients were prescribed an ACE inhibitor/angiotensin II receptor blockers, 278 (86.9%) a loop diuretic, 260 (81.3%) spironolactone, 234 (73.1%) digoxin, 98 (30.6%) a calcium channel blocker, 49 (15.3%) hydralazine/isosorbide, 25 (7.8%) a thiazide diuretic, and only 9 (2.7%) a beta blocker.

13.3.4.2 Health outcomes

Median length of stay was 9 days and was similar for men and women. In-hospital case-fatality was 3.4% and 3.8% for men and women, respectively. Thereafter, 30 ,

Table 13.4 Patients' 12-lead ECG and echocardiography findings.

	Women (n = 136)	Men (n = 184)	All (n = 320)
Aortic root diameter (cm)	2.90±0.39	3.24±0.50	3.10±0.50
AF	18 (13.2%)	23 (12.5%)	41 (12.8%)
Corrected QT (ms)	450.3±35.5	457.5±35.5	454.8±35.4
LVH on 12-lead ECG	136 (100%)	173 (94.3%)	309 (96.5%)
ECG LVH with strain pattern	49 (36.4%)	87 (47.2%)	138 (43.0%)
LVEF (%)	44.5±16.3	41.8±16.6	42.9±16.5
Fractional shortening (%)	18.7±8.6	17.4±8.7	17.9±8.7
LV mass index (g/ht)	81.1±28.0	96.7±41.8	90.4±37.7
Interventricular septal wall thickness in diastole (cm)	1.28±0.29	1.40±0.41	1.35±0.37
Interventricular septal wall thickness in systole (cm)	1.48±034	1.67±0.55	1.60±0.85
LV internal diameter in diastole (cm)	5.08±1.40	5.84±1.47	5.52±1.49
Left atrial area	24.8±7.36	27.7±8.3	26.6±8.1
LV filling pattern (n=262)			
Systolic HF	59.1%	69.9%	182 (69.5%)
Diastolic HF	40.9%	30.1%	96 (36.6%)
Impaired relaxation	27.2%	26.4%	70 (26.7%)
Moderate-to-severe aortic regurgitation	46.7%	43%	125 (47.7%)
Moderate-to-severe MR	80.3%	78%	207 (79.0%)
Moderate-to-severe tricuspid regurgitation	63.9%	58.2%	159 (60.7%)
Pseudo-normalized filling	45.6%	45.3%	119 (45.4%)
Restrictive filling	27.2%	28.3%	73 (27.9%)
LV geometry (n=263)			
Concentric hypertrophy	41.7%	43.2%	42.6
Concentric remodelling	12.0%	3.9%	19 (7.2%)
E/A ratio	1.95±1.35	2.11±1.52	2.05±1.45
Eccentric hypertrophy	42.6%	48.4%	121 (46.0%)
Mitral A-wave	0.57±0.28	0.50±0.23	0.53±0.25
Mitral E-wave	0.85±0.32	0.80±0.28	0.82±0.29
Normal geometry	3.7%	4.5%	11 (4.2%)
LV internal diameter systole (cm)	4.15±1.31	4.86±1.43	4.57±1.49
LV mass (g)	283.9±100.4	376.4±140.8	338.4±133.6
LV posterior wall thickness diastole (cm)	1.15±0.35	1.22±0.30	1.19±0.36
LV posterior wall thickness systole (cm)	1.65±0.37	1.66±0.38	1.65±0.37
QRS duration (ms)	104.4±25.5	113.1±23.9	109.8±24.7
QT interval (ms)	358.8±54.6	368.5±36.6	364.8±44.3
Relative wall thickness	0.47±0.15	0.44±0.15	0.45±0.15

90-, and 180-day case-fatality was 0.9% (95% CI 0.2–3.5), 3.5% (95% CI 1.7–7.3), and 11.7% (95% CI 7.8–17.5), respectively. Rehospitalization rates at 30 days, 90 days, and 180 days were 4.2% (95% CI 2.3–7.6), 5.6% (95% CI, 3.3–9.5), and 7.3% (95% CI 4.5–11.7), respectively. Compared with patients who survived at

180 days, those who died were more likely to be NYHA Class III or IV (86.7% versus 38.7%, p<.001), to have lower systolic BP (130.7±20.9mmHg versus 144.1±32.4 mm Hg, p=.030), lower diastolic BP (80.0±13.7 versus 89.3±18.9, p=.044), lower pulse pressure (42.7±13.3mm Hg versus 53.5±12.1mm Hg, p=.009), and a higher serum creatinine (2.2±2.6 versus 1.2±1.0, p=.005). After multiple logistic regression analysis, only serum creatinine was an independent predictor of mortality at 180 days (adjusted OR, 1.76; 95% CI 1.17–2.64). The only significant difference in rehospitalization status was serum potassium level (higher in those readmitted to hospital).

13.3.5 Study interpretation

This study was the first study on hypertensive HF in Nigeria. The condition was found to be particularly prevalent in middle-aged individuals, with only 46% of the study patients being aged >60 years. Patterns of severe LV remodeling, comorbid conditions, and frequent functional valvular dysfunction were particularly frequent in de novo HF patients. As observed earlier in this chapter, late presentation to tertiary care could explain the alarmingly high prevalence of hypertensive HF, as individuals with elevated BP levels are frequently unaware of their condition and can sustain organ damage without preventive treatment. A high proportion of patients were prescribed spironolactone, or ACE inhibitor/angiotensin II receptor blockers therapy, but use of hydralazine/isosorbide and beta blockers was low, perhaps due to disease severity, edema, or low BP levels at presentation, or poverty (as patients pay out of pocket). The low rates of stroke in Nigeria relative to those observed in developed countries may be partially due to the fact that most individuals at risk of stroke secondary to untreated hypertension develop hypertensive HF first and die before they experience a stroke. Such competing risks are complex and require further investigation. In comparison with European and North American cohorts with HF, the overall demographic and clinical profile (in addition to associated mortality and morbidity rates) of the current cohort highlights some similarities but many profound differences. The predominance of hypertensive HF, late presentations, and the age of those affected are crucial factors in considering what evidence should be applied to improve health outcomes in this context. Overall, these findings highlight a gap in our knowledge of the burden of HF. They provide an opportunity for future interventions to focus on educating the Nigerian population as well as training the physicians in local medical clinics to combat hypertension and hypertensive heart disease, a similar opportunity being evident throughout the African continent.

13.3.6 Study limitations

As this study was conducted in a tertiary care facility, it may not have captured all HF cases in the population. Biomarkers in this study were not assessed due to cost constraints. Finally, some of the newer parameters for assessing diastolic function were not used in this study.

13.3.7 Study conclusions

In conclusion, Nigerians who develop hypertensive HF experience high economic loss and disability-adjusted life-years, as they are commonly in their most productive years from a social and economic perspective. Late presentations are common among individuals with elevated BP levels due to lack of awareness and/or education. Nigerian communities should be educated in hypertensive HF prevention, early detection, treatment, and management.

CHAPTER 14

Chronic heart failure

Okechukwu Samuel Ogah[1], Anastase Dzudie[2], Dike Bevis Ojji[3], and Mahmoud Sani[4]

[1] University College Hospital, Ibadan, Oy, Nigeria
[2] Hospital General de Douala, Douala, Littoral, Cameroon
[3] University of Abuja Teaching Hospital, Abuja, Nigeria
[4] Bayero University Kano/Aminu Kano Teaching Hospital, Kano, Nigeria

14.0 Introduction

While there is a growing body of literature focusing on acute presentations of HF in sub-Saharan Africa, there is, perhaps understandably, a lesser focus on chronic HF, regarding both long-term management and outcomes. This chapter focuses on two seminal reports (one from Cameroon and the other from Nigeria) that provide important insights into not only the prevalence of HF in high-risk patient populations (unfortunately, population data are limited) but also the economic burden of HF. It is only with such knowledge that blueprints for the cost-effective primary and secondary prevention of HF in the unique African context can be applied.

14.1 Chronic HF among adults treated for hypertension in a cardiac referral hospital in Cameroon

Dzudie A, Kengne, Mbahe S, Menanga A, Kenflack M, Kingue S. Chronic heart failure, selected risk factors and comorbidities among adults treated for hypertension in a cardiac referral hospital in Cameroon. *European Journal of Heart Failure* 2008; 10:367–372. [98]

14.1.1 Study background

As noted in Chapter 13, reflecting its disproportionate impact in the developing world [99], hypertension is the most common form of noncommunicable disease in many African countries, and Cameroon is no exception [100,101]. A clustering of risk factors including type 2 diabetes, cigarette smoking, and obesity among those of African ancestry increases the probability of end-organ damage (i.e., renal disease, stroke, and HF) [102]. Although there is some (limited) information on the link

---

The Heart of Africa: Clinical Profile of an Evolving Burden of Heart Disease in Africa, First Edition.
Edited by Simon Stewart, Karen Sliwa, Ana Mocumbi, Albertino Damasceno, and Mpiko Ntsekhe.
© 2016 John Wiley & Sons, Ltd. Published 2016 by John Wiley & Sons, Ltd.

between hypertension and stroke in the African context (see Chapter 11) [103,104], at the time of this study there were limited equivalent data on the development of chronic HF (noting the distinction between the acute manifestations of the syndrome outlined in Chapter 12); this was particularly true in Cameroon.

14.1.2 Study aims

The primary aim of this study was to examine the prevalence and characteristics of chronic HF among patients captured by the Hypertension Register from the outpatient department of the Yaounde General Hospital in Cameroon.

14.1.3 Study methods
14.1.3.1 Patient enrollment

Between 1995 and 2005, the Yaounde General Hospital was the main referral center for CVD cases in Cameroon, comprising patients from the capital city Yaounde and the wider country (population of approximately 15 million people). The hospital provides comprehensive, tertiary level facilities and management for high-level cases. Note that without a social security system, the cost of medical care was the responsibility of the patients and their relatives. As noted, this study focused on patients registered in the hypertension clinic of the hospital (typically attending a consultation twice a year, at which their medications were reviewed). Each patient was clinically profiled by trained nurses annually where possible. This included standardized BP measurements, 12-lead ECG, renal function assessment, fasting blood glucose, and serum electrolytes. Echocardiography was also performed based on clinical presentation. Clinical data were stored in a formal register. As part of the study, patients receiving treatment for hypertension in the clinic between February 1995 and January 2005 were evaluated for evidence of HF. The clinical notes of those with HF were reviewed for additional details, including sociodemographic profile and multimorbidity. Of 1,218 hypertensive patients registered during this period, 151 (12.4%) adult patients were identified as presenting with clinical HF or asymptomatic LV dysfunction; 4 (2.6%) patients with CHD were subsequently excluded in addition to 3 (2%) patients with VHD and 4 (2.6%) with missing echocardiographic data. Complete data were therefore available for 140 (92.7%) patients. This study received approval from the relevant ethics committee.

14.1.4 Study findings
14.1.4.1 Demographic and clinical characteristics

The overall prevalence of chronic HF in this hypertensive cohort of patients was 11.5%—rising from 7.2% in the first two years of the study to 12.4% in the final two years. As depicted in Table 14.1, HF patients were relatively young (mean age 55 years) with a predominance of men. Overall, 62 (44.2%) patients were NYHA Class III–IV, and 70 (50%) displayed echocardiographic evidence of LVH. The main form of HF was HFrEF (64%), with a residual 14% exhibiting asymptomatic LV systolic dysfunction. Isolated diastolic dysfunction occurred in 23% of patients.

Table 14.1 Patients' demographic and clinical characteristics according to sex.

	Women (n = 54)	Men (n = 86)	All (n = 140)
Demographic Characteristics			
Age (years)	52.5 ± 10.6	58.7 ± 14.6	54.9 ± 12.6
Risk Factors			
Current Smoker	2 (3.7%)	16 (18.6%)	18 (12.9)
Dyslipidaemia	11 (20.4%)	10 (11.6%)	21 (15.0%)
BMI (kg/m²)	26.3 ± 4.1	23.3 ± 5.1	24.7 ± 4.7
Obesity	7 (13.0%)	9 (10.5%)	16 (11.4%)
Systolic BP (mm Hg)	152 ± 32	177 ± 41	164 ± 21
Diastolic BP (mm Hg)	93 ± 23	102 ± 15	98 ± 14.6
Controlled Hypertension	15 (27.8%)	17 (19.8%)	32 (22.9%)
Severe Hypertension	27 (50.0%)	31 (36.1%)	58 (41.4%)
NYHA Class			
I - II	37 (68.5%)	41 (47.7%)	78 (55.7%)
III - IV	29 (53.7%)	33 (38.4%)	62 (44.3%)
HF profile			
All systolic HF	38 (70.4%)	52 (60.5%)	90 (64.3%)
Asymptomatic LV Dysfunction	7 (13.0%)	13 (15.1%)	20 (14.3%)
Isolated Diastolic HF	19 (35.2%)	13 (15.1%)	32 (22.9%)
LVH	39 (72.2%)	31 (36.1%)	70 (50.0%)

Overall there were minimal differences between men and women, although significantly more women (p = 0.05) displayed isolated diastolic dysfunction (i.e. HFpEF). There were also minimal differences in BP levels and renal dysfunction between those with HFrEF and those with HFpEF (diastolic dysfunction).

14.1.4.2 Pharmacological management

Most patients were prescribed a combination of a diuretic (87.1%), ACE inhibitor/ angiotensin II receptor blockers (68.6%), and/or calcium channel blocker (48.6%); beta blockers (11.1%) and centrally acting BP-lowering drugs (4.1%) were less common. Mean BP was 165/98 mm Hg and patients had been treated for an average of 7 years. At the last evaluation, 22.8% of patients had optimal BP control.

14.1.4.3 Risk factors

There were no sex differences in BMI profiles (11% obese), and dyslipidemia was evident in 15% of patients, with similar profiles in men and women. Smoking was more prevalent in men (18.6% versus 9.3%, p = 0.007).

14.1.4.4 Comorbidities

Figure 14.1 shows the distribution of comorbidities according to sex. No sex-related differences were observed in this regard; however, there were high levels of renal dysfunction and anemia among women and concurrent disease states

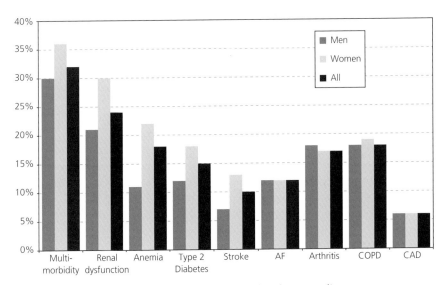

Figure 14.1 Pattern of concurrent morbidity in the study cohort according to sex.

such as chronic obstructive pulmonary disease (COPD) and arthritis, with minimal levels (just over 5%) of underlying CAD.

14.1.5 Study interpretation

These data provide important insights into the prevalence of chronic HF in a hypertensive outpatient cohort in sub-Saharan Africa, with around 12% of individuals affected by the syndrome. Affected individuals were relatively young (middle-aged) and more likely to be male, with a clustering of risk factors and multimorbidity. Beyond the data presented in other parts of this section, these findings are particularly notable for exploring the prevalence of HF and asymptomatic LV dysfunction in patients with treated hypertension. The 11.5% prevalence of HF reported in this cohort is consistent with the 10.5% found by another Nigerian study [105], and both are likely to be an underestimate of the true prevalence of HF in this patient population. Isolated diastolic dysfunction in this cohort was similar to contemporary Caucasian population-based cohort studies [106] but higher than that (12.6%) described in another Nigerian series [107]. Renal dysfunction was revealed in one quarter of cases, representing a classic finding for this kind of cohort. This high frequency of renal dysfunction among a relatively young population is worthy of comment, with potential contributing factors including medication, low cardiac output, and the severe nature of hypertension among individuals of African ancestry. Numerous studies have demonstrated this to be an independent predictor of subsequent morbidity and mortality risk in patients with HF [108,109]. Diabetes, also evident but not highly prevalent in this cohort, likewise conveys an increased risk of poor outcomes; its prevalence being similar to that described in a hospitalized series of patients in Senegal [34]. Other noncardiovascular conditions such as COPD are progressively being recognized as important contributors to HF outcomes, and this may be particularly significant in the context of RHF (see Chapter 15) [110]. As reported in the Heart of Soweto Study [111], AF (found in 13% of this relatively young population) is becoming increasingly important in the context of HF, and given the age profile of the cohort, its prevalence and potential impact should be regarded as being relatively high.

14.1.6 Study limitations

Due to the retrospective nature of the study and the characteristics of the study population (which are likely to favor patients self-selected by symptoms from the total hypertension population), these data may provide imprecise estimates of the prevalence of hypertensive heart failure in the target population. As such, these factors may limit the generalizability of study findings.

14.1.7 Study conclusions

In conclusion, these data provide important insights into the prevalence of chronic HF in a particularly at-risk patient cohort. As noted in the original report, given the high prevalence of hypertension and other risk factors for HF in the Cameroon population at large [112], these findings are indicative of a future increase in the incidence of major target organ damages such as HF, kidney impairment, and stroke (often in the same individual). Primary and secondary prevention strategies alike are required to mitigate the future burden of chronic HF in Cameroon and wider sub-Saharan Africa.

14.2 The Economic burden of HF in Nigeria: Insights from the Abeokuta HF Registry Cohort

Ogah OS, Stewart S, Onwujekwe OE, Falase AO, Adebayo SO, Olunuga T, Sliwa K. Economic burden of heart failure: investigating outpatient and inpatient costs in Abeokuta, Southwest Nigeria. *PLoS One* **2014; 9(11):e113032. [113]**

14.2.1 Study background

Until recently, little was known about the emerging problem of noncommunicable forms of HF supplementing traditional pathways to the syndrome in sub-Saharan Africa. A series of studies from South Africa [22,30] and Nigeria [16,87,97] (previously outlined in Chapter 6 and this section of the book) have added to historical reports on the syndrome by demonstrating very clearly that the etiology, natural history, and profile of chronic HF (i.e., more women and younger individuals affected in the prime of their life) diverge from high-income countries where the literature traditionally arises. It is now estimated that HF is responsible for 7%–10% of medical admissions in the region [16,97,114]. Significantly, given its potentially enormous cost implications (related both to direct health care costs and to the financial strain on affected individuals and their families), there is virtually no data on the economic burden of HF in sub-Saharan African countries and major populaces such as Nigeria.

14.2.2 Study aims

Given the paucity of data to describe the cost of HF both in its acute and chronic forms, this study was designed to determine the scope and cost of health care resources directed toward the treatment of HF in Abeokuta, Nigeria. Estimates were derived from a large and representative cohort of affected cases. Data were extrapolated to estimate the annual cost of HF in the region to inform health care policy toward efficient use of resources to mitigate the individual and societal impact of the syndrome.

14.2.3 Study methods
14.2.3.1 Patient enrollment

Study data were derived from the Federal Medical Centre, Abeokuta, Ogun State, southwest Nigeria. The Federal Medical Centre Abeokuta is a tertiary referral institution that receives patients from primary and secondary health facilities within and outside the state. All managed patients are given monthly appointments for clinical review as well as for refill of their medications. Patients pay out of pocket, and many are unable to buy medication that will cover longer periods. Significantly, patients are often cared for by their relatives, and health care costs in the city of Abeokuta and in most parts of Nigeria are typically borne by the patient as out-of-pocket expenses, given the limited access within the Nigerian population to social health insurance [115,116]. However, there are typically strong family and community bonds to care for the sick.

Data were derived from the Abeokuta HF registry. As described in more detail in Chapter 13, this was a hospital-based, prospective, observational registry that ran from January 2009 to December 2010, established to determine the current clinical profile of HF in the city as well as to assess typical clinical outcomes and health care costs (the focus of this report) associated with HF. In brief, all cases of HF presenting to the hospital were captured in the database. As noted in the original report, the study cohort was broadly representative of the population. During the study period, HF was responsible for 9% of total medical admissions [16], a figure that is consistent with equivalent reports from other parts of Africa [30,75,114].

14.2.3.2 Estimating health care expenditure

Costs were divided into two forms of activity: (a) direct health care costs associated with HF management and (b) indirect costs. The former comprised hospitals' inpatient costs (e.g., cost of medical and nursing care, investigations, and pharmacotherapy). It also included the cost of surgical procedures and hospital transfer costs). Personnel costs included the opportunity cost of medical care, nursing, and ancillary support by other health workers (derived from Federal Government of Nigeria salary scales). For indirect costs, the days of lost work due to HF disability/illness (productivity loss) were calculated and the minimum wage used to monetize them.

14.2.3.3 Inpatient and outpatient costs

The standard costing table (unit costs) of the Federal Medical Centre, Abeokuta, for the year 2010 was used to compute the cost of consultations, hospital admissions, medical consumables, medical investigations, and pharmacotherapy. Outpatient costs were based on the costs associated (patients discharged alive) with monthly appointments for clinical review as well as refilled medications.

14.2.3.4 Specific costs

The cost of pharmacotherapy was based on the hospital's price list (purchase price plus a 10% dispensing fee). The frequency of use of the various categories of drugs was based on the findings from the HF registry. The most frequent dosage was used for cost calculation. The cost of all laboratory and diagnostic tests was based on the price list of the hospital in 2010. The rate of consumption of these items was also garnered from the HF registry. The costs of surgeries and procedures were obtained from the most active surgical institutions in the region and were multiplied by the frequency of those surgeries and procedures.

14.2.3.5 Estimation of indirect costs

A human capital approach was applied with average annual earnings based on occupational group and average daily earnings then calculated per patient. The product of the working days lost and average daily earnings provided the productivity losses associated with HF in the study, and these were assigned monetary values.

14.2.3.6 Cost analyses

All available costs (as detailed above) were computed for the year 2010. An annual, prevalence-based approach was employed in estimating the cost of the resources used for the management of HF [117–120]. Health care costs were then expressed in the local currency—naira—and converted to US dollars (US$) (at a rate of 150 Nigerian naira to US$1 in 2010).

14.2.4 Study findings

Table 14.2 provides a summary of the clinical and demographic characteristics of the study cohort from which all HF-related health care activities and extrapolated costs were derived. The mean age was 58 years with just under half (46.9%) of the patients being female. Significantly, around one-third were aged ≤55 years and therefore in the prime of their potential working life.

14.2.4.1 Summary of inpatient and outpatient care cost

The total cost of inpatient care was estimated at N34,996,477 or US$301,230, comprising N17,899,977 (50.9%, $US114,600) and N17,806,500 (49.1%, $US118,710) for direct and indirect costs, respectively. Direct costs were responsible for 61% of inpatient care costs. Approximately 40% of the direct cost was due to surgery/procedures. Hospitalization, medical investigations, drug therapy, and transportation accounted for 20%, 24%, 15%, and 1% of costs, respectively.

Outpatient care was estimated at N41,292,368 or US$275,282. Direct and indirect costs were N20,963,168 (US$139,754) and N20,329,200 (US$135,528), respectively, comprising 51% and 49% of total outpatient care costs. Transportation, medications, clinic visits, and medical investigations contributed 46%, 44%, 5%, and 5% respectively to these costs.

14.2.4.2 Total costs

The total estimated cost of health care attributable to HF in Abeokuta for the year 2010 was N76,288,845 or US$508,595. This translated to a cost of N319,200 or US$2,128 per patient per year. The proportional contribution of inpatient and

Table 14.2 HF patients' demographic characteristics in 2010.

	All (n = 239)
Demographic Characteristics	
Women	112 (46.9%)
Age profile	
Mean age (years)	58.0 ± 15.1
Aged 45–54 years	40 (16.7%)
Aged 55–64 years	59 (24.7%)
Aged 65–74 years	63 (26.4%)
Aged ≥75-years	33 (13.8%)
Married	168 (70.3%)
No formal education	88 (36.8%)
Unemployed	20 (8.4%)
Unskilled labour	146 (61.1%)
Resident of Abeokuta city	138 (57.7%)
Resident within Ogun State	53 (22.7%)
Resident outside Ogun State	48 (20.1%)
Monthly Income (Naira)	
Unemployed*	18000 (US$120)
Unskilled labour	90,000 (US$600)
Skilled labour	240,000 (US$1600)
Professional	480,000 (US$3200)
Pensioner/Retiree	330,000 (US$2200)
Aetiology of HF	
Hypertensive HF	195 (81.6%)
Dilated CMO	14 (5.9%)
Comorbidities	
Hypertension	185 (77.4%)
Osteoarthritis	49 (20.5%)
AF	37 (15.5%)
Type 2 Diabetes	24 (10.0%)

*Allocated minimum wage in the country.

outpatient costs was 46% and 54%, respectively. The contribution of various components to the total cost of HF to the region from an inpatient and outpatient perspective is summarized in Figure 14.2 and Figure 14.3, respectively.

14.12.5 Study interpretation

As described in the original report, this study represents the first systematic attempt to estimate the cost of HF in Nigeria (a major populace of sub-Saharan Africa) and the wider African continent. Costs were derived from an individual perspective, while the total cost per annum overall was calculated from a societal perspective. During the study period, 9% of total medical admissions were attributed to HF, a figure similar to earlier reports from other parts of Africa [30,75,114]. Overall, the total cost of HF or cost per patient per year (evenly distributed between inpatient and outpatient care) is enormous considering the context of a developing economy where out-of-pocket expenses are the main means of health care financing. A large proportion of estimated direct cost for inpatient care was attributable to surgical and medical procedures, while outpatient medications and transfers were responsible for 90% of the direct cost of outpatient care. This cost burden is not markedly dissimilar from reports derived from high-income countries [116,118,120,121]. Alternatively, the distribution of cost of HF in this setting is different from that observed in high income countries [117,118,121,122] but similar to one report from Brazil [120]. Significantly, there have been no reports from Africa with which to compare these findings. The contribution of hospital care cost in these countries ranged from 53% to 75%. Cost of outpatient care was in the range of 4% to 31% while the cost of drug therapy was between 6% and 8% of the total cost of care. The pattern of heart diseases as well as the level of technological development influence the mode of care, in addition to the utilization of sophisticated and expensive medical equipment, procedures, and consumables that are obviously needed for the care of HF patients. The consumption of these is higher in high-income countries than in this setting. This is clearly highlighted by the impact of surgery or procedures on the cost of hospital care. The few cases

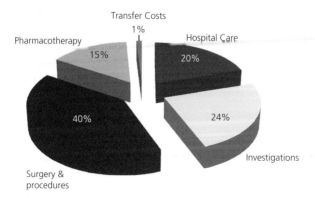

Figure 14.2 Components of direct inpatient costs.

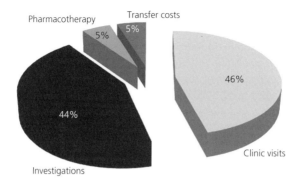

Figure 14.3 Components of direct outpatient costs.

receiving surgery for valvular diseases or coronary interventions (out of the many that needed it) escalated the cost of hospital care in Nigeria. It is important to note that because of the younger age of affected individuals, HF in the Nigerian setting is associated with longer disability-adjusted life-years. By extension, this equates to a huge cost to the whole of society. With the changing demographic and epidemiological landscape in Nigeria coupled with the rising burden of cardiovascular risk factors and noncommunicable diseases (especially hypertension) in the country, the rate of HF is predicted to rise. Preventive measures are therefore critically needed but place an enormous strain on an already resource-poor health care system. The high cost of surgical interventions and procedures is out of the reach of the average Nigerian. Moreover, there is a need for a functional, effective, and efficient social health insurance system in Nigeria and other countries such as Cameroon (see Section 14.1 above). Unfortunately, most of those afflicted by HF are poor and are unlikely to sustain the treatment of their illness for an extended period. There is also a need to develop community-based HF care in Nigeria and other parts of sub-Saharan Africa, as this will reduce the cost of outpatient care, which is largely influenced by the substantial cost of frequent transport to and from the health facility for specialist HF management.

14.2.6 Study limitations

A few limitations are worth noting. First, as this study was conducted in a tertiary care facility, it is possible that mild cases may have been missed. Second, cost based on the severity of HF was not assessed, nor were age and sex-specific cost analysis. Third, the cost of comorbidities were not included, nor the cost due to alternative medicines, over-the-counter purchases, capital cost, and indirect cost by caregivers as well as the general cost to society.

14.2.7 Study conclusions

These seminal data, representing a first of a kind in the African context, show the profound impact and importance of HF as a major public health problem in a developing economy such as Nigeria. Unfortunately, the country is still battling with communicable diseases. As described in Soweto, South Africa (see Chapter 6), there is an obvious confluence or crossroads of communicable and noncommunicable disease in vulnerable populations with limited health care resources and personal wealth. The annual individual cost of HF is high, coupled with the fact that out-of-pocket expenses in Nigeria compose close to two-thirds of health care costs. There is urgent need, therefore, to reduce HF-related expenditure and cost through the control of known risk factors for the syndrome (see Section 3). As outlined in Chapter 13, this particularly applies to elevated BP levels in many rural and urban communities due to epidemiological transition and a movement away from traditional lifestyles that previously protected individuals from noncommunicable diseases. At the same time there is an imperative to reduce hospital as well as outpatient care costs through the development of community-based HF care programs that have the potential to reduce the high levels of recurrent hospital stay and case-fatality already seen in this population [123,124].

CHAPTER 15

Pulmonary hypertension and right heart failure

Anastase Dzudie[1], Friedrich Thienemann[2], Okechukwu Samuel Ogah[3], Dike Bevis Ojji[4], and Mahmoud Sani[5]

[1] Hospital General de Douala, Douala, Littoral, Cameroon
[2] University of Cape Town, Cape Town, South Africa
[3] University College Hospital, Ibadan, Oyo, Nigeria
[4] University of Abuja Teaching Hospital, Abuja, Nigeria
[5] Bayero University Kano/Aminu Kano Teaching Hospital, Kano, Nigeria

15.0 Introduction

Recent years have brought increasing awareness of the clinical significance of PH and cor pulmonale (RV dysfunction and RHF arising from pathological changes in the pulmonary vasculature/system) in Africa. This applies equally to the recognition of the importance of PH and RHF as both a primary diagnosis and as a poor prognostic marker for those primarily affected by left-sided HF [125,126]. However, data on the precursors and risk factors of those conditions are limited. As described in chapter 6, the largest study on PH/RHF in Africa was derived from the Heart of Soweto Study in South Africa, in which 2,505 cases presented with de novo HF during 2006 and 2008. Of these, 697 (28%) patients were diagnosed with PH/RHF, with PH/RHF as the primary diagnosis in 50% of cases. The majority presented with dyspnea and a mean right ventricular systolic pressure (RVSP) >50 mmHg. Left heart disease (31%), COPD and TB (26%), and PH (20%) due to HIV-related PH (HIV-PH), adult CHD, or idiopathic PH were the most common causes of RHF [127] in the Heart of Soweto cohort. Investigating the prevalence of PH in RHD, a review of 1,312 echocardiographic studies at a tertiary center in Nigeria found evidence of RHD in 10% of cases; in 80% of these, secondary PH was present [128]. The same center described an echocardiographic series of 80 HF admissions; in the 53 cases with PH, the most common causes were hypertensive heart disease (25%), PPCMO (25%), dilated CMO (17%), and RHD (13%) [129]. A study from Uganda, meanwhile, reported a 33% prevalence of PH in 309 patients with newly diagnosed RHD [130]. Investigating the prevalence of CVD in HIV-infection, a Nigerian study found HIV-PH in 1 of 100 patients [131], while an echocardiographic series of 102 HIV patients presenting with cardiac symptoms in

The Heart of Africa: Clinical Profile of an Evolving Burden of Heart Disease in Africa, First Edition.
Edited by Simon Stewart, Karen Sliwa, Ana Mocumbi, Albertino Damasceno, and Mpiko Ntsekhe.
© 2016 John Wiley & Sons, Ltd. Published 2016 by John Wiley & Sons, Ltd.

Tanzania revealed PH in 13% [132]. PH was also present in 7% of long-term survivors in a cohort from Zimbabwe with vertically acquired HIV infection [133]. Hemolytic anemia is a known risk factor for PH; a screening study of patients with sickle-cell disease (SCD) in Nigeria found a PH prevalence of 25% [134], while an Egyptian study reported that patients with β-thalassemia were at risk for PH [135]. Another study from Egypt revealed PH in 9% of patients seropositive for schistosomal antibodies. Finally, a Sudanese group described 14 consecutive cases of PH in previously treated pulmonary TB, concluding that PH can occur after resolution of TB [136]. Combined, these data suggest that left heart disease, chronic lung disease, RHD, HIV-infection, schistosomiasis, and SCD may be the most common underlying causes of PH in the African context.

15.1 A prospective registry of PH in Africa: The landmark PAPUCO study

Thienemann F, Dzudie A, Mocumbi AO, Blauwet L, Sani MU, Karaye KM, et al. Rationale and design of the Pan African Pulmonary Hypertension Cohort (PAPUCO) study: implementing a contemporary registry on pulmonary hypertension in Africa. *BMJ Open* 2014; 4(10):e005950. [137]

15.1.1 Study aim and objectives
Given the paucity of African data on PH/RHF (<1% of published reports) in the context of its potentially rising burden, the PAPUCO study aims to describe the presentation, etiologies, comorbidities, and natural course of PH in Africa, as well as its diagnosis and therapeutic management. Specific secondary objectives are to determine the overall 6-month survival rate in PH/RHF and the 24-month survival rate in HIV-related PAH, and to compare 6-month survival rates between different diagnostic groups of PH (including PAH) while also determining the predictors of mortality across those groups. More broadly, the PAPUCO registry endeavours to develop sustainable clinical and research capacity across the African continent as well as raising awareness of PH and its risk factors.

15.1.2 Study methods
15.1.2.1 Study design and setting
The PAPUCO study is a prospective observational registry on PH with nine actively recruiting specialist centers in four countries in sub-Saharan Africa (see Figure 15.1). The registry aims to recruit 250 patients with newly diagnosed PH based on echocardiography (noting a research report based on the successful achievement of this target will be submitted for publication in the last quarter of 2015). All participating centers are public health care institutions, and the majority of patients will represent socioeconomic disadvantaged populations with restricted access to health care. Center eligibility criteria include (a) availability of echocardiography and training in assessing right heart function, (b) experience in diagnosing PH according to WHO classification (see Table 15.1), (c) experience in

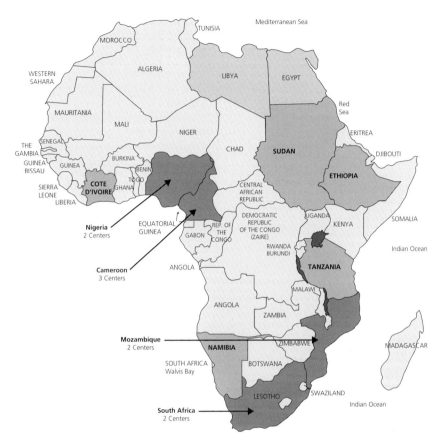

Figure 15.1 Country participation in the PAPUCO registry. Adapted from Thienemann et al., 2014 [137].

clinical management of patients with RHF, and (d) resources to review patients at 6-month follow-up. All participating centers obtained ethical approval from their local ethics committee review board.

15.1.2.2 Patient enrollment
Consecutive patients per center will be included if newly diagnosed with PH according to prespecified clinical and echocardiographic criteria (see below), able or likely to return for 6-month follow-up, at least 18 years old (except for pediatric centers in Mozambique and Nigeria), and consented in writing to participate in the registry.

15.1.2.3 Definition of PH
For the purpose of this registry, PH is defined as >35 mmHg RVSP on transthoracic echocardiography in the absence of pulmonary stenosis and acute RHF; it is usually accompanied by dyspnea, fatigue, peripheral edema, and other cardiovascular symptoms, and there are possibly ECG and chest x-ray

Table 15.1 WHO classification for pulmonary hypertension [138].

Pulmonary Hypertension Group Description	Clinical Correlate
Group 1: PAH	HIV-related PAH, schistosomiasis, drugs/toxins
Group 2: Pulmonary hypertension due to left heart disease	Mitral stenosis due to RHD, hypertensive VHD, PPCMO, VHD
Group 3: Pulmonary hypertension due to lung diseases and/or hypoxemia	COPD, posttuberculous lung bronchiectiasis, interstitial lung disease
Group 4: Chronic thromboembolic pulmonary hypertension	Chronic pulmonary embolism
Group 5: Pulmonary hypertension with unclear or multifactorial mechanisms	EMF, chronic hemolytic anemia (SCD)

changes in keeping with PH [138]. The WHO classification system for PH will be applied to describe the different etiologies of PH presentation. Once definitive assessment and treatment has been applied, specific data are documented for each patient: (a) all major cardiovascular diagnoses according ICD-10 coding, (b) up to six noncardiovascular diagnoses according to ICD-10 coding, and (c) prescribed pharmacological therapy.

15.1.2.4 The PAPUCO research platform

A tailor-made database was developed to fulfill the study requirements. Open-source technology was used to develop the web-based system (www.papuco.org) that allows investigators to collect, store, analyze, report on, and export clinical research data in various formats. Simple and user friendly, the system anonymizes personal patient data, which are stored as electronic case report forms on a secure, encrypted, and backed-up server. It provides hierarchic permissions and validation at the point of data entry. Multimedia data formats (including echocardiographic images) can be uploaded on the platform, allowing storage of complete clinical records, which guarantees completeness of data. Tools for education, training, and communication are installed within the web portal, and documents such as paper case report forms, informed consent forms, study information sheets, and patient education sheets on PH are available for download. The platform has been developed to cater for mobile Internet connectivity available in most parts of Africa and represents a unique research platform far beyond a simple web-based database.

15.1.2.5 Diagnostic algorithm and data collection in the PAPUCO registry

A diagnostic algorithm to diagnose PH in resource-limited settings without access to right heart catheterization (Figure 15.2) has been developed following the guidelines for the diagnosis of PH in the African context. Key information collected includes information on socioeconomic background, medical history, comorbidities, cardiac risk factors, and environmental exposures. The clinical

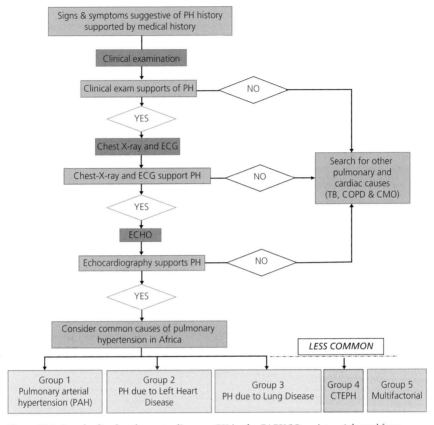

Figure 15.2 Standardized pathway to diagnose PH in the PAPUCO registry. Adapted from Thienemann et al., 2014 [137].

aspects of the assessment include symptom scoring, a full clinical examination, and functional tests including WHO functional class and 6-minute walk test [139,140]. Further investigations are at the discretion of the treating physician and typically include pulmonary function tests, radio nucleotide perfusion scans, chest x-ray, chest CT, and right heart catheterization if available. HF treatment and comedication, hospitalization, and mortality data will also be collected.

15.1.3 Study findings

At the time of publication of this book, the findings from this landmark study were not far from being published, the collaboration having successfully reached its goal of collecting data on >250 cases of PH across a range of African countries and in adult and pediatric patients. Any future editions of this book will, of course, provide the specific details.

15.1.4 Study interpretation

Newly released guidelines on the management of PH [141] provide an important contrast and backdrop to the future findings of the PAPUCO study given the emphasis on right heart catheterization (as opposed to the heavy reliance on clinical presentation and echocardiography in the African context) and the extremely expensive/niche first-line therapeutics that impose a burden on even the richest of countries. Establishing a definitive diagnosis of PH is an enormous challenge when relying on bedside tools, including history and physical examination. Right heart catheterization is indeed the gold standard to diagnose and confirm PH, but performing this procedure in all patients with dyspnea would be costly, apply excessive risk, and be impractical in any cost-constrained environment such as sub-Saharan Africa. The question of a better test that is widely available and supplies accuracy, safety, simplicity, and cost-effectiveness therefore becomes vital, particularly in an African-specific context. Echocardiography is more readily available in Africa and provides an estimate of RVSP, functional and morphologic cardiac sequelae of PH, and identification of possible cardiac causes. However, the accuracy of RVSP determination by echocardiography remains open to question, with some contemporary studies suggesting that echocardiography may not accurately estimate pulmonary arterial pressures [142,143]. Possible explanations for this inaccuracy include the presence of sufficient tricuspid regurgitation to produce a Doppler envelope and appropriate gain adjustments [142,143]. An undergained spectral signal will tend to result in underestimation of pulmonary pressures, while an overgained signal might significantly overestimate the measurement. Furthermore, careful adjustment of the transducer position and the use of color-flow Doppler are critical in order to reduce the Doppler angle and to obtain the maximal regurgitant flow velocity. Moreover, in the case of severe tricuspid regurgitation, the potential for laminar flow is high, invalidating the application of the Bernoulli equation. Volume status and systemic BP are other confounding factors. Finally, although it is commonly assumed the highest value of right atrial pressure is 15 mm Hg, values commonly exceed this in clinical practice. In the first systematic review and meta-analysis addressing the diagnostic accuracy of echocardiography for PH, the correlation of pulmonary arterial systolic pressure by echocardiography compared with right heart catheter was revealed to be reasonable, with a summary correlation coefficient of 0.70 (95% CI 0.67–0.73) [144]. The diagnostic accuracy of echocardiography to detect PH was also acceptable with a summary sensitivity and specificity of 83% (95% CI 73–90) and 72% (95% CI 53–85), respectively. Furthermore, pulmonary pressure measurements provided by echocardiography in experienced hands have been demonstrated as a strong predictor of mortality [145]. Finally, easily obtainable echocardiographic parameters such as E/A ratio and left atrial size can reliably distinguish between PH due to lung disease and PH due to left heart disease, allowing for rapid triage of patients for right heart catheterization if required. The results of the PAPUCO study will largely rely on echocardiography and will need to be evaluated using the best available resources in a resource-poor environment.

15.1.5 Study limitations

As with all observational registries, the PAPUCO initiative is reliant upon the flow of cases through participating centers and the systematic application of standardized clinical profiling. The risk of selection bias remains ever present in this situation. More important, from a PAH perspective, is the selective (if available) use of right heart catheterization. As always there are pragmatic considerations to be made when deriving a clinical diagnosis in limited resource settings—not applying a diagnosis (and treatment) is not an option.

15.1.6 Study conclusions

The PAPUCO study represents an important step in understanding the prevalence and clinical spectrum (including outcomes) of PH/RHF from a uniquely African standpoint. It joins such initiatives as the THESUS-HF study (see Chapter 12) in illuminating the burden of HF from a pan-African perspective. The ability to derive practical guidelines to inform the management and future pragmatic treatment trials of PH/RHF will surely arise, thereby improving what are otherwise likely to be very poor health outcomes in mainly young and disadvantaged individuals with limited resources to cope with a devastating condition.

S6.2 An increasingly complex picture of HF in Africa

As described in various parts of this book (particularly Section 3), profound sociodemographic and economic change on the African continent (particularly in the form of epidemiological transition) has transformed the landscape of heart disease and its most common chronic manifestatio—HF. This change is best summarized in Falase and Ogah's [7] comparison of underlying causes of HF presentations in patients of African ancestry to the University College Hospital in Ibadan, Nigeria, between the late 1960s and 2010 (see Figure S6.1 and Figure S6.2).

As was thoroughly illustrated in Chapters 12, 13, and 14, acute and chronic manifestations of HF are predominantly driven by hypertensive heart disease. Conversely, HF cases due to ischemic CMO remain at historical lows, despite the prospect of more cases as African lifestyles begin to mirror those of Western countries. The Heart of Soweto Study first published in 2006 [30] made a key contribution to our understanding of the current spectrum of HF in urban African communities in epidemiological transition. It highlighted in particular the importance of maintaining detailed case presentations records underpinned by echocardiography and standardized case reporting. However, these data are limited both in scope and geographic representation. As the insights from data derived from a wide body of research across Western countries attest, it is clear that Africa needs a more wide-scale and consistent approach to monitoring the evolving burden of HF, in addition to developing its own evidence base to improve health outcomes. Fortunately, this process has commenced (even as this book was written and went to press other important studies, such as those published by Makubi and colleagues from Tanzania were published [146,147]) and will continue to expand as pan-African collaborations are initiated and begin to inform clinicians and health administrators alike on how to combat an evolving burden of HF in sub-Saharan Africa. In Chapter 12, the pattern of acute forms of HF, as captured by the international THESUS-HF Registry, was described. Chapter 13 concentrated on the contribution and pattern of hypertensive HF in an array of African countries (from Cameroon to Nigeria and then South Africa). Although there has been a natural tendency to focus on hospitalized cases of HF (predominantly acute episodes of HF) in a resource-poor, tertiary health care–dominated system, it is important to acknowledge that HF is primarily a chronic condition. In this context, Chapter 14 examined the pattern and cost of chronic HF from an individual to societal perspective. Finally, Chapter 15 broadly surveyed the pattern of RHF/cor pulmonale and PAH in the sub-Saharan African setting. Importantly, given the paucity of data that can be derived from European, pan-Pacific, and North American registries (typically reporting far fewer cases derived from right-sided heart disease [37,148–150] this chapter describes a pan-African initiative to better understand this important contributor to HF cases on the continent. Rather than purporting to present definitive data on RHF in Africa, therefore, Chapter 15 concludes fittingly with the illustration of an increasingly common phenomenon—the creation of pan-African collaborations to derive robust, representative, and meaningful clinical data that will inform public health policy and clinical practice initiatives across the African continent for decades to come.

In summary, therefore, HF (as with all forms of heart disease) on the African continent has reached a historically important turning point that will exert a profound effect on African communities from an individual to a whole society perspective, particularly given its propensity to strike both men and women in the prime of life.

References

1 Hung J, Teng TH, Finn J, Knuiman M, Briffa T, Stewart S, et al. Trends from 1996 to 2007 in incidence and mortality outcomes of heart failure after acute myocardial infarction: a population-based study of 20,812 patients with first acute myocardial infarction in Western Australia. *J Am Heart Assoc.* 2013;2(5):e000172.

2 Jhund PS, Macintyre K, Simpson CR, Lewsey JD, Stewart S, Redpath A, et al. Long-term trends in first hospitalization for heart failure and subsequent survival between 1986 and 2003: a population study of 5.1 million people. *Circulation.* 2009;119(4):515–23.

3 Mozaffarian D, Benjamin EJ, Go AS, Arnett DK, Blaha MJ, Cushman M, et al. Heart disease and stroke statistics—2015 update: a report from the American Heart Association. *Circulation.* 2015;131(4):e29–322.

4 Stewart S, Ekman I, Ekman T, Oden A, Rosengren A. Population impact of heart failure and the most common forms of cancer: a study of 1 162 309 hospital cases in Sweden (1988 to 2004). *Circ Cardiovasc Qual Outcomes.* 2010;3(6):573–80.

5 Teng TH, Katzenellenbogen JM, Thompson SC, Sanfilippo FM, Knuiman M, Geelhoed E, et al. Incidence of first heart failure hospitalisation and mortality in Aboriginal and non-Aboriginal patients in Western Australia, 2000–2009. *Int J Cardiol.* 2014;173(1):110–7.

6 Dudas K, Lappas G, Stewart S, Rosengren A. Trends in out-of-hospital deaths due to coronary heart disease in Sweden (1991 to 2006). *Circulation.* 2011;123(1):46–52.

7 Falase AO, Ogah OS. Cardiomyopathies and myocardial disorders in Africa: present status and the way forward. *Cardiovasc J Afr.* 2012;23(10):552–62.

8 Myers GA. *African Cities: Alternative Visions of Urban Theory and Practice.* London: Zed Books, 2011.

9 Abubakar IR. Abuja city profile. *Cities.* 2014;41:81–91.

10 Iro I. *Demographic pressure and the application of GIS in land reforms: The case of restoration of Abuja Master Plan and sanitization of cadastral and land registry.* Map Middle East Conference on GIS Development; 2007; Dubai, UAE.

11 Wen LS, Oshiomogho JI, Eluwa GI, Steptoe AP, Sullivan AF, Camargo CA, Jr. Characteristics and capabilities of emergency departments in Abuja, Nigeria. *Emerg Med J.* 2012;29(10): 798–801.

12 Oyewale TO, Mavundla TR. Socioeconomic factors contributing to exclusion of women from maternal health benefit in Abuja, Nigeria. *Curationis.* 2015;38(1):E1–E11.

13 Amune T, Alade E, Farzan A. Descriptive analysis of cardiac services provision in urban Nigeria. 2010. https://apha.confex.com/apha/138am/webprogram/Paper221712.html (Accessed February 2016).

14 Solanke MO. Socio-economic characteristics of urban residents and intra-urban trip generation: an illustration from Abeokuta, Ogun State, Nigeria. *EJESM.* 2015;8(5):593–605.

15 National Population Commission. *National Population Census.* Abuja, Nigeria: National Population Commission, 2006.

16 Ogah OS, Stewart S, Falase AO, Akinyemi JO, Adegbite GD, Alabi AA, et al. Contemporary profile of acute heart failure in Southern Nigeria: data from the Abeokuta Heart Failure Clinical Registry. *JACC Heart Fail.* 2014;2(3):250–9.

17 Cotter G, Metra M, Milo-Cotter O, Dittrich HC, Gheorghiade M. Fluid overload in acute heart failure: redistribution and other mechanisms beyond fluid accumulation. *Eur J Heart Fail.* 2008;10(2):165–9.

18 Gaziano TA. Cardiovascular disease in the developing world and its cost-effective management. *Circulation.* 2005;112(23):3547–53.

19 Mebazaa A, Gheorghiade M, Pina IL, Harjola VP, Hollenberg SM, Follath F, et al. Practical recommendations for prehospital and early in-hospital management of patients presenting with acute heart failure syndromes. *Crit Care Med.* 2008;36(1 Suppl):S129–39.

20 Ntusi NB, Mayosi BM. Epidemiology of heart failure in sub-Saharan Africa. *Expert Rev Cardiovasc Ther.* 2009;7(2):169–80.

21 Damasceno A, Cotter G, Dzudie A, Sliwa K, Mayosi BM. Heart failure in sub-saharan Africa: time for action. *J Am Coll Cardiol.* 2007;50(17):1688–93.

22 Sliwa K, Wilkinson D, Hansen C, Ntyintyane L, Tibazarwa K, Becker A, et al. Spectrum of heart disease and risk factors in a black urban population in South Africa (the Heart of Soweto Study): a cohort study. *Lancet.* 2008;371(9616):915–22.

23 Mayosi BM. Contemporary trends in the epidemiology and management of cardiomyopathy and pericarditis in sub-Saharan Africa. *Heart.* 2007;93(10):1176–83.

24 Mayosi BM, Burgess LJ, Doubell AF. Tuberculous pericarditis. *Circulation.* 2005;112(23):3608–16.

25 Mayosi BM, Flisher AJ, Lalloo UG, Sitas F, Tollman SM, Bradshaw D. The burden of non-communicable diseases in South Africa. *Lancet.* 2009;374(9693):934–47.

26 Sliwa K, Carrington M, Mayosi BM, Zigiriadis E, Mvungi R, Stewart S. Incidence and characteristics of newly diagnosed rheumatic heart disease in urban African adults: insights from the heart of Soweto study. *Eur Heart J.* 2010;31(6):719–27.

27 Sliwa K, Fen J, Elkayam U. Peripartum cardiomyopathy. *Lancet.* 2006;368(9536):687–93.

28 Fezeu L, Minkoulou E, Balkau B, Kengne AP, Awah P, Unwin N, et al. Association between socioeconomic status and adiposity in urban Cameroon. *Int J Epidemiol.* 2006;35(1):105–11.

29 Damasceno A, Mayosi BM, Sani M, Ogah OS, Mondo C, Ojji D, et al. The causes, treatment, and outcome of acute heart failure in 1006 Africans from 9 countries. *Arch Intern Med.* 2012;172(18):1386–94.

30 Stewart S, Wilkinson D, Hansen C, Vaghela V, Mvungi R, McMurray J, et al. Predominance of heart failure in the Heart of Soweto Study cohort: emerging challenges for urban African communities. *Circulation.* 2008;118(23):2360–7.

31 Amoah AG, Kallen C. Aetiology of heart failure as seen from a national cardiac referral centre in Africa. *Tropical Cardiology.* 2000;93:11–8.

32 Freers J, Mavania-Kizza H, Ziegler JL, Rutakingirwa M. Echocardiographic diagnosis of heart disease in Uganda. *Trop Doct.* 1996;26(3):125–8.

33 Kingue S, Dzudie A, Menanga A, Akono M, Ouankou M, Muna W. A new look at adult chronic heart failure in Africa in the age of the Doppler echocardiography: experience of the medicine department at Yaounde General Hospital. *Ann Cardiol Angeiol (Paris).* 2005;54(5):276–83.

34 Thiam M. Cardiac insufficiency in the African cardiology milieu. *Bull Soc Pathol Exot.* 2003;96(3):217–8.

35 McMurray JJ, Adamopoulos S, Anker SD, Auricchio A, Bohm M, Dickstein K, et al. ESC guidelines for the diagnosis and treatment of acute and chronic heart failure 2012: the Task Force for the Diagnosis and Treatment of Acute and Chronic Heart Failure 2012 of the European Society of Cardiology. Developed in collaboration with the Heart Failure Association (HFA) of the ESC. *Eur J Heart Fail.* 2012;14(8):803–69.

36 Adams KF, Jr., Fonarow GC, Emerman CL, LeJemtel TH, Costanzo MR, Abraham WT, et al. Characteristics and outcomes of patients hospitalized for heart failure in the United States: rationale, design, and preliminary observations from the first 100,000 cases in the Acute Decompensated Heart Failure National Registry (ADHERE). *Am Heart J.* 2005;149(2):209–16.

37 Nieminen MS, Brutsaert D, Dickstein K, Drexler H, Follath F, Harjola VP, et al. EuroHeart Failure Survey II (EHFS II): a survey on hospitalized acute heart failure patients: description of population. *Eur Heart J.* 2006;27(22):2725–36.

38 Zannad F, Mebazaa A, Juilliere Y, Cohen-Solal A, Guize L, Alla F, et al. Clinical profile, contemporary management and one-year mortality in patients with severe acute heart failure syndromes: the EFICA study. *Eur J Heart Fail.* 2006;8(7):697–705.

39 Hunt SA, Abraham WT, Chin MH, Feldman AM, Francis GS, Ganiats TG, et al. 2009 Focused update incorporated into the ACC/AHA 2005 Guidelines for the Diagnosis and Management of Heart Failure in Adults A Report of the American College of Cardiology Foundation/American Heart Association Task Force on Practice Guidelines Developed in Collaboration With the International Society for Heart and Lung Transplantation. *J Am Coll Cardiol.* 2009;53(15):e1–e90.

40 Taylor AL, Ziesche S, Yancy C, Carson P, D'Agostino R, Jr., Ferdinand K, et al. Combination of isosorbide dinitrate and hydralazine in blacks with heart failure. *N Engl J Med.* 2004;351(20):2049–57.

41 Ogah OS, Davison BA, Sliwa K, Mayosi BM, Damasceno A, Sani MU, et al. Gender differences in clinical characteristics and outcome of acute heart failure in sub-Saharan Africa: results of the THESUS-HF study. *Clin Res Cardiol.* 2015;104(6):481–90.

42 Fonarow GC, Abraham WT, Albert NM, Stough WG, Gheorghiade M, Greenberg BH, et al. Age- and gender-related differences in quality of care and outcomes of patients hospitalized with heart failure (from OPTIMIZE-HF). *Am J Cardiol.* 2009;104(1):107–15.

43 Galvao M, Kalman J, DeMarco T, Fonarow GC, Galvin C, Ghali JK, et al. Gender differences in in-hospital management and outcomes in patients with decompensated heart failure: analysis from the Acute Decompensated Heart Failure National Registry (ADHERE). *J Card Fail.* 2006;12(2):100–7.

44 Nieminen MS, Harjola VP, Hochadel M, Drexler H, Komajda M, Brutsaert D, et al. Gender related differences in patients presenting with acute heart failure: results from EuroHeart Failure Survey II. *Eur J Heart Fail.* 2008;10(2):140–8.

45 Tsuchihashi-Makaya M, Hamaguchi S, Kinugawa S, Goto K, Goto D, Furumoto T, et al. Sex differences with respect to clinical characteristics, treatment, and long-term outcomes in patients with heart failure. *Int J Cardiol.* 2011;150(3):338–9.

46 Ferrari R, Bohm M, Cleland JG, Paulus WJ, Pieske B, Rapezzi C, et al. Heart failure with preserved ejection fraction: uncertainties and dilemmas. *Eur J Heart Fail.* 2015; 17(7):665–71.

47 McMurray JJ, Adamopoulos S, Anker SD, Auricchio A, Bohm M, Dickstein K, et al. ESC Guidelines for the diagnosis and treatment of acute and chronic heart failure 2012: the Task Force for the Diagnosis and Treatment of Acute and Chronic Heart Failure 2012 of the European Society of Cardiology. Developed in collaboration with the Heart Failure Association (HFA) of the ESC. *Eur Heart J.* 2012;33(14):1787–847.

48 Dzudie A, Milo O, Edwards C, Cotter G, Davison BA, Damasceno A, et al. Prognostic significance of ECG abnormalities for mortality risk in acute heart failure: insight from the Sub-Saharan Africa Survey of Heart Failure (THESUS-HF). *J Card Fail.* 2014;20(1):45–52.

49 Jessup M, Abraham WT, Casey DE, Feldman AM, Francis GS, Ganiats TG, et al. 2009 focused update: ACCF/AHA Guidelines for the Diagnosis and Management of Heart Failure in Adults: a report of the American College of Cardiology Foundation/American Heart Association Task Force on Practice Guidelines. Developed in collaboration with the International Society for Heart and Lung Transplantation. *Circulation.* 2009;119(14):1977–2016.

50 Khan NK, Goode KM, Cleland JG, Rigby AS, Freemantle N, Eastaugh J, et al. Prevalence of ECG abnormalities in an international survey of patients with suspected or confirmed heart failure at death or discharge. *Eur J Heart Fail*. 2007;9(5):491–501.

51 De Bacquer D, De Backer G, Kornitzer M, Blackburn H. Prognostic value of ECG findings for total, cardiovascular disease, and coronary heart disease death in men and women. *Heart*. 1998;80(6):570–7.

52 Mason JW, Ramseth DJ, Chanter DO, Moon TE, Goodman DB, Mendzelevski B. Electrocardiographic reference ranges derived from 79,743 ambulatory subjects. *J Electrocardiol*. 2007;40(3):228–34.

53 Sliwa K, Lee GA, Carrington MJ, Obel P, Okreglicki A, Stewart S. Redefining the ECG in urban South Africans: electrocardiographic findings in heart disease–free Africans. *Int J Cardiol*. 2013;167(5):2204–9.

54 Cygankiewicz I, Zareba W, Vazquez R, Vallverdu M, Gonzalez-Juanatey JR, Valdes M, et al. Heart rate turbulence predicts all-cause mortality and sudden death in congestive heart failure patients. *Heart Rhythm*. 2008;5(8):1095–102.

55 Abdel-Qadir HM, Tu JV, Austin PC, Wang JT, Lee DS. Bundle branch block patterns and long-term outcomes in heart failure. *Int J Cardiol*. 2011;146(2):213–8.

56 Hebert K, Quevedo HC, Tamariz L, Dias A, Steen DL, Colombo RA, et al. Prevalence of conduction abnormalities in a systolic heart failure population by race, ethnicity, and gender. *Ann Noninvasive Electrocardiol*. 2012;17(2):113–22.

57 Tabrizi F, Englund A, Rosenqvist M, Wallentin L, Stenestrand U. Influence of left bundle branch block on long-term mortality in a population with heart failure. *Eur Heart J*. 2007;28(20):2449–55.

58 Hummel SL, Skorcz S, Koelling TM. Prolonged electrocardiogram QRS duration independently predicts long-term mortality in patients hospitalized for heart failure with preserved systolic function. *J Card Fail*. 2009;15(7):553–60.

59 Wang NC, Maggioni AP, Konstam MA, Zannad F, Krasa HB, Burnett JC, Jr., et al. Clinical implications of QRS duration in patients hospitalized with worsening heart failure and reduced left ventricular ejection fraction. *JAMA*. 2008;299(22):2656–66.

60 Kolo PM, Opadijo OG, Omotoso AB, Balogun MO, Araoye MA, Katibi IA. Prevalence of QTc prolongation in adult Nigerians with chronic heart failure. *West Afr J Med*. 2008;27(2):69–73.

61 Hawkins NM, Wang D, McMurray JJ, Pfeffer MA, Swedberg K, Granger CB, et al. Prevalence and prognostic implications of electrocardiographic left ventricular hypertrophy in heart failure: evidence from the CHARM programme. *Heart*. 2007;93(1):59–64.

62 Mosterd A, Hoes AW. Clinical epidemiology of heart failure. *Heart*. 2007;93(9):1137–46.

63 Sidney S, Rosamond WD, Howard VJ, Luepker RV, National Forum for Heart D, Stroke P. The "heart disease and stroke statistics—2013 update" and the need for a national cardiovascular surveillance system. *Circulation*. 2013;127(1):21–3.

64 Cowie MR, Mosterd A, Wood DA, Deckers JW, Poole-Wilson PA, Sutton GC, et al. The epidemiology of heart failure. *Eur Heart J*. 1997;18(2):208–25.

65 Cleland JG, Swedberg K, Cohen-Solal A, Cosin-Aguilar J, Dietz R, Follath F, et al. The Euro Heart Failure Survey of the EUROHEART survey programme. A survey on the quality of care among patients with heart failure in Europe. The Study Group on Diagnosis of the Working Group on Heart Failure of the European Society of Cardiology. The Medicines Evaluation Group Centre for Health Economics University of York. *Eur J Heart Fail*. 2000;2000(2):123–32.

66 Cleland JG, Swedberg K, Follath F, Komajda M, Cohen-Solal A, Aguilar JC, et al. The EuroHeart Failure survey programme: a survey on the quality of care among patients with heart failure in Europe. Part 1: patient characteristics and diagnosis. *Eur Heart J*. 2003;24(5):442–63.

67 Cowie MR, Wood DA, Coats AJ, Thompson SG, Poole-Wilson PA, Suresh V, et al. Incidence and aetiology of heart failure: a population-based study. *Eur Heart J.* 1999;20(6):421–8.

68 Redfield MM, Jacobsen SJ, Burnett JC, Jr., Mahoney DW, Bailey KR, Rodeheffer RJ. Burden of systolic and diastolic ventricular dysfunction in the community: appreciating the scope of the heart failure epidemic. *JAMA.* 2003;289(2):194–202.

69 Antony KK. Pattern of cardiac failure in Northern Savanna Nigeria. *Trop Geogr Med.* 1980;32(2):118–25.

70 Parry EH, Davidson NM, Ladipo GO, Watkins H. Seasonal variation of cardiac failure in northern Nigeria. *Lancet.* 1977;1(8020):1023–5.

71 Ladipo GO. Cardiac failure at Ahmadu Bello University Hospital, Zaria. *Nigerian Med J.* 1978;8:96–9.

72 Adams KF, Jr., Uddin N, Patterson JH. Clinical predictors of in-hospital mortality in acutely decompensated heart failure: piecing together the outcome puzzle. *Congest Heart Fail.* 2008;14(3):127–34.

73 Ogah OS, Akinyemi RO, Adesemowo A, Ogbodo EI. A two-year review of medical admissions at the emergency unit of a Nigerian tertiary health facility. *Afr J Biomed Res.* 2012;15:59–63.

74 Ogah OS, Okpechi I, Chukwuonye, II, Akinyemi JO, Onwubere BJ, Falase AO, et al. Blood pressure, prevalence of hypertension and hypertension related complications in Nigerian Africans: a review. *World J Cardiol.* 2012;4(12):327–40.

75 Oyoo GO, Ogola EN. Clinical and socio demographic aspects of congestive heart failure patients at Kenyatta National Hospital, Nairobi. *East Afr Med J.* 1999;76(1):23–7.

76 Kuule JK, Seremba E, Freers J. Anaemia among patients with congestive cardiac failure in Uganda and its impact on treatment outcomes. *S Afr Med J.* 2009;99:876–80.

77 Tchoumi JCT, Ambassa JC, Kingue S, Giamberti A, Cirri S, Frigiola A, et al. Occurrence, aetiology and challenges in the management of congestive heart failure in sub-Saharan Africa: experience of the Cardiac Centre in Shisong, Cameroon. *Pan Afr Med J.* 2011;8:11.

78 Kearney PM, Whelton M, Reynolds K, Muntner P, Whelton PK, He J. Global burden of hypertension: analysis of worldwide data. *Lancet.* 2005;365(9455):217–23.

79 Stewart S, Libhaber E, Carrington M, Damasceno A, Abbasi H, Hansen C, et al. The clinical consequences and challenges of hypertension in urban-dwelling black Africans: insights from the Heart of Soweto Study. *Int J Cardiol.* 2011;146(1):22–7.

80 Addo J, Smeeth L, Leon DA. Hypertension in sub-saharan Africa: a systematic review. *Hypertension.* 2007;50(6):1012–8.

81 Stewart S, Wilkinson D, Becker A, Askew D, Ntyintyane L, McMurray JJ, et al. Mapping the emergence of heart disease in a black, urban population in Africa: the Heart of Soweto Study. *Int J Cardiol.* 2006;108(1):101–8.

82 Libhaber EN, Libhaber CD, Candy GP, Sliwa K, Kachope J, Hlatshwayo NM, et al. Effect of slow-release indapamide and perindopril compared with amlodipine on 24-hour blood pressure and left ventricular mass in hypertensive patients of African ancestry. *Am J Hypertens.* 2004;17(5 Pt 1):428–32.

83 Skudicky D, Sareli P, Libhaber E, Candy G, Radevski I, Valtchanova Z, et al. Relationship between treatment-induced changes in left ventricular mass and blood pressure in black african hypertensive patients: results of the Baragwanath Trial. *Circulation.* 2002; 105(7):830–6.

84 Inglis SC, Stewart S, Papachan A, Vaghela V, Libhaber C, Veriava Y, et al. Anaemia and renal function in heart failure due to idiopathic dilated cardiomyopathy. *Eur J Heart Fail.* 2007;9(4):384–90.

85 Tibazarwa K, Ntyintyane L, Sliwa K, Gerntholtz T, Carrington M, Wilkinson D, et al. A time bomb of cardiovascular risk factors in South Africa: results from the Heart of Soweto Study "Heart Awareness Days." *Int J Cardiol.* 2009;132(2):233–9.

86 Stewart S, Carrington M, Pretorius S, Methusi P, Sliwa K. Standing at the crossroads between new and historically prevalent heart disease: effects of migration and socio-economic factors in the Heart of Soweto cohort study. *Eur Heart J*. 2011;32(4):492–9.

87 Ojji D, Stewart S, Ajayi S, Manmak M, Sliwa K. A predominance of hypertensive heart failure in the Abuja Heart Study cohort of urban Nigerians: a prospective clinical registry of 1515 de novo cases. *Eur J Heart Fail*. 2013;15(8):835–42.

88 van der Sande MA. Cardiovascular disease in sub-Saharan Africa: a disaster waiting to happen. *Neth J Med*. 2003;61(2):32–6.

89 Mosley WH, Bobadilla JL, Jamison DT. *The Health Transition: Implications for Health Policy in Developing Countries*. New York: World Bank, 1993.

90 Unwin N. Non-communicable disease and priorities for health policy in sub-Saharan Africa. *Health Policy Plan*. 2001;16(4):351–2.

91 ALLHAT Collaborative Research Group. Major cardiovascular events in hypertensive patients randomized to doxazosin vs chlorthalidone: the antihypertensive and lipid-lowering treatment to prevent heart attack trial (ALLHAT). *JAMA*. 2000;283(15):1967–75.

92 Ogah OS, Sliwa K, Akinyemi JO, Falase AO, Stewart S. Hypertensive heart failure in Nigerian Africans: insights from the Abeokuta Heart Failure Registry. *J Clin Hypertens (Greenwich)*. 2015;17(4):263–72.

93 Danaei G, Finucane MM, Lin JK, Singh GM, Paciorek CJ, Cowan MJ, et al. National, regional, and global trends in systolic blood pressure since 1980: systematic analysis of health examination surveys and epidemiological studies with 786 country years and 5.4 million participants. *Lancet*. 2011;377(9765):568–77.

94 Mancia G, Fagard R, Narkiewicz K, Redon J, Zanchetti A, Bohm M, et al. 2013 ESH/ESC Guidelines for the management of arterial hypertension: the task force for the management of arterial hypertension of the European Society of Hypertension (ESH) and of the European Society of Cardiology (ESC). *J Hypertens*. 2013;31(7):1281–357.

95 Modesti PA, Agostoni P, Agyemang C, Basu S, Benetos A, Cappuccio FP, et al. Cardiovascular risk assessment in low-resource settings: a consensus document of the European Society of Hypertension Working Group on Hypertension and Cardiovascular Risk in Low Resource Settings. *J Hypertens*. 2014;32(5):951–60.

96 Ogah OS. Hypertension in Sub-Saharan African populations: the burden of hypertension in Nigeria. *Ethn Dis*. 2006;16(4):765.

97 Ojji DB, Alfa J, Ajayi SO, Mamven MH, Falase AO. Pattern of heart failure in Abuja, Nigeria: an echocardiographic study. *Cardiovasc J Afr*. 2009;20(6):349–52.

98 Dzudie A, Kengne AP, Mbahe S, Menanga A, Kenfack M, Kingue S. Chronic heart failure, selected risk factors and co-morbidities among adults treated for hypertension in a cardiac referral hospital in Cameroon. *Eur J Heart Fail*. 2008;10(4):367–72.

99 Lawes CM, Vander Hoorn S, Law MR, Elliott P, MacMahon S, Rodgers A. Blood pressure and the global burden of disease 2000. Part II: estimates of attributable burden. *J Hypertens*. 2006;24(3):423–30.

100 Lawes CM, Vander Hoorn S, Law MR, Elliott P, MacMahon S, Rodgers A. Blood pressure and the global burden of disease 2000. Part 1: estimates of blood pressure levels. *J Hypertens*. 2006;24(3):413–22.

101 Opie LH, Seedat YK. Hypertension in sub-Saharan African populations. *Circulation*. 2005;112(23):3562–8.

102 Mendez GF, Cowie MR. The epidemiological features of heart failure in developing countries: a review of the literature. *Int J Cardiol*. 2001;80(2–3):213–9.

103 Connor MD, Walker R, Modi G, Warlow CP. Burden of stroke in black populations in sub-Saharan Africa. *Lancet Neurol*. 2007;6(3):269–78.

104 Kengne AP, Anderson CS. The neglected burden of stroke in Sub-Saharan Africa. *Int J Stroke.* 2006;1(4):180–90.

105 Ayodele OE, Alebiosu CO, Salako BL, Awoden OG, Abigun AD. Target organ damage and associated clinical conditions among Nigerians with treated hypertension. *Cardiovasc J S Afr.* 2005;16(2):89–93.

106 Vasan RS, Larson MG, Benjamin EJ, Evans JC, Reiss CK, Levy D. Congestive heart failure in subjects with normal versus reduced left ventricular ejection fraction: prevalence and mortality in a population-based cohort. *J Am Coll Cardiol.* 1999;33(7):1948–55.

107 Oyati IA, Danbauchi SS, Alhassan MA, Isa MS. Diastolic dysfunction in persons with hypertensive heart failure. *J Natl Med Assoc.* 2004;96(7):968–73.

108 Bibbins-Domingo K, Lin F, Vittinghoff E, Barrett-Connor E, Grady D, Shlipak MG. Renal insufficiency as an independent predictor of mortality among women with heart failure. *J Am Coll Cardiol.* 2004;44(8):1593–600.

109 Cohen N, Gorelik O, Almoznino-Sarafian D, Alon I, Tourovski Y, Weissgarten J, et al. Renal dysfunction in congestive heart failure, pathophysiological and prognostic significance. *Clin Nephrol.* 2004;61(3):177–84.

110 Le Jemtel TH, Padeletti M, Jelic S. Diagnostic and therapeutic challenges in patients with coexistent chronic obstructive pulmonary disease and chronic heart failure. *J Am Coll Cardiol.* 2007;49(2):171–80.

111 Sliwa K, Carrington MJ, Klug E, Opie L, Lee G, Ball J, et al. Predisposing factors and incidence of newly diagnosed atrial fibrillation in an urban African community: insights from the Heart of Soweto Study. *Heart.* 2010;96(23):1878–82.

112 Kengne AP, Awah PK, Fezeu L, Mbanya JC. The burden of high blood pressure and related risk factors in urban sub-Saharan Africa: evidences from Douala in Cameroon. *Afr Health Sci.* 2007;7(1):38–44.

113 Ogah OS, Stewart S, Onwujekwe OE, Falase AO, Adebayo SO, Olunuga T, et al. Economic burden of heart failure: investigating outpatient and inpatient costs in Abeokuta, Southwest Nigeria. *PLoS One.* 2014;9(11):e113032.

114 Laabes EP, Thacher TD, Okeahialam BN. Risk factors for heart failure in adult Nigerians. *Acta Cardiol.* 2008;63(4):437–43.

115 Lawanson AO, Olaniyan O, Soyibo A. National Health Accounts estimation: lessons from the Nigerian experience. *Afr J Med Med Sci.* 2012;41(4):357–64.

116 Soyibo A, Olaniyan O, Lawanson OA. National health accounts: Structure, trends and sustainability of health expenditure in Nigeria. *Afr. J. Econ. Pol.* 2007;14(1).

117 Stewart S, Jenkins A, Buchan S, McGuire A, Capewell S, McMurray JJ. The current cost of heart failure to the National Health Service in the UK. *Eur J Heart Fail.* 2002;4(3):361–71.

118 Ryden-Bergsten T, Andersson F. The health care costs of heart failure in Sweden. *J Intern Med.* 1999;246(3):275–84.

119 Czech M, Opolski G, Zdrojewski T, Dubiel JS, Wizner B, Bolisega D, et al. The costs of heart failure in Poland from the public payer's perspective. Polish programme assessing diagnostic procedures, treatment and costs in patients with heart failure in randomly selected outpatient clinics and hospitals at different levels of care: POLKARD. *Kardiologia polska.* 2013;71(3):224–32.

120 Araujo DV, Tavares LR, Verissimo R, Ferraz MB, Mesquita ET. [Cost of heart failure in the Unified Health System]. *Arq Bras Cardiol.* 2005;84(5):422–7.

121 Writing Group Members, Lloyd-Jones D, Adams RJ, Brown TM, Carnethon M, Dai S, et al. Heart disease and stroke statistics—2010 update: a report from the American Heart Association. *Circulation.* 2010;121(7):e46–e215.

122 Fagnani F, Buteau L, Virion JM, Briancon S, Zannad F. [Management, cost and mortality of a cohort of patients with advanced heart failure (the EPICAL study)]. *Therapie.* 2001;56(1):5–10.

123 Stewart S, Carrington MJ, Horowitz JD, Marwick TH, Newton PJ, Davidson PM, et al. Prolonged impact of home versus clinic-based management of chronic heart failure: extended follow-up of a pragmatic, multicentre randomized trial cohort. *Int J Cardiol.* 2014;174(3):600–10.

124 Maru S, Byrnes J, Carrington MJ, Chan YK, Thompson DR, Stewart S, et al. Cost-effectiveness of home versus clinic-based management of chronic heart failure: Extended follow-up of a pragmatic, multicentre randomized trial cohort: The WHICH? study (Which Heart Failure Intervention Is Most Cost-Effective & Consumer Friendly in Reducing Hospital Care). *Int J Cardiol.* 2015;201:368–75.

125 Boudestein LC, Rutten FH, Cramer MJ, Lammers JW, Hoes AW. The impact of concurrent heart failure on prognosis in patients with chronic obstructive pulmonary disease. *Eur J Heart Fail.* 2009;11(12):1182–8.

126 Hawkins NM, Petrie MC, Jhund PS, Chalmers GW, Dunn FG, McMurray JJ. Heart failure and chronic obstructive pulmonary disease: diagnostic pitfalls and epidemiology. *Eur J Heart Fail.* 2009;11(2):130–9.

127 Stewart S, Mocumbi AO, Carrington MJ, Pretorius S, Burton R, Sliwa K. A not-so-rare form of heart failure in urban black Africans: pathways to right heart failure in the Heart of Soweto Study cohort. *Eur J Heart Fail.* 2011;13(10):1070–7.

128 Sani MU, Mukhtar-Yola M, Karaye KM. Spectrum of congenital heart disease in a tropical environment: an echocardiography study. *J Natl Med Assoc.* 2007;99(6):665–9.

129 Karaye KM, Saidu H, S. BM, Yahaya IA. Prevalence, clinical characteristics and outcome of pulmonary hypertension among admitted heart failure patients. *Ann Afr Med.* 2013;12(4):197–204.

130 Okello E, Wanzhu Z, Musoke C, Twalib A, Kakande B, Lwabi P, et al. Cardiovascular complications in newly diagnosed rheumatic heart disease patients at Mulago Hospital, Uganda. *Cardiovasc J Afr.* 2013;24(3):80–5.

131 Olusegun-Joseph DA, Ajuluchukwu JN, Okany CC, Mbakwem AC, Oke DA, Okubadejo NU. Echocardiographic patterns in treatment-naive HIV-positive patients in Lagos, southwest Nigeria. *Cardiovasc J Afr.* 2012;23(8):e1–6.

132 Chillo P, Bakari M, Lwakatare J. Echocardiographic diagnoses in HIV-infected patients presenting with cardiac symptoms at Muhimbili National Hospital in Dar es Salaam, Tanzania. *Cardiovasc J Afr.* 2012;23:90–7.

133 Ferrand RA, Luethy R, Bwakura F, Mujuru H, Miller RF, Corbett EL. HIV infection presenting in older children and adolescents: a case series from Harare, Zimbabwe. *Clin Infect Dis.* 2007;44(6):874–8.

134 Aliyu ZY, Gordeuk V, Sachdev V, Babadoko A, Mamman AI, Akpanpe P, et al. Prevalence and risk factors for pulmonary artery systolic hypertension among sickle cell disease patients in Nigeria. *Am J Hematol.* 2008;83(6):485–90.

135 Mokhtar GM, Tantawy AA, Adly AA, Ismail EA. Clinicopathological and radiological study of Egyptian beta-thalassemia intermedia and beta-thalassemia major patients: relation to complications and response to therapy. *Hemoglobin.* 2011;35(4):382–405.

136 Ahmed AE, Ibrahim AS, Elshafie SM. Pulmonary hypertension in patients with treated pulmonary tuberculosis: analysis of 14 consecutive cases. *Clin Med Insights Circ Respir Pulm Med.* 2011;5:1–5.

137 Thienemann F, Dzudie A, Mocumbi AO, Blauwet L, Sani MU, Karaye KM, et al. Rationale and design of the Pan African Pulmonary hypertension Cohort (PAPUCO) study: implementing a contemporary registry on pulmonary hypertension in Africa. *BMJ Open.* 2014;4(10):e005950.

138 Galie N, Hoeper MM, Humbert M, Torbicki A, Vachiery JL, Barbera JA, et al. Guidelines for the diagnosis and treatment of pulmonary hypertension: the Task Force for the Diagnosis and Treatment of Pulmonary Hypertension of the European Society of Cardiology (ESC) and the European Respiratory Society (ERS), endorsed by the International Society of Heart and Lung Transplantation (ISHLT). *Eur Heart J.* 2009;30(20):2493–537.

139 Henry WL, DeMaria A, Gramiak R, King DL, Kisslo JA, Popp RL, et al. Report of the American Society of Echocardiography Committee on Nomenclature and Standards in Two-dimensional Echocardiography. *Circulation.* 1980;62(2):212–7.

140 World Health Organization. WHO International Classification of Diseases (ICD). World Health Organization, 1994.

141 Authors/Task Force Members, Galie N, Humbert M, Vachiery JL, Gibbs S, Lang I, et al. 2015 ESC/ERS Guidelines for the diagnosis and treatment of pulmonary hypertension: The Joint Task Force for the Diagnosis and Treatment of Pulmonary Hypertension of the European Society of Cardiology (ESC) and the European Respiratory Society (ERS). Endorsed by: Association for European Paediatric and Congenital Cardiology (AEPC), International Society for Heart and Lung Transplantation (ISHLT). *Eur Heart J.* 2015.

142 Fisher MR, Forfia PR, Chamera E, Housten-Harris T, Champion HC, Girgis RE, et al. Accuracy of Doppler echocardiography in the hemodynamic assessment of pulmonary hypertension. *Am J Respir Crit Care Med.* 2009;179(7):615–21.

143 Penning S, Robinson KD, Major CA, Garite TJ. A comparison of echocardiography and pulmonary artery catheterization for evaluation of pulmonary artery pressures in pregnant patients with suspected pulmonary hypertension. *Am J Obstet Gynecol.* 2001;184(7):1568–70.

144 Janda S, Shahidi N, Gin K, Swiston J. Diagnostic accuracy of echocardiography for pulmonary hypertension: a systematic review and meta-analysis. *Heart.* 2011;97(8):612–22.

145 Damy T, Goode KM, Kallvikbacka-Bennett A, Lewinter C, Hobkirk J, Nikitin NP, et al. Determinants and prognostic value of pulmonary arterial pressure in patients with chronic heart failure. *Eur Heart J.* 2010;31(18):2280–90.

146 Makubi A, Hage C, Lwakatare J, et al. Contemporary aetiology, clinical characteristics and prognosis of adults with heart failure observed in a tertiary hospital in Tanzania: the prospective Tanzania Heart Failure (TaHeF) study. *Heart.* 2014;100(16):1235–41.

147 Makubi A, Hage C, Lwakatare J, et al. Prevalence and prognostic implications of anaemia and iron deficiency in Tanzanian patients with heart failure. *Heart.* 2015;101(8):592–9.

148 Atherton JJ, Hayward CS, Wan Ahmad WA, Kwok B, Jorge J, Hernandez AF, et al. Patient characteristics from a regional multicenter database of acute decompensated heart failure in Asia Pacific (ADHERE International–Asia Pacific). *J Card Fail.* 2012;18(1):82–8.

149 Harjola VP, Follath F, Nieminen MS, Brutsaert D, Dickstein K, Drexler H, et al. Characteristics, outcomes, and predictors of mortality at 3 months and 1 year in patients hospitalized for acute heart failure. *Eur J Heart Fail.* 2010;12(3):239–48.

150 West R, Liang L, Fonarow GC, Kociol R, Mills RM, O'Connor CM, et al. Characterization of heart failure patients with preserved ejection fraction: a comparison between ADHERE-US registry and ADHERE-International registry. *Eur J Heart Fail.* 2011;13(9):945–52.

Abbreviations

ACCESS	Acute Coronary Events—a Multinational Survey of Current Management Strategies
ACE	Angiotensin-converting enzyme
ACS	Acute coronary syndrome
ADP	Adenosine diphosphate
AF	Atrial fibrillation
AHF	Acute heart failure
AIDS	Acquired immune deficiency syndrome
AMI	Acute myocardial infarction
ApoB	Apolipoprotein B
ApoA1	Apolipoprotein A-1
BMI	Body mass index
BP	Blood pressure
CABG	Coronary artery bypass graft
CAD	Coronary artery disease
CDC	Centers for Disease Control and Prevention
CHD	Congenital heart disease
CHF	Congestive heart failure
CI	Confidence interval
CMO	Cardiomyopathy
COPD	Chronic obstructive pulmonary disease
CRIBSA	Cardiovascular Risk in Black South Africans
CTEPH	Chronic Thromboembolic Pulmonary Hypertension
CVD	Cardiovascular disease
ECG	Electrocardiogram
EMF	Endomyocardial fibrosis
HAART	Highly active antiretroviral therapy
HDL	High-density lipoprotein
HF	Heart failure
HFpEF	Heart failure with preserved ejection fraction
HFrEF	Heart failure with reduced ejection fraction
HIV	Human immuno-deficiency virus
IHD	Ischemic heart disease
IMPI	Investigation of the Management of Pericarditis
IQR	Interquartile range
IV	Intravenous

The Heart of Africa: Clinical Profile of an Evolving Burden of Heart Disease in Africa, First Edition.
Edited by Simon Stewart, Karen Sliwa, Ana Mocumbi, Albertino Damasceno, and Mpiko Ntsekhe.
© 2016 John Wiley & Sons, Ltd. Published 2016 by John Wiley & Sons, Ltd.

LDL	Low-density lipoprotein
LMIC	Low- and middle-income countries
LV	Left ventricular
LVEF	Left ventricular ejection fraction
LVH	Left ventricular hypertrophy
MI	Myocardial infarction
MR	Mitral regurgitation
NSTEMI	Non-ST segment elevation myocardial infarction
NYHA	New York Heart Association
OR	Odds ratio
PAH	Pulmonary arterial hypertension
PH	Pulmonary hypertension
PAPUCO	Pan African Pulmonary Hypertension Cohort
PCI	Percutaneous coronary intervention
PPCMO	Peripartum cardiomyopathy
REMEDY	The Global Rheumatic Heart Disease Registry
RHD	Rheumatic heart disease
RHF	Right heart failure
RNA	Ribonucleic Acid
RV	Right ventricular
RVSP	Right ventricular systolic pressure
SABPA	Sympathetic Activity and Ambulatory Blood Pressure in Africans
SCD	Sickle Cell Disease
STEMI	ST segment elevation myocardial infarction
STROBE	Strengthening the Reporting of Observational Studies in Epidemiology
TB	Tuberculosis
THESUS-HF	The Sub-Saharan Africa Survey of Heart Failure
THUSA	Transition and Health during Urbanisation of South Africans
TIA	Transient ischemic attack
VHD	Valvular heart disease
WHO	World Health Organization

Index

Note: Page references in *italics* refer to Figures; those in **bold** refer to Tables

The Heart of Africa: Clinical Profile of an Evolving Burden of Heart Disease in Africa, First Edition.
Edited by Simon Stewart, Karen Sliwa, Ana Mocumbi, Albertino Damasceno, and Mpiko Ntsekhe.
© 2016 John Wiley & Sons, Ltd. Published 2016 by John Wiley & Sons, Ltd.